CRASH COURSE
Muscles, Bones and Skin
SECOND EDITION

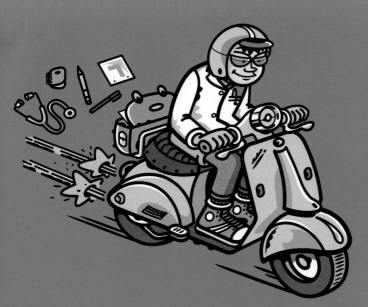

Series editor
Daniel Horton-Szar
BSc (Hons) MBBS (Hons)
GP Registrar
Northgate Medical Practice
Canterbury
Kent

Faculty advisor
Sam Jacob
MBBS MS
Senior Lecturer
Department of Biomedical Science
University of Sheffield
Western Bank
Sheffield

Muscles, Bones and Skin

SECOND EDITION

Sîan Knight

BMedSci
University of Nottingham Medical School
Clifton Boulevard
Nottingham

First edition authors
Sona V Biswas, Rehana Iqbal

M Mosby

London • Edinburgh • New York • Philadelphia • St Louis • Sydney • Toronto 2003

MOSBY
An affliliate of Elsevier Science Limited

Commissioning Editor	**Alex Stibbe**
Project Manager	**Frances Affleck**
Project Development Manager	**Duncan Fraser**
Designer	**Andy Chapman**
Cover Design	**Kevin Faerber**
Illustration Manager	**Mick Ruddy**

First edition 1998
Second edition 2003

ISBN 0723432910

British Library Cataloguing in Publication Data
A catalogue record for this book is available from the British Library

Library of Congress Cataloging in Publication Data
A catalog record for this book is available from the Library of Congress

Note
Medical knowledge is constantly changing. As new information becomes available,
changes in treatment, procedures, equipment and the use of drugs become
necessary. The author, editors and the publishers have taken care to ensure that the
information given in this text is accurate and up to date. However, readers are
strongly advised to confirm that the information, especially with regard to drug
usage, complies with the latest legislation and standards of practice.

Typeset by SNP Best-set Typesetter Ltd., Hong Kong
Printed in Spain

The publisher's policy is to use paper manufactured from sustainable forests

The
Publisher's
policy is to use
**paper manufactured
from sustainable forests**

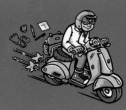

Preface

Medical school can be stressful at the best of times, so learning the huge amount of material necessary to pass exams can sometimes seem like an impossible task. In *Crash Course: Muscles, Bones and Skin* we've broken the topics down into manageable chunks whilst still comprehensively covering both the pre-clinical and clinical aspects of rheumatology, orthopaedics and dermatology. A new section on communication skills gives practical advice on taking an effective history and a hefty Self-assessment section will help identify weak areas of knowledge.

As medical students, the authors of the *Crash Course* books have already been there, done it, and most importantly, passed the exams. This means the books focus on the stuff you need to know, rather than the stuff that other textbooks think you should know—you've probably realised the difference by now! I hope you find *Crash Course Muscles, Bones and Skin* a useful revision tool, and that all your exams go well.

Sîan Knight

Traditionally I would advise preclinical students to read big books to get a full understanding of anatomical details and physiological mechanisms. However, with recent changes to the medical curriculum and the advent of integrated medical courses there is a need for books with comprehensive but concise coverage of many medical topics. *Crash Course: Muscles, Bones and Skin* meets this requirement.

The text is presented in a pithy, digestible form for easy comprehension. The anatomy, physiology, pathology and pharmacology of muscles, bones and skin have been fully integrated and are supplemented with many illustrations. This user-friendly book will help students master the basic sciences of the musculoskeletal system and skin and to appreciate their relevance to medical practice.

Dr Sam Jacob
Faculty Advisor

In the six years since the first editions were published, there have been many changes in medicine, and in the way it is taught. These second editions have been largely rewritten to take these changes into account, and keep *Crash Course* up to date for the twenty-first century. New material has been added to include recent research and all pharmacological and disease management information has been updated in line with current best practice. We've listened to feedback from hundreds of students who have been using *Crash Course* and have improved the structure and layout of the books accordingly: pathology material has been closely integrated with the relevant basic medical science; there are more MCQs and the clarity of text and figures is better than ever.

The principles on which we developed the series remain the same, however. Medicine is a huge subject, and the last thing a student needs when exams are looming is to waste time assembling information from different sources, and wading through pages of irrelevant detail. As before, *Crash Course* brings you all the information you need, in compact, manageable volumes that integrate basic medical science with clinical practice. We still tread the fine line between producing clear, concise text and providing enough detail for those aiming at distinction. The series is still written by medical students with recent exam experience, and checked for accuracy by senior faculty members from across the UK.

I wish you the best of luck in your future careers!

Dr Dan Horton-Szar
Series Editor (Basic Medical Sciences)

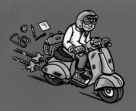

Acknowledgements

Thanks to Cynthia and Merve for the last 25 years; to Jason, for a blissful three; to Amanda and Bec for their fussing, clucking, and general concern; to Mat and all at Impact, for their support and the offers of help which must have been torture to their non-medical souls.

Thanks also to the wonderful people at Mosby for their patience and support.

Figure acknowledgements

Fig 1.6, 4.5, 4.11, 4.19, 4.22A, 5.30, 5.31 and 5.32 redrawn with permission from P G Bullough and V J Vigorita. Orthopaedic Pathology, 3rd edition. TMIP, 1997

Figs 2.8B, 2.9, 2.10, 2.22, 4.6, 4.9A–C and 6.3 reproduced with permission from A Stevens and J Lowe. Human Histology, 2nd edition. Mosby, 1997. Fig 2.8B also courtesy of T Gray

Figs 3.1, 3.7 and 5.1 reproduced with permission from R M H McMinn, P Gaddum-Rosse, R T Hutchings and B M Logan. McMinn's Functional and Clinical Anatomy. TMIP, 1995

Figs 4.1, 11.6 and 11.9 reproduced with permission from J A Gosling, P F Harris, J R Humpherson, I Whitmore and P L T Wilan. Human Anatomy, Color Atlas and Text, 3rd edition. TMIP, 1996

Fig 4.3 adapted with permission from P G Bullough, V J Vigorita and W F Enneking. Atlas of Orthopaedic Pathology. Gower Medical Publishing, 1984

Figs 4.13, 4.21, 5.6 and 5.7 reproduced with permission from A Stevens and J Lowe. Pathology. Mosby, 1991

Figs 5.10, 5.11, 5.18, 5.21, 5.28 and 5.29 redrawn with permission from O Epstein, G D Perkin, D P deBono and J Cookson. Clinical Examination, 2e. Mosby, 1997

Plates 1–24 reproduced with permission from G White. Levene's Color Atlas of Dermatology, 2nd edition. Mosby, 1997

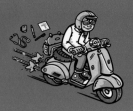

Contents

Contents

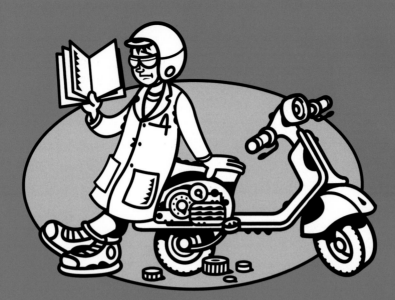

BASIC MEDICAL SCIENCE OF MUSCLES, BONES AND SKIN

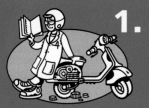

1. Musculoskeletal System —an overview

Introduction

The musculoskeletal system comprises muscles, bones and joints. It makes up most of the body's mass and performs several essential functions, including:

- The maintenance of body shape.
- The support and protection of soft tissue structures.
- Movement.
- Breathing.
- The storage of calcium and phosphate in bone.

Connective tissue

Most of the musculoskeletal system is made up of connective tissue such as bone and cartilage. Connective tissue comprises specialized cells embedded in an extracellular matrix of collagen, elastin and structural proteoglycans. In bone, this matrix is mineralized and rigid.

Muscle

There are three types of muscle: skeletal, cardiac and smooth muscle (Fig. 1.1).

- Skeletal muscle—striated muscle controlled by the nervous system. Most muscle in the body is of this type.
- Cardiac muscle—striated muscle of the heart.
- Smooth muscle—non-striated muscle controlled by a variety of chemical mediators. Smooth muscle is important in the function of most tissues, e.g. blood vessels, the gastrointestinal and reproductive tracts.

Energy stored in tissues as ATP is converted by muscle tissue into mechanical energy. This produces movement or tension.

The contraction of muscle requires stimulation. The type of stimulation varies: for example, skeletal muscle is activated by motor neurons, cardiac muscle initiates its own contractions and smooth muscle is activated by a variety of chemical mediators. Stimulation of muscle causes protein filaments within its cells, called actin and myosin, to interact and thus produce a contractile force.

The skeleton

The skeleton consists of bone, cartilage and fibrous ligaments (p. 59). A joint is the site at which bones are attached to each other. The range of movement at the joint, and whether a joint is rigid or flexible, depends on how the bones meet.

Bone

Bone is rigid and forms most of the skeleton. It functions as a supportive framework for the musculoskeletal system, and the bony sites for muscle attachment provide the mechanical basis for locomotion. Other functions of bone include mineral storage in its matrix and formation of blood cells (haemopoiesis) within the marrow.

Cartilage

Cartilage is a resilient tissue that provides semi-rigid support in some parts of the skeleton. Cartilage is also a component of some types of joint. Most bone is formed within a cartilaginous template during development.

Ligaments, tendons and aponeuroses

Ligaments, tendons and aponeuroses are fibrous tissues that connect the various components of the musculoskeletal system.

- Ligaments are flexible bands that connect bones or cartilage together, strengthening and stabilizing joints.
- Tendons are connections between muscle and bone.
- An aponeurosis may be considered as a broad, sheet-like tendon.

Joints

Joints are composite structures between bones. They may also include cartilage and fibrous connective tissue. There are several types of joint (p. 91). The strength of a joint and the range of movement it allows depend upon its position and function.

Properties of the three different muscle types

	Skeletal	Cardiac	Smooth
histological appearance	cross-striated, multinucleated muscle fibres	cross-striated, single nucleated muscle fibres containing intracellular discs	non-striated, spindle cells with a single nucleus
site	skeletal covering	muscular component of the heart	found in wall of blood vessel, airways and walls of hollow organs
cell size	50–60 µm in diameter, up to 10 cm long	15 µm in diameter, 100 µm long	2–10 µm in diameter, 20–400 µm long
control	voluntary/reflex; controlled by somatic nervous system	self-regulated by pacemaker cells; heart rate can be altered by autonomic nervous system	involuntary control or regulation by inherent contraction initiation (visceral smooth muscle)
nature of contraction	rapid contraction and relaxation	spontaneous and rhythmical contraction	slow and sustained contraction
function	voluntary movement of skeleton and posture maintenance	contractions pump blood around the body	related to the structure, e.g. regulation of blood vessel diameter, hair erection, etc.

Fig. 1.1 Properties of the three different types of muscle.

Control of the musculoskeletal system

The musculoskeletal system is controlled by the nervous system to produce coordinated movements and locomotion. There are a number of elements to this control. These include:

- Efferent motor neurons, which activate groups of muscle fibres to produce contraction.
- Afferent feedback from stretch receptors in muscles and tendons, and sensory nerve endings in joints and skin, allowing coordination of movement.
- Neural pathways within the spinal cord, which coordinate the action of related muscle groups (agonist–antagonist pairs, for example) and also initiate repetitive actions, such as walking ('central pattern generator').

For further information about central control of movement and locomotion, refer to *Crash Course: Nervous System, 2nd edn.*

Skin

Structure

The skin is composed of three layers: an outer protective epidermis, an inner connective tissue dermis, and a fatty subcutaneous layer (Fig. 1.2). It is characterized by a tough keratinized surface which protects underlying tissues from the external environment.

The thickness of skin varies depending on its location on the body. The epidermis is usually around 0.1 mm thick, though this increases to between 0.8 and 1.4 mm in places such as the soles of the feet and the palms of the hands where it undergoes repeated trauma. The dermis follows this pattern, ranging from 0.6 mm thickness on the eyelids to 3 mm on the palms and soles. The subcutaneous layer (subcutis) of the skin is much thicker than the above layers and has a different thickness distribution: it is

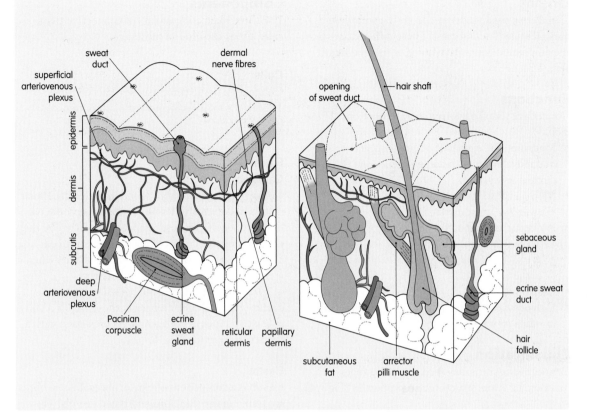

Fig. 1.2 The structure of the skin. (Adapted with permission from *Dermatology: an Illustrated Colour Text*, 2nd edn, by D.J. Gawkrodger, Churchill Livingstone, 1997.)

thickest on the abdomen, where it reaches depths of 3 cm.

Functions

The skin performs many functions on top of its main protective role, including thermoregulation, synthesis of vitamin D and various hormones, and the perception of sensation, temperature and pain.

Skin derivatives

There are many derivatives of skin, including hair, nails, sebaceous glands and sweat glands, which will also be discussed within this book. These structures are so named because they have developed from cells derived from the epidermis. They perform important functions in both the protection and homeostasis of the skin.

Pathology

Because of the skin's exposure to the external environment, it is open to insults caused by infection and infestation. These will be covered later in the book (Chapter 8), as will the clinical manifestations caused by the usual gamut of pathology: inflammation, tumours, genetic disorders, systemic disease and drug-induced disorders.

Connective tissue

Definition

Connective tissue is a basic type of tissue. It comprises cells embedded in an extracellular matrix of ground substance and fibres. Connective tissue is characterized by a high matrix:cell ratio.

Origins

Connective tissue is derived from the embryonic mesoderm and neural crest. These differentiate into the embryonic connective tissue or mesenchyme (Fig. 1.3).

Functions

Connective tissue performs several functions. These include:

- Mediating the exchange of nutrients and metabolic products between tissues and the circulatory system.
- Mechanical support, both physical as well as allowing for muscle attachment.
- Packaging, as connective tissue encloses and lies between other specialized tissues.
  - A metabolic role, allowing fat storage in adipose tissue.
- Insulation.
- Defence and repair; some cells are involved in the immune response.

Classification

Connective tissue is classified according to its function, location, structure and properties (Fig 1.4).

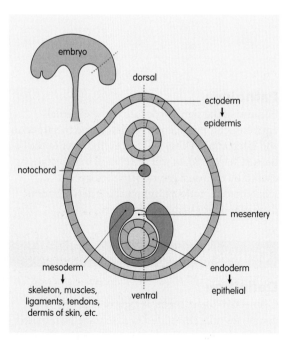

Fig. 1.3 The three primitive embryonic layers and their derivative structures.

Components

The three main components of connective tissue are cells, fibres and ground substance.

Cells

Connective tissue comprises several cell types. These cells each perform a certain function (Fig. 1.5).

Fibres
Collagen

Collagen is the main fibre found in the extracellular matrix of connective tissue. Collagen is produced from tropocollagen, a substance synthesized by the endoplasmic reticulum of matrix-secreting cells. Tropocollagen becomes modified to collagen when it is released into the extracellular matrix.

Collagen comprises three helical polypeptide chains (Fig. 1.6). Differences in these chains result in at least 15 types of collagen molecules, each with a particular function (Fig. 1.7).

Elastin

Elastin is a component of elastic fibres. Elastic fibres are found in the skin, lung and blood vessels. They are thinner than collagen and are arranged in random sheets.

Elastin is produced from proelastin, a substance synthesized by matrix-secreting cells. Proelastin becomes modified to elastin by the cell's Golgi apparatus, when it is released into the extracellular matrix.

Structural proteoglycans

Structural proteoglycans provide a ground substance surrounding the cells and fibres of connective tissue. They comprise protein chains bound to branched polysaccharides and form fibres such as fibronectin and laminin. Some structural proteoglycans are found on the surface of cells, where their functions include cell–cell recognition, adhesion and migration.

Communication between cells and their environment is facilitated by the stuctural proteoglycans which function as cell adhesion molecules. In doing so, they regulate a large number of cell functions, including proliferation, gene expression, apoptosis and differentiation. In future, modifying the actions of adhesion molecules may well be the key to treating illnesses such as cancer.

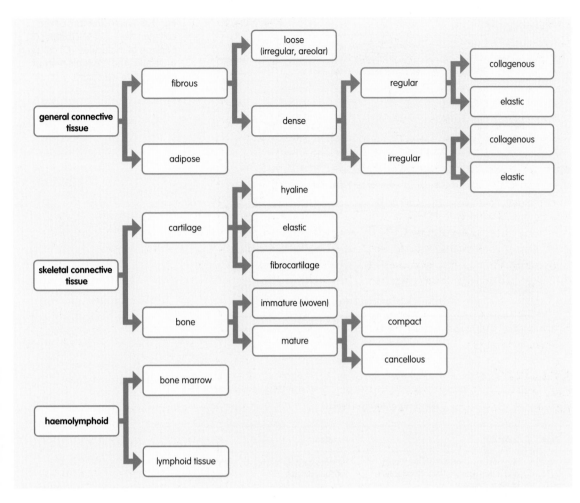

Fig. 1.4 Classification of connective tissue.

	Connective tissue cell types and functions	
	Cell type	**Functions**
fixed cells	fibroblasts, chondroblasts, osteoblasts, osteoclasts	synthesis and maintenance of matrix
	adipocytes	fat metabolism
	mast cells	release of histamine
	mesenchymal cells	mature cell precursors
transient cells	white blood cells	immune response
	melanocytes	pigmentation

Fig. 1.5 Connective tissue cell types and their functions.

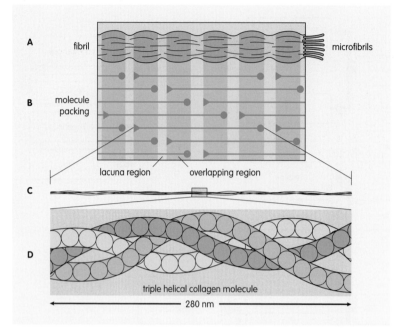

Fig. 1.6 Microstructure of the collagen fibril. (A) Microfibril; (B) packing of molecules; (C) collagen molecule; and (D) triple helix of polypeptide (α) chains.

	Functions of collagen types	
Type	**Location**	**Function**
I	skin, tendon, ligaments, bone, fascia and organ capsules (accounts for 90% of body collagen)	provides variable mechanical support (loose or dense)
II	hyaline and elastic cartilage, notochord, and intervertebral discs	provides shape and resistance to pressure
III	connective tissue of organs (liver, lymphoid organs, etc.), blood vessels, and fetal skin	forms reticular networks
IV	basement membrane of epithelial and endothelial cells	provides support and a filtration barrier
V	basement membrane of smooth and skeletal muscle cells	provides support (other functions poorly understood)

Fig. 1.7 Functions of the different types of collagen.

- List the components of the musculoskeletal system.
- What are the general functions of the musculoskeletal system?
- Describe the stimulation of skeletal, cardiac and smooth muscle.
- List the general functions of the skin.
- Name the three layers of the skin.
- Define connective tissue.
- List the functions of connective tissue.
- Give a simple classification of connective tissue.
- Describe the components of connective tissue.

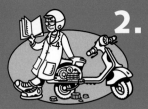

2. Skeletal Muscle

Comparison of the three types of muscle

Muscle is a tissue made up of contractile cells. These cells are capable of producing movement or tension. Other examples of contractile cells include myoepithelial cells (see p. 57) and myofibroblasts, found in connective tissue.

Three types of muscle tissue are found in the human body: skeletal, cardiac and smooth (Fig. 2.1). Cardiac and smooth muscle will be discussed in more detail in Chapter 3.

Skeletal muscle

The alternative names for skeletal muscle are striated (from its histological appearance) or voluntary (from the mechanism by which contraction is controlled).

Sites

The majority of muscle found within the body is skeletal (Fig. 2.2). It is found in the limbs, thorax, abdominal wall, pelvis and face.

Control

Contraction of skeletal muscle tends to be either voluntary or reflex, and is controlled by the somatic nervous system.

Histological appearance

Skeletal muscle cells are long and thin, and are therefore often referred to as muscle fibres. The cells are multinucleated and appear cross-striated under light microscopy.

Cell size

Skeletal muscle cells are 50–60 μm in diameter (range 10–100 μm) and up to 10 cm long.

Nature of contraction

Rapid contraction and relaxation of skeletal muscle occurs as a twitch. The nature of the stimulus is important because, if the muscle is stimulated rapidly and repetitively, contractions may summate to produce smooth and sustained contractions.

Function

Skeletal muscle has an important role in voluntary movement of the skeleton and maintenance of posture. It is also involved in the movement of the tongue and the globe of the eye.

Cardiac muscle

The alternative name for cardiac muscle is myocardium.

Sites

Myocardium forms the muscular component of the heart (Fig. 2.1), lying between the pericardium and endocardium (Fig. 3.1; p. 50).

Control

Contraction of myocardium is regulated by pacemaker cells within the tissue. The autonomic nervous system can modify contraction of myocardium by altering heart rate and therefore the duration and strength of contraction.

Histological appearance

As with skeletal muscle, longitudinal and transverse striations are seen under light microscopy. However, cardiac cells are smaller and branched and have single central nuclei. Intercellular junctions are often seen; these are called intercalated discs.

 Cardiac muscle is a type of striated muscle and its properties can be considered to lie between those of smooth and skeletal muscle.

Cell size

Myocardium cells are 15 μm in diameter and 100 μm long.

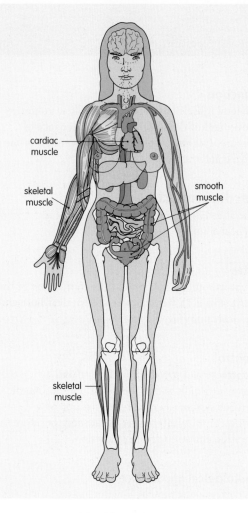

cardiac muscle

skeletal muscle

smooth muscle

skeletal muscle

Fig. 2.1 Location of the different muscle types in the human body.

Nature of contraction

Myocardium undergoes spontaneous and rhythmical contractions. These contractions are always brief twitches followed by a long refractory period. This enables cardiac muscle to relax, allowing the heart to fill with blood. Because of the long refractory period after each brief twitch, summation of contractions does not occur.

Function

Myocardium pumps deoxygenated blood to the lungs and oxygenated blood to the body tissues.

Smooth muscle

The alternative name for smooth muscle is involuntary muscle, named after the mechanism by which contraction is controlled.

Smooth muscle can be divided into visceral (single unit or syncytial) or multi-unit types. Most smooth muscle is of the visceral type.

Sites

Single-unit smooth muscle is found in small blood vessels, the ducts of secretory glands, and the walls of hollow organs of the gastrointestinal and urogenital systems (Fig. 2.1). Multi-unit smooth muscle is found in large blood vessels, large airways, the eye and hair follicles.

Control

Smooth muscle contraction is always under involuntary control. In the case of visceral smooth muscle, initiation of contraction is inherent (caused by pacemaker cells within the smooth muscle tissue, which discharge in an irregular pattern) and can be modified by hormones, local metabolites and the autonomic nervous system. Multi-unit smooth muscle, however, is neurogenic (the initiation of each contraction is under the control of the autonomic nervous system).

Histological appearance

Smooth muscle is less organized than skeletal muscle and myocardium, and no striations are seen under light microscopy. The cells are spindle-shaped and have large, single, central nuclei.

Cell size

Smooth muscle cells are 2–10 μm in diameter and 20–400 μm long. Cell size varies, depending on location; e.g. cells of 20 μm are found in small blood vessels while cells up to 400 μm in length are found in the uterus.

Nature of contraction

Low-force contraction of smooth muscle occurs with relatively little energy expenditure. In the case of multi-unit smooth muscle, individual muscle fibres contract via the same mechanism as in skeletal muscle. In visceral smooth muscle, however, the whole muscle mass contracts and not individual

Fig. 2.2A Anterior view of major muscle groups in the body. (Courtesy of Dr K.M.Backhouse.)

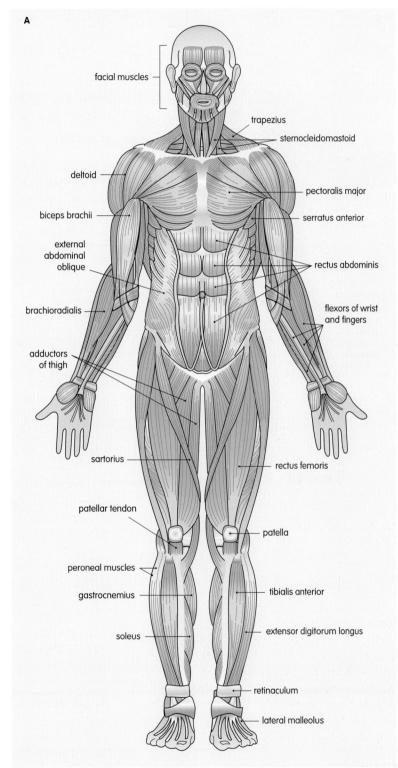

A

facial muscles

trapezius

sternocleidomastoid

deltoid

pectoralis major

biceps brachii

serratus anterior

external abdominal oblique

rectus abdominis

brachioradialis

flexors of wrist and fingers

adductors of thigh

sartorius

rectus femoris

patellar tendon

patella

peroneal muscles

gastrocnemius

tibialis anterior

soleus

extensor digitorum longus

retinaculum

lateral malleolus

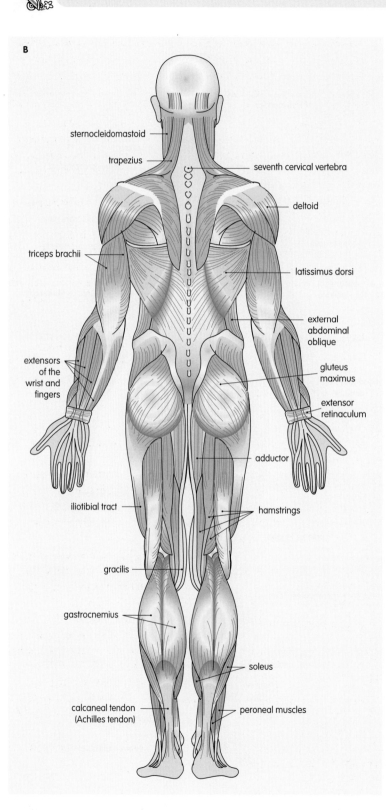

Fig. 2.2B Posterior view of major muscle groups in the body. (Courtesy of Dr K.M. Backhouse.)

sternocleidomastoid

trapezius

seventh cervical vertebra

deltoid

triceps brachii

latissimus dorsi

external abdominal oblique

extensors of the wrist and fingers

gluteus maximus

extensor retinaculum

adductor

iliotibial tract

hamstrings

gracilis

gastrocnemius

soleus

calcaneal tendon (Achilles tendon)

peroneal muscles

muscle fibres, meaning that contraction is slow and sustained.

Function

The functions of smooth muscle are related to the structure in which they are found, e.g. the smooth muscle component of blood vessels regulates blood flow by altering the diameter of the blood vessels.

Multi-unit smooth muscle is involved in the alteration of pupil size by contraction of iris muscles, and accommodation by contraction of the ciliary muscle. Multi-unit smooth muscle is also responsible for 'goose bumps', which result from contraction of muscle at the base of each hair follicle.

Skeletal and multi-unit smooth muscle may be referred to as neurogenic muscle, i.e. muscle in which contraction arises as a result of nerve stimulation.
Cardiac and visceral smooth muscle may be referred to as myogenic muscle, i.e. they require no nerve stimulation for contraction that arises from within the muscle owing to the presence of pacemaker cells.

Skeletal muscle

The contraction generated by a muscle depends on:
- The length of the muscle fibres.
- The volume/number of muscle fibres.
- The rate at which fibre length changes.

The range of movement produced by a muscle is proportional to the length of the muscle fibres, whereas the bulkier the muscle the greater the force it will generate. This can be illustrated by the following example. Consider two pieces of muscle tissue, of equal volume. One is long and narrow, the other short but broad in cross-section. The long muscle will allow a greater degree of shortening but, because of its narrow cross-section, it cannot generate much force of contraction. By contrast, the

shorter muscle cannot contract over any great length but, because its cross-section incorporates many muscle fibres, it generates a large force of contraction.

Muscles assume a variety of shapes, depending on the type of contraction involved. For example, a multipennate arrangement results in a large number of short fibres attached to a single tendon, and the force of contraction is great and concentrated on the tendon (Fig. 2.3).

Muscle groups are arranged in pairs which consist of:
- A functional group in which one muscle is the main participant and the other muscles help to perform a movement, e.g. flexion at the elbow joint is due to the action of biceps with the help of brachialis, brachioradialis and the forearm flexor muscles.
- An antagonistic group in which muscles oppose the movement of the functional group, e.g. triceps, assisted by anconeus, antagonizes the action of biceps by causing extension at the elbow (Fig. 2.4).

A muscle can belong to more than one group, e.g. latissimus dorsi is involved in both adduction and extension of the shoulder joint.

Each end of a muscle is usually attached to bone. The origin, or head, is the attachment site at which there is little movement when the muscle performs its main action (see Fig. 2.5). The insertion is the more mobile attachment site.

The terms proximal and distal attachment may be more appropriate as, depending on movement, the origin (proximal attachment) may be more mobile than the insertion (distal attachment).

Muscles are attached to bone by fibrous connective tissue, although not all skeletal muscle is attached to bone; for instance, the tongue has neither bony proximal nor distal attachments. In addition, rings of skeletal muscle or sphincters, e.g. the external urethral sphincter that controls passage of urine from the bladder to the urethra, do not attach to bone.

Other structures associated with skeletal muscle are:

Tendons:
A tendon is an inelastic, flexible cord consisting of closely packed collagen fibres, which attaches muscle to bone.

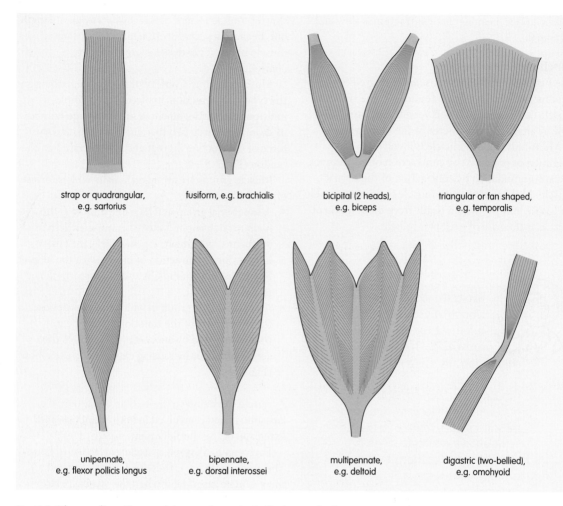

strap or quadrangular, e.g. sartorius

fusiform, e.g. brachialis

bicipital (2 heads), e.g. biceps

triangular or fan shaped, e.g. temporalis

unipennate, e.g. flexor pollicis longus

bipennate, e.g. dorsal interossei

multipennate, e.g. deltoid

digastric (two-bellied), e.g. omohyoid

Fig. 2.3 Fibre configurations and shapes of muscles in the human body.

Aponeuroses:

An aponeurosis is a thin sheet of fibrous connective tissue attaching muscle to bone. It is found in muscles that have a wide attachment area to bone, e.g. the anterior abdominal wall. An aponeurosis sheet is, in essence, a broad tendon.

Sesamoid bones:

A sesamoid bone is a small bone found within the tendons of certain muscles, e.g. the patella, and some bones in the hand and foot. Its presence may correlate with sites susceptible to wear and tear. The bone may also provide extra leverage.

Microstructure of skeletal muscle
Arrangement of muscle tissue

Whole muscle consists of fibres that are arranged in bundles called fasciculi. Connective tissue lies between the individual muscle fibres and fasciculi, and in addition there is a dense connective tissue coat surrounding the whole muscle (Fig. 2.5).

Skeletal muscle has a rich blood supply. The blood vessels and nerves divide and extend throughout the perimysium (the collagen connective tissue that surrounds fasciculi).

Smaller fasciculi are found in muscles involved in fine movement; hence the size of fasciculi is suggestive of function.

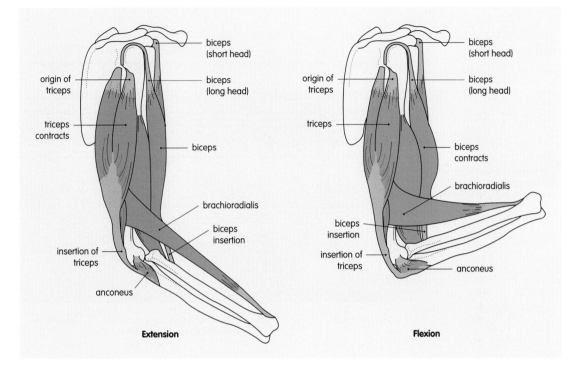

Fig. 2.4 Arrangement of muscles in antagonistic pairs demonstrated at the elbow joint.

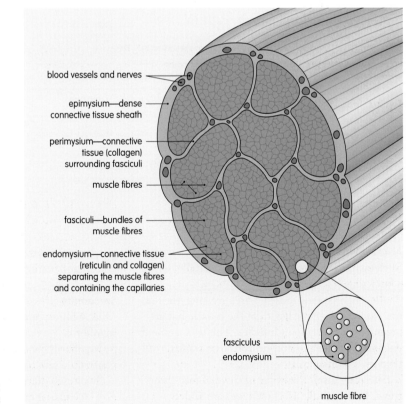

Fig. 2.5 Cross-section of whole muscle showing the arrangement of muscles into fasciculi and fibres surrounded by connective tissue.

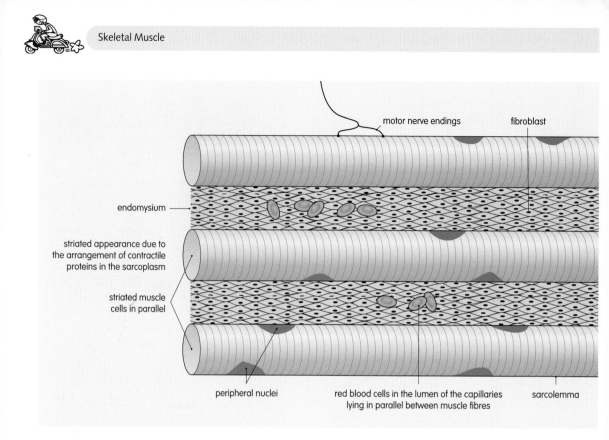

endomysium

striated appearance due to
the arrangement of contractile
proteins in the sarcoplasm

striated muscle
cells in parallel

motor nerve endings

fibroblast

peripheral nuclei

red blood cells in the lumen of the capillaries
lying in parallel between muscle fibres

sarcolemma

Fig. 2.6 Longitudinal section showing the arrangement of skeletal muscle fibres within a fasciculus.

Classification of different types of skeletal muscle fibres			
Fibre type	Colour	Speed and force of twitch	Resistance to fatigue
I	red (because of myoglobin)	slow, only 10% of force of type IIb	high (fatigue resistant)
IIa	intermediate	fast, but force and speed less than type IIb	intermediate (fatigue resistant)
IIb	white	fast and high force	low (fatigues after repeated stimulation), fast fatiguable

Fig. 2.7 Classification of the different types of skeletal muscle fibres.

Microenvironment of skeletal muscle

Skeletal muscle fibres are arranged in parallel within a fasciculus (Fig. 2.6).

Although skeletal muscle fibres are long, they do not extend the whole length of the muscle but are organized as overlapping bundles. This arrangement enables the force of a contraction to be transmitted throughout the muscle.

Skeletal muscle fibres can be divided into three types: I, IIa and IIb. All three types are widely distributed throughout the muscle (Fig. 2.7). The properties of the different types of muscle fibres are considered in more detail on p. 33 (Fig. 2.25).

Sarcomere

Muscle fibres, or myofibres, are cells containing myofibrils.

Myofibrils consist of myofilaments arranged in contractile units called sarcomeres.

Two types of myofilaments occur:
• Thick filaments, mainly composed of myosin protein.

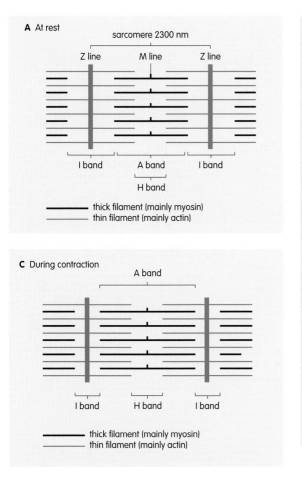

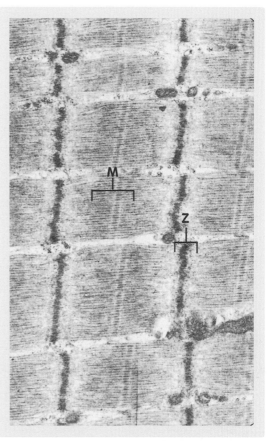

Fig. 2.8 Arrangement of contractile proteins in the sarcomere at rest and during contraction. At rest (A), the H and I bands represent areas in which the thick and thin filaments do not overlap. The Z line anchors the actin filaments and the M line anchors the myosin filaments. The pattern of actin and myosin filaments is demonstrated clearly on the electron micrograph (B). During contraction (C), the Z lines 'slide' closer together, causing shortening of muscle. The A band remains constant in width but the I and H bands shorten. (M, M line; Z, Z line.) (Electron micrograph courtesy of Dr T. Gray.)

- Thin filaments, mainly composed of actin protein.

It is the organization of these myofilaments that leads to the striated appearance of skeletal muscle (Figs 2.8 and 2.9).

Cellular structure of muscle fibre

A muscle fibre is a specialized cell (Fig. 2.10) that comprises:
- A sarcolemma or cell membrane.
- Sarcoplasm or cytoplasm.
- A sarcoplasmic reticulum or endoplasmic reticulum.

Each muscle fibre cell has multiple peripheral nuclei, glycogen granules and mitochondria that lie in the sarcoplasm between myofibrils. They contain T-tubules—channels that extend from the sarcolemma of the muscle fibre and surround each muscle fibre at the junction of the A and I band, the AI junction. T-tubules ensure that all sarcomere contractions are synchronized.

Sarcoplasmic reticulum runs longitudinally along myofibrils and wraps around groups of myofibrils. In regions of T-tubules, the sarcoplasmic reticulum forms terminal cisternae.

Within the muscle, triads are an important structure which consist of a T-tubule with

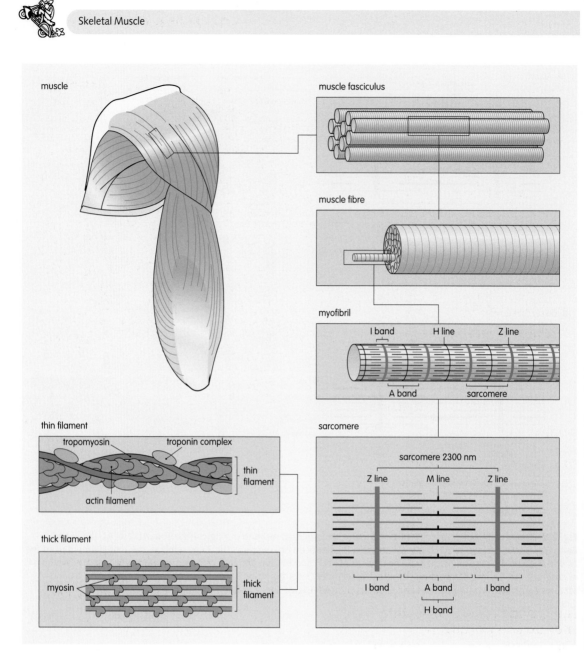

Fig. 2.9 Organization of skeletal muscle.

sarcoplasmic reticulum on either side. Depolarization (p. 23) is transmitted through the T-tubule, causing release of Ca^{2+} into the sarcoplasm. Ca^{2+} in the sarcoplasm triggers muscular contraction.

Replacement of muscle fibres

Satellite cells are small spindle-shaped cells that lie between the sarcolemma and basal lamina in adult skeletal muscle; they are visible under electron microscopy.

If muscle damage occurs but the basal lamina remains intact, several events occur:
- Satellite cells proliferate to form myoblasts.
- Myoblasts fuse to form myotubules around which myofibrils assemble.
- New muscle fibres form in which the nuclei are centrally, rather than peripherally, placed.

If the basal lamina becomes damaged, fibroblasts are activated to repair the tissues, with resulting scar formation.

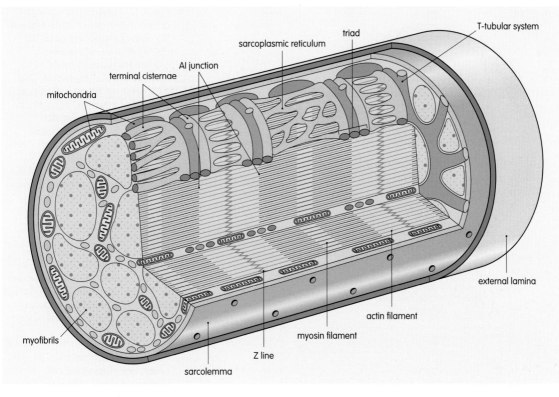

Fig. 2.10 Components of the muscle fibre.

Cellular physiology of skeletal muscle

Ion balance and the resting membrane potential

There are differences in the ionic composition of the intracellular fluid (ICF) and extracellular fluid (ECF) of muscle cells (Fig. 2.11). These differences are due to:

- The selective permeability of the cell membrane to K⁺ and Cl⁻.
- The presence of large intracellular impermeant anions from amino acid metabolism. These cause movement of Cl⁻ extracellularly and K⁺ intracellularly.
- Relative cell membrane impermeability to Na⁺.

Resting membrane potential

The resting membrane potential (RMP) is the difference in voltage between the inside and the

Distribution of ions in the ICF and ECF of muscle cells		
Ion	ICF (mmol/L)	ECF (mmol/L)
Na⁺	12	145
K⁺	155	4
H⁺	13×10^{-5}	3.8×10^{-5}
Ca²⁺	8	1.5
Cl⁻	3.8	12.0
HCO₃⁻	8	27
A⁻	155	0

Fig. 2.11 Distribution of ions in the intracellular fluid (ICF) and extracellular fluid (ECF) of muscle cells. A⁻, Organic impermeant anions. (Adapted with permission from *Review of Medical Physiology*, 17th edn, by W.F. Ganong, Appleton & Lange, 1995.)

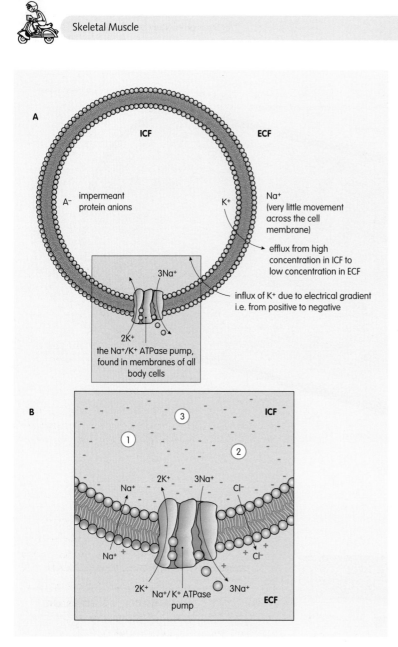

Fig. 2.12 Factors involved in the determination and maintenance of the resting membrane potential (RMP). K^+ is the key player. (A) The Na^+ pump is found in membranes of all body cells. The mechanism of action is as follows: removal of 3 Na^+ and entry of 2 K^+, expending 1 ATP molecule; phosphorylation of the protein subunits produces a conformational change and binding of Na^+; dephosphorylation results in binding of K^+ and reversion of the protein to its original shape. The cycle is repeated 100 times per second. Other contributors to RMP are shown in (B).
1. There is a passive leakage of a small amount of Na^+ from ECF to ICF along a concentration gradient.
2. Passive movement of Cl^- from ICF to ECF along an electrical gradient.
3. Presence of impermeant protein anions (A^-).
(Note that the bulk of the solution is electrochemically neutral. The excess ions close to the cell membrane are a small proportion. However, they are significant enough to cause movements across the cell membrane.) (ICF, intracellular fluid; ECF, extracellular fluid.)

outside of the cell at rest, normally a value of –90 mV in muscle cells. This separation of charge across the cell membrane creates the potential to do work and is a result of the differences in the distribution and permeabilities of ions across the cell membrane (Fig. 2.12).

The movement of ions across the cell membrane which causes the voltage difference is caused by:

- A concentration gradient that favours K^+ efflux.
- An electrostatic gradient that favours K^+ influx.

The main ion responsible for the RMP is K^+. However, the RMP is not equal to the equilibrium potential of potassium (E_K) owing to:

- Small concentration of Na^+ leaking from ECF to ICF.
- Diffusion of Cl^-.
- Presence of protein impermeant ions (A^-).
- The activities of the Na^+/K^+ pump.

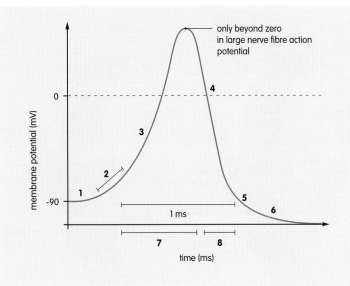

Fig. 2.13 Phases of the action potential (AP). (1) Resting membrane potential; (2) initial slow depolarization of cell in response to stimulus; (3) opening of voltage-gated Na+ channels when threshold is reached; (4) repolarization, i.e. opening of voltage-gated K+ channels; (5) return to resting membrane potential (–90 mV); (6) hyperpolarization due to 'excessive' K+ efflux; (7) absolute refractory period (AP may not be initiated); (8) relative refractory period (greater stimulus than normal to initiate the AP).

Na+/K+ ATPase pump

Sites: The Na+/K+ ATPase pump is found in the membranes of all body cells (Fig. 2.12).
Functions: The functions of the Na+/K+ ATPase pump are:

- Maintenance of cell volume.
- Co-transport and counter-transport of other solutes.
- Contribution to RMP (by maintaining the necessary electrostatic gradient; RMP is mainly due to passive K+ efflux).
- Maintenance of the intracellular environment.

Mechanism of action: The removal of 3Na+ and entry of 2K+ expends an ATP molecule. Phosphorylation of the ATP protein subunits results in a conformational change and binding of Na+, whereas dephosphorylation results in K+ binding, which causes the protein to revert back to its original shape. This cycle is repeated 100 times per second (Fig. 2.13).

Electrochemical equilibrium

Electrochemical equilibrium (E) of K+ is achieved when the forces acting in both directions are equal so that there is no net movement of K+.

Equilibrium potential

Equilibrium potential is the voltage required to stop the diffusion of a permeant ion across the cell membrane. It can be calculated from the Nernst equation, given that the ion is permeable to the cell membrane, and assuming that the Nernst potential is the potential inside the membrane and that the potential outside the membrane is zero.

$$E_{ion} = \frac{\pm 61 \log[ion]_{ECF}}{\log[ion]_{ICF}}$$

E, equilibrium potential of the ion; 61, a constant which takes into account the valency of the ion (Z), the absolute temperature (T), the gas constant (R) and the electrical constant (F); [ion], the ion concentration in mmol/l. Note that E_K is –95 mV, which is close to the value of the RMP of a muscle cell, implying that the cell membrane is mainly permeable to K+.

Effects of Na+ and K+ channels on the membrane potential
Depolarization

Depolarization results from the opening of Na+ channels and a Na+ influx. It results in a membrane potential that is less negative than the RMP.

Hyperpolarization

Hyperpolarization occurs upon closure of Na+ channels and opening of K+ channels, causing a K+ efflux which restores, and may exceed, the normal RMP. This results in a membrane potential which is more negative than the RMP.

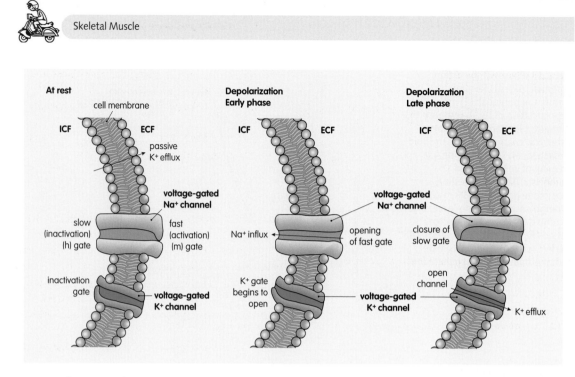

Fig. 2.14 Changes in voltage-activated channels during an action potential derived from studies using the voltage clamp and selective channel blockers. (ICF, intracellular fluid; ECF, extracellular fluid.)

Action potential

An action potential (AP) is a transient depolarization of the cell membrane beyond a critical level or 'threshold potential' (Fig. 2.14). When there is slow depolarization of a cell in response to a stimulus, an AP is generated at the threshold potential via the triggering of voltage-gated ion channels. It is an important means of transmitting information through the nervous system and initiating contraction of muscle cells. The size and duration of the AP within different cell types is variable.

Initiation of the AP

APs are usually initiated:
• At synapses—specialized junctions between cells.
• By the passage of current from one cell to another via gap junctions.

Either of these stimuli activate a slow depolarization of the cell membrane, which reaches the critical threshold level and thus generates an AP. The all-or-none law states that once an AP has been initiated, the size is constant for a given type of cell and will not be affected by altering the stimuli strength.

Ionic basis of the AP

Both Na$^+$ and K$^+$ movements across the cell membrane are important (Fig. 2.14). At rest, the voltage-activated Na$^+$ and K$^+$ channels are closed, although K$^+$ moves passively along a concentration gradient through the cell membrane.

Early phase of depolarization

During the early phase of depolarization, the fast gate (m-gate) of a voltage-gated Na$^+$ channel opens and the slow gate (h-gate) starts to close. As the slow gate takes longer to close, there is an influx of Na$^+$. This influx results in the activation of more Na$^+$ channels via a feedback mechanism.

The voltage-activated K$^+$ channel starts to open slowly.

Late phase of depolarization

During the late phase of depolarization, the slow gate of a voltage-gated Na$^+$ channel is closed and there is no more influx of Na$^+$. The slow gate re-opens when RMP is reached, i.e. when the fast gate is closed.

The K$^+$ channel is open and remains so until RMP is restored. Closure of the K$^+$ channel is slow, meaning that hyperpolarization may occur following an AP.

Propagation of the AP

An AP occurring at any one site on the cell membrane causes voltage changes in the adjacent parts of the membrane; these allow the AP to propagate in both directions. These changes can be explained by the local circuit theory (Fig. 2.15).

Saltatory conduction

Saltatory conduction occurs in myelinated nerve fibres (Fig. 2.16). The local circuit theory still applies but the current can leave the axon only at nodes of Ranvier. This results in a greater conduction velocity because the current density at the nodes is greater, so depolarization is more rapid.

The circuit of current can travel a number of internodal lengths and still be able to depolarize a node to threshold. This produces a large safety factor.

Conduction velocity

In nerves the conduction velocity (CV) ranges from 100 m/s to less than 1 m/s.

Factors affecting conduction velocity are:

- Fibre diameter, i.e. myelin sheath, large nerve fibres: increasing the fibre diameter increases the conduction velocity.

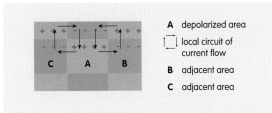

A	depolarized area
	local circuit of current flow
B	adjacent area
C	adjacent area

Fig. 2.15 Local circuit theory. The local circuit of current may cause sufficient depolarization in B and/or C to initiate an action potential. This can then be propagated in the same way.

- Temperature: increasing temperature increases the conduction velocity. However, above 40°C the conduction velocity decreases until there is 'heat block'.
- Strength of local circuits: stronger local circuits result in a greater conduction velocity.

The synapse

The junction at which nerve cells communicate with each other is called a synapse.

Synapses can be electrical, i.e. direct transmission of current from presynaptic cell to target cell through ion channels, or chemical, i.e. release of a chemical that binds to protein receptors on the target cell membrane, causing direct or indirect opening of ion channels (Fig. 2.17).

Transmission of a signal at a chemical synapse involves:

- An AP propagated at the presynaptic nerve terminal.
- Depolarization of the nerve terminal.
- Voltage-activated Ca^{2+} channels open, causing an influx of Ca^{2+}.
- Vesicles in the active zone fusing with the presynaptic membrane, releasing neurotransmitter by exocytosis.
- The neurotransmitter binding to protein receptors in the postsynaptic membrane.
- Changes in the postsynaptic membrane, leading to depolarization or hyperpolarization of the target cell.

Electrical synapses correspond to gap junctions between certain cells (e.g. neurons, cardiac muscle cells, smooth muscle cells, epithelial cells). Transmission of a signal at an electrical synapse involves:

Fig. 2.16 Saltatory conduction in myelinated nerve fibres. The current is only able to leave at the nodes of Ranvier. In this way, the circuit of current can be thought of as 'jumping' from node to node, allowing a greater speed of conduction.

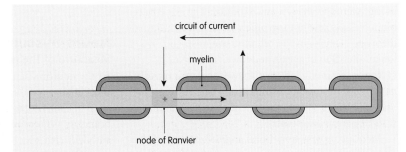

Comparison of electrical and chemical synapses		
Property	**Electrical**	**Chemical**
site	nerves, heart, smooth muscle, liver, epithelium	most of synapses in body, including skeletal muscle and brain
structures seen at synapse	gap junctions	presynaptic vesicles and mitochondria, postsynaptic receptors
mechanism of transmission	ionic current	chemical messenger
cytoplasmic continuity between presynaptic and postsynaptic cell	yes	no
synaptic cleft	3.5 nm	20–40 nm
nature of transmission	rapid, usually excitatory effect on target cell	synaptic delay 1–5 ms, excitatory or inhibitory effect on target cell
plasticity	no	yes
amplification of signal	no	yes

Fig. 2.17 Comparison of electrical and chemical synapses. (Adapted with permission from *Human Physiology and Mechanisms of Disease*, 8th edn, by A.C. Guyton, W.B. Saunders, 1991.)

- Depolarization of the presynaptic membrane.
- Direct flow of current through gap junction ion channels to target cell.
- Depolarization of the target cell.

Local anaesthetics

Local anaesthetics are drugs that are used to provide temporary relief of pain. They are weak bases: 90% are un-ionized and can cross the cell membrane but are not very effective at blocking the Na^+ channels, while 10% are ionized and block the Na^+ channels from inside the axon when the channels are open.

The more common local anaesthetics include lignocaine, bupivacaine, prilocaine, benzocaine and cocaine.

Vasoconstrictors (e.g. adrenaline) are often administered with local anaesthetics. The constricted blood vessels prevent too much local anaesthetic diffusing away from the relevant site, resulting in a longer duration of action and lower chance of systemic toxicity. However, the vasoconstrictors are never used in sites with small blood vessels (e.g. fingers, ears), owing to the risk of tissue ischaemia resulting from vasospasm.

Mechanism of action: Local anaesthetics block Na^+ channels to prevent depolarization and propagation of APs. The un-ionized form crosses the cell membrane and 10% ionizes in the cytoplasm. This ionized form then blocks open Na^+ channels from within. Nerve fibres with a small diameter are more easily blocked; hence, local anaesthetics can prevent the sensation of pain without affecting touch.

Use dependency: The more a nerve is stimulated the greater the block achieved, as the Na^+ channels are blocked when open.

Adverse effects: Local anaesthetics can affect the cardiovascular system by causing hypotension or cardiac arrest, or the central nervous system (CNS) by causing restlessness, sleepiness, convulsions and respiratory depression. Anaphylaxis can also occur.

Neuromuscular junction
Structure of the neuromuscular junction

At the neuromuscular junction (NMJ, Fig. 2.18) each muscle fibre is innervated by one motor nerve. The axon of each motor neuron divides into many branches as it enters the muscle, each branch forming an NMJ with a single muscle fibre. Each muscle fibre has only one NMJ.

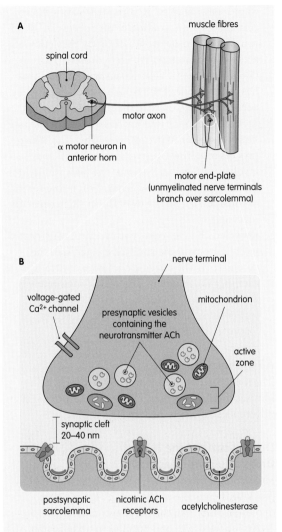

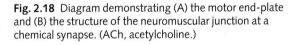

Fig. 2.18 Diagram demonstrating (A) the motor end-plate and (B) the structure of the neuromuscular junction at a chemical synapse. (ACh, acetylcholine.)

Presynaptic nerve terminal
Vesicles
At the presynaptic nerve terminal, acetylcholine (ACh) is synthesized in the cytoplasm and then stored in vesicles (about 10 000 molecules per vesicle) with an ATP molecule. At rest, 85% of ACh is stored in the vesicles and 15% is present in the cytoplasm.

Mitochondria
Numerous mitochondria provide energy for the uptake of choline and synthesis of ACh.

Active zones
Active zones are specialized regions of the presynaptic membrane. They are sites of neurotransmitter release and are positioned so they lie opposite a junctional fold in the postsynaptic membrane.

Voltage-activated Ca^{2+} channels
Voltage-activated Ca^{2+} channels are believed to be adjacent to active zones. The channels open in response to an AP. The associated influx of Ca^{2+} causes the vesicles to move to the active zone.

Although the overall intracellular concentration of Ca^{2+} is relatively low, remember that there is a high concentration of Ca^{2+} in the sarcoplasmic reticulum.

Postsynaptic membrane
Motor end-plate
The motor end-plate is a specialized region of the muscle fibre membrane at which the terminal branches of the motor nerve communicate with the muscle fibre.

Junctional folds
Junctional folds are folds in the motor end-plate upon which nicotinic ACh receptors (nicAChR) are located. These folds increase the surface area upon which the transmitter can act.

Basal lamina
The basal lamina is connective tissue lying between the nerve terminal and muscle fibre membrane. Large quantities of the enzyme acetylcholinesterase

The nerve terminal invaginates into the muscle fibre near its midpoint to form a depression in the muscle membrane, termed the synaptic trough (gutter). However, the nerve terminal does not cross the muscle membrane.

The synaptic cleft is:
- The space between the nerve terminal and the muscle membrane.
- Occupied by connective tissue and ECF.

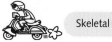

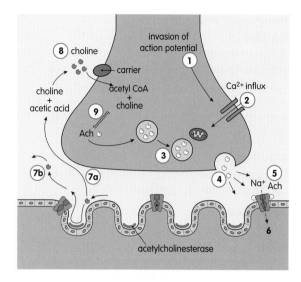

Fig. 2.19 Events at the neuromuscular junction upon arrival of a nerve action potential. Refer to text for an explanation of the sequence (which occurs in 10–15 ms). (ACh, acetylcholine.)

are found here, particularly at the bases of the junctional folds.

Nicotinic ACh receptor

The nicAChR consists of five protein subunits (2α, 1β, 1γ and 1δ). The binding of two ACh molecules (one to each of the two α subunits) induces a conformational change and the channel opens. The channel is permeable to both K^+ and Na^+. However, concentration gradients favour Na^+ influx.

When a nerve AP arrives at the NMJ a sequence of events, lasting 10–15 ms, takes place. This sequence is numbered to correspond to Fig. 2.19, as follows:

1. The AP arrives at the nerve terminal.
2. The voltage-activated Ca^{2+} channels open, allowing Ca^{2+} influx.
3. Ca^{2+} influx attracts presynaptic vesicles to the active zones.
4. Vesicles fuse to the presynaptic membrane and release ACh in 'packets' by the process of exocytosis.
5. ACh diffuses across the synaptic cleft to bind to nicAChR on the junctional folds. There is activation of channels and an influx of Na^+ occurs.
6. Na^+ influx depolarizes the muscle. This is called an end-plate potential (epp). The epp depolarizes adjacent regions of the muscle membrane. Upon reaching threshold, an AP occurs in the muscle fibre.

7. Rapid removal of ACh from the synaptic trough terminates the activation of the receptors. This removal occurs in two ways: (a) by the action of acetylcholinesterase, which hydrolyses ACh to choline and acetic acid; (b) a small amount that has diffused out of the trough is broken down by pseudocholinesterase in the plasma.
8. Uptake of choline into nerve terminals is the rate-limiting step of ACh synthesis. This is an active process requiring the hydrolysis of ATP, and involves two carrier systems: the high affinity–low capacity mechanism, which is responsible for 90% of the uptake, and the low affinity–high capacity mechanism.
9. Recycled choline reacts with acetyl CoA (formed in the mitochondria and transported into the cytoplasm). The enzyme choline acetyltransferase catalyses the reaction. The vesicle membrane is also recycled by endocytosis from the nerve terminal membrane. ACh is again stored in 'packets' in the nerve terminal.

AP in skeletal muscle

The ionic basis of the AP in skeletal muscle is the same as the AP in nerves. However, there are certain differences between the two (Fig. 2.20).

Drugs acting at the NMJ
Drugs acting presynaptically

Hemicholinium acts presynaptically at the NMJ by blocking the uptake of choline. There is a slow depletion of ACh in the nerve terminal.

Aminoglycosides and botulinum toxin inhibit ACh release.

Drugs enhancing transmission

Anticholinesterases enhance transmission at the NMJ by increasing the time that ACh is present in the synaptic cleft.

Mechanism of action: Anticholinesterases inhibit acetylcholinesterase. There are three main types of anticholinesterases: short-acting (up to 15 min) drugs such as edrophonium (these bind reversibly to the active site of the enzyme); intermediate-acting drugs, e.g. pyridostigmine and neostigmine (these bind covalently to the enzyme); and long-acting drugs, e.g. organophosphorus compounds (these form strong covalent bonds with the active site; they are often referred to as irreversible, as the enzyme is inactivated for a long period of time; they have no clinical use, but are used in chemical weapons).

Fig. 2.20 Comparison of the action potential (AP) in skeletal muscle with that in nerves.

Comparison of the action potential of skeletal muscle with nerve		
Property	**Skeletal muscle AP**	**Nerve AP**
RMP	−80 to −90 mV	−40 mV (small nerves) to −90 mV (large nerves)
duration	1–5 ms	<1 ms
spread of AP to interior	T-tubule system	depolarization of membrane is sufficient
conduction velocity	3–5 m/s	<1–100 ms, depends on a number of factors (see page 22)

Indications: Edrophonium assists in the diagnosis of myasthenia gravis (p. 40). An intravenous injection leads to short-term improvement in muscle strength. Treatment involves the use of intermediate-acting anticholinesterases. Anticholinesterases reverse competitive neuromuscular block after surgery.

Adverse effects: Side effects of anticholinesterases include paradoxical depolarizing neuromuscular block; convulsions, coma and respiratory arrest if a lipid-soluble anticholinesterase (e.g. physostigmine) is used; symptoms associated with the parasympathetic nervous system, as ACh is the neurotransmitter acting on muscarinic receptors.

Drugs acting postsynaptically

Neuromuscular-blocking drugs are either competitive or depolarizing.

Competitive drugs

Tubocurarine and gallamine are examples of competitive neuromuscular-blocking drugs.

Mechanism of action: Neuromuscular-blocking drugs compete with ACh for binding sites on the ACh receptor in the postsynaptic membrane. There is no opening of the ion channel when they bind, therefore AP generation in muscle is less likely. Their action is reversed by anticholinesterases and enhanced by general anaesthetics.

Indications: Neuromuscular-blocking drugs are used in surgery to relax skeletal muscles and for electroconvulsive therapy.

Adverse effects: Side effects of neuromuscular-blocking drugs include a decrease in blood pressure owing to blockage of autonomic nicotinic receptors, and anaphylaxis.

Depolarizing drugs

Suxamethonium is an example of a depolarizing drug.

Mechanism of action: Depolarizing drugs are nicotinic agonists with blockage occurring because of prolonged membrane depolarization and desensitization of nicotinic receptors. Their action is potentiated by anticholinesterases.

Indications: Depolarizing drugs are used in surgery to relax skeletal muscles, and for electroconvulsive therapy. Although competitive blockers are more widely used, depolarizing drugs tend to be used for brief procedures.

Adverse effects: As initial stimulation occurs before blockage, asynchronous muscle fibre twitches may result in muscle pains following the use of depolarizing drugs. Other side effects include bradycardia due to action on muscarinic receptors.

Excitation–contraction coupling

Excitation–contraction coupling refers to the events that occur from initiation of an AP in the sarcolemma, contraction of muscle and subsequent relaxation.

Initiation of an AP in muscle fibre

The end-plate potential (epp) resulting from a single neuronal AP is usually greater in amplitude than that required to initiate an AP in muscle fibre. For this reason the NMJ is said to have a very high 'safety factor'.

Propagation of an AP into muscle fibre via T-tubules

An AP is propagated into muscle fibre via T-tubules in a sequence of events (the following numbers refer to Fig. 2.21).

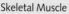

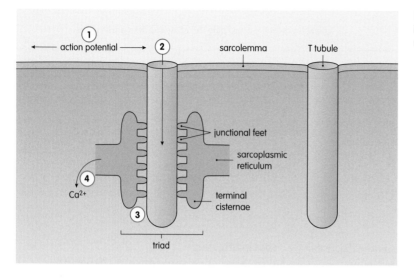

Fig. 2.21 Sarcoplasmic release of intracellular Ca^{2+}. The numbers refer to the text.

1. Bidirectional propagation of the AP occurs along the sarcolemma. This causes excitation of muscle fibre along its whole length so that all sarcomeres contract simultaneously.
2. The AP is then propagated into the muscle fibre via the T-tubule. There are two T-tubules per sarcomere. These encircle the myofibril at the AI junction. T-tubules communicate with the extracellular space.
3. The sarcoplasmic reticulum on both sides of the T-tubule communicates with the T-tubule via junctional feet. Depolarization of the T-tubule results in a signal from the T-tubule to the sarcoplasmic reticulum terminal cisternae.
4. Ca^{2+} channels then open in the sarcoplasmic reticulum and Ca^{2+} moves along a concentration gradient into the sarcoplasm around the myofibrils.

Muscle contraction

Two types of molecule—thick and thin filaments—are involved in the muscle contraction (Fig. 2.22).

Thick filament

Myosin: This is the main component of thick filament. It is a much larger protein than actin and consists of a tail, neck and head (cross-bridge) region.

The head region possesses ATPase activity and can attach to specific binding sites on the actin molecule; the neck region is flexible, which is necessary for attachment and detachment to the actin filament, and the tail region provides strength.

Thin filament

Actin: This is the main component of thin filament. It is capable of binding five other proteins.

Tropomyosin: This is a structural protein found bound to actin filaments. Each tropomyosin is bound to seven actin filaments.

Tropomyosin 'covers' the myosin-binding sites on the actin filament, thereby preventing a myosin–actin interaction.

Troponin: This protein consists of a complex of three subunits: T, which binds one tropomyosin; C, which has a high affinity for Ca^{2+}; and I, which has a high affinity for actin (hence the attachment of tropomyosin to actin).

The binding of Ca^{2+} causes a change in shape and movement of the associated tropomyosin. This uncovers the myosin-attachment site on actin.

α-Actinin: This protein is found in the Z band.

Mechanism of contraction
Huxley's cross-bridge cycle

Huxley's cross-bridge cycle demonstrates the shortening of the sarcomere caused by the sliding of the actin filaments. The numbers correspond to Fig. 2.23 as follows:

1. In the resting state the myosin-attachment sites on the actin molecule are covered by tropomyosin.
2. An increase in intracellular Ca^{2+} results in the binding of Ca^{2+} to troponin C. The binding of Ca^{2+} causes a conformational change in the troponin complex, resulting in movement of the

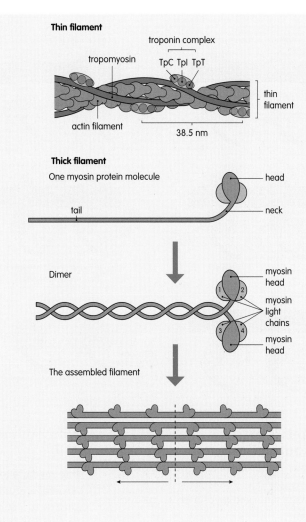

Fig. 2.22 Different arrangement of contractile proteins in thin filament and thick (myosin) filament

tropomyosin and uncovering of the myosin-binding sites.
3. The myosin head attaches to an actin molecule and releases the phosphate group.
4. This attachment causes the myosin head to tilt towards its tail, thereby pulling the actin filament in that direction. Tilting of the head causes release of ADP.
5. A molecule of ATP binds to the myosin head. This causes detachment of the head from the actin.
6. The ATPase action of the myosin head cleaves ATP, resulting in a myosin head with attached ADP and phosphate. The energy derived from this process causes straightening (or

'untilting') of the head, preparing it for reattachment.

The whole process is repeated. In this way the myosin head 'walks' along the actin filament. This is the basis of the 'walk along' theory.

Relaxation of muscle
Relaxation of muscle is Ca^{2+}-dependent. Upon repolarization of the muscle fibre, Ca^{2+} is actively pumped back into the sarcoplasmic reticulum. The concentration of Ca^{2+} drops and it is no longer bound to troponin.
   The myosin-binding sites become 'covered' by tropomyosin again, preventing further 'walking'.

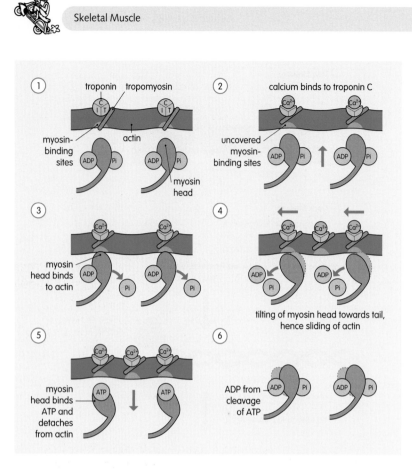

Fig. 2.23 Interaction of myosin heads with thin filaments during contraction. The numbers refer to the text.

Bioenergetics of muscle contraction

Muscle contraction results in energy expenditure during:

- Interaction of actin and myosin filaments during contraction.
- Pumping of Ca^{2+} from the sarcoplasm back into the sarcoplasmic reticulum after contraction.
- Restoration of the intracellular ionic environment after muscle contraction, because of the actions of the Na^+/K^+ pump.

Sources of energy
Short term
Sarcoplasm: ATP molecules are present in sarcoplasm. These would be expended within the first 2 s of contraction if they were not replaced.

Creatine phosphokinase: As a substrate, creatine phosphokinase contains high-energy phosphate bonds, which can be used to phosphorylate ADP to ATP by the enzyme creatine kinase. It is located in the Z line.

Myokinase: The enzyme myokinase catalyses the transfer of a phosphate group from one ADP molecule to another to form ATP and the by-product AMP.

Intermediate term
Anaerobic glycolysis: This causes the breakdown of glucose to lactate and pyruvate with the release of energy, which is used to convert ADP to ATP. ATP is generated at double the rate of oxidative phosphorylation. See *Crash Course: Metabolism and Nutrition* for more detail.

Anaerobic glycolysis is predominant in type II muscle fibres, which have few mitochondria but many glycogen granules.

This is an intermediate-term source of energy only, as lactate and pyruvate accumulate in the cell.

Long term
Oxidative phosphorylation: This is an aerobic process in which ATP is liberated from fats, carbohydrates and protein. See *Crash Course: Metabolism and Nutrition* for more information.

Energy can be provided for longer periods (a few hours) than with glycolysis.

Type I muscle fibres are suited to oxidative phosphorylation as they have numerous mitochondria and lipid droplets.

Fig. 2.24 Components of the myofibre cytoskeleton and their linkage with the extracellular matrix. (Adapted with permission from *Muscle and Nerve* by J. Wiley and Sons, 1994.)

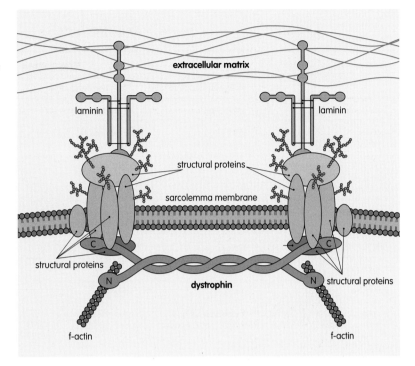

Myofibre cytoskeleton

The myofibre cytoskeleton is essential to the mechanical stability and function of muscle. The proteins present in the myofibre cytoskeleton are dystrophin and bridging glycoproteins.

Actin filaments are linked to dystrophin, which in turn is linked to a number of glycoproteins that extend to the surface of the sarcolemma. These glycoproteins link to laminin in the basement membrane (Fig. 2.24).

The myofibre cytoskeleton forms a link between the inside of the cell and the extracellular matrix. (The extracellular matrix supports the muscle fibre, decreasing the likelihood of tearing upon contraction.) Duchenne muscular dystrophy is an example of a condition resulting from abnormalities in the myofibre cytoskeleton (p. 41).

Functions of skeletal muscle

Motor unit

The motor unit refers to the motor neuron and all the muscle fibres innervated by it.

Each motor neuron may innervate many muscle fibres, but a single muscle fibre receives input from only one motor neuron.

The number of muscle fibres innervated by a motor neuron is known as the innervation ratio. A smaller number of muscle fibres per motor neuron is present in muscles involved in fine, precise movements, e.g. ocular muscles, while a larger number is seen in muscles involved in gross movements, e.g. maintaining posture.

The muscle fibres innervated by a single motor neuron are spread out within the muscle.

The muscle fibres within a motor unit are of the same type and contract simultaneously.

There are three different types of motor units (Fig. 2.25).

Orderly recruitment

Small motor neurons innervate slow muscle fibres (type I) whereas fast muscle fibres (types IIa and IIb) are innervated by larger motor neurons. This is referred to as the **size principle**.

Smaller motor neurons require a smaller excitatory input for activation. During reflex or voluntary movement for a given excitatory input, it is the slow units that are activated first. This results in an orderly recruitment of muscle fibres, with activation of slow units first, followed by fast fatigue-resistant units and finally fast fatiguable units. This is important *in vivo* as it allows movement to be graded

Properties of different motor unit types			
Property	Motor unit type		
	slow, resistant to fatigue	fast, non-fatiguable	fast, fatiguable
fibre diameter	small (type I)	intermediate (type IIa)	large (type IIb)
force of contraction	low	intermediate	high
myosin–ATPase activity (indicates rate of ATP hydrolysis and therefore speed of twitch)	low	low	high
source of energy	oxidative phosphorylation	oxidative phosphorylation and some anaerobic glycolysis	anaerobic glycolysis
glycogen content	low	intermediate	high
mitochondria	many	many	few
capillaries	many	many	few
function	fine movement and maintenance of posture	sustained activity	brief strong contractions, e.g. jumping

Fig. 2.25 Properties of different motor unit types.

by altering the level of excitatory input rather than having to select different fibre types.

Effects of denervation and reinnervation on motor units

Denervation of a motor unit results in atrophy of the muscle fibres within that unit. There may also be fibrillations on the electromyogram, shown as fine, irregular contractions of individual fibres, and an increase in sensitivity to circulating ACh.

Clinically, the signs of a lower motor neuron lesion are seen. These include a decrease in muscle tone, decrease in power and diminished reflexes.

Some of the muscle fibres are replaced by fibrous and fatty tissue. However, this fibrous tissue shortens and contractures may form.

Other muscle fibres may be reinnervated by collaterals from the remaining adjacent motor neurons. This results in:

- Possible alteration of the fibre type, as it is the motor neuron that determines the fibre type. In this way there may be areas of muscle containing fibres of only one type. This is termed fibre clumping and produces characteristic waveforms on a diagnostic electromyogram (EMG).
- Larger motor units.

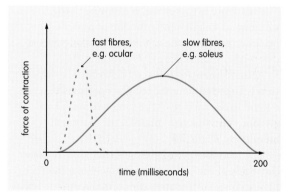

Fig. 2.26 Duration of contraction in different muscles demonstrated by isometric tests.

Muscle mechanics
Isometric contraction

Isometric contraction occurs in muscle with a constant length.

Isometric tests can be used to compare force against duration of contraction of different muscles (Figs 2.26 and 2.27).

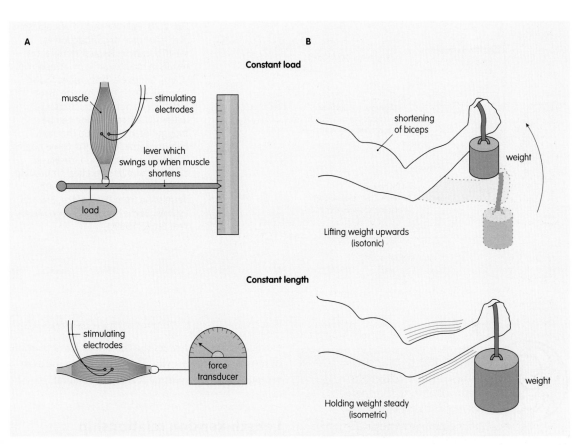

Fig. 2.27 (A) Measurement of isotonic and isometric contractions. (Modified from *Human Physiology and Mechanisms of Disease*, 8th edn by A.C. Guyton, W.B. Saunders, 1992.) (B) Situations involving isotonic and isometric contractions. (Adapted with permission from *Review of Medical Physiology*, 17th edn, by W.F. Ganong, Appleton Lange, 1995.)

Isotonic contraction

Isotonic contraction occurs in muscle with a constant tension. The length of the muscle changes while maintaining constant tension.

Isotonic tests can be used to compare the speed of shortening of different muscle types (Fig. 2.27).

Sarcoplasmic Ca²⁺ concentration and muscle twitch

Every AP in skeletal muscle results in a similar amount of Ca^{2+} release. Hence, under isometric conditions, the force of the twitch resulting from a single AP will remain the same.

Unlike myocardium, the strength of contraction in skeletal muscle is not dependent on sarcoplasmic Ca^{2+} concentration as each AP results in sufficient Ca^{2+} release to produce the maximal response.

Maximal response in skeletal muscle, however, is not seen with a single AP because:
- Series elasticity occurs whereby structural components (e.g. tendons, cross-bridges) of the muscle are elastic and lengthen when force is generated; therefore initial shortening of muscle is slow.
- Sarcoplasmic Ca^{2+} is rapidly pumped back into the sarcoplasmic reticulum following an AP, thereby ending the response.

Force of contraction in skeletal muscle may be increased by maintaining the sarcoplasmic Ca^{2+} concentration by repetitive stimulation. This would result in greater shortening as the initial twitch would be involved in stretching of the elastic elements with no 'wasting' of force upon subsequent twitches as the elastic elements are already stretched (Fig. 2.28).

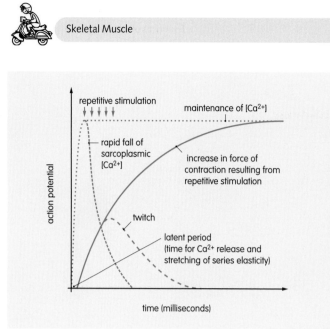

Fig. 2.28 Relationship of sarcoplasmic [Ca^{2+}] to force of contraction in skeletal muscle. Repeat stimulation results in maintenance of intracellular [Ca^{2+}]. Series elasticity refers to the inherent elasticity of muscle tissue, including its non-contractile C/T matrix. The latent period can be thought of as 'taking up the slack' before contraction of the tissue begins. In repetitive stimulation the elastic elements remain stretched, improving muscle efficiency. (Adapted with permission from *Physiology*, 3rd edn, by R.M. Berne and M.N. Levy, Mosby Year Book, 1993.)

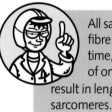

All sarcomeres in a muscle fibre contract at the same time, otherwise shortening of one sarcomere would result in lengthening of adjacent sarcomeres.

Maintained muscle contractions

Twitch is a single contraction resulting from a single AP. It is a submaximal response.

Unfused tetanus occurs when muscle is repetitively stimulated such that there is insufficient time for complete relaxation between each twitch. As a result, the successive mechanical responses fuse, with an additive effect on force of contraction. This is called summation of twitches (Fig. 2.29).

Fused tetanus results from summation of twitches. However, there is no relaxation of muscle between each stimulus, resulting in fusion of consecutive twitches and a smooth sustained contraction.

Summation of twitches is an important means of varying the force of contraction. Therefore, increasing the frequency of stimulation is an important means of modulating force of contraction (see Fig. 2.29).

Tetany is spasm and twitching of skeletal muscle due to low levels of extracellular Ca^{2+}. A decrease in extracellular Ca^{2+} lowers the threshold for activation of muscle and nerve cells. This is not the same as a tetanus, which is a normal feature of skeletal muscle.

Length–tension relationship

The force or tension a muscle fibre generates depends on the length of the sarcomere (Fig. 2.30). There is an optimum range of lengths at which the force generated is at its maximum. This can be explained by the sliding filament theory—if a sarcomere is stretched, the overlap between actin and myosin is reduced and there are fewer actin–myosin interactions and lower force. Alternatively, if the sarcomere is shortened, the thin filaments overlap and the number of actin–myosin interactions are again reduced.

In a whole muscle the total tension developed is the sum of active tension and passive tension.

- Total tension results from isometric contraction of muscle in response to a maximal stimulus.
- Passive tension results from stretching of the muscle in the absence of contraction and occurs owing to the elastic forces of connective tissue, blood vessels, etc.
- Active tension is the increase in tension resulting from muscular contraction. This is determined by subtracting passive tension from total tension. Most muscles in the body are at the optimum length for maximum tension.

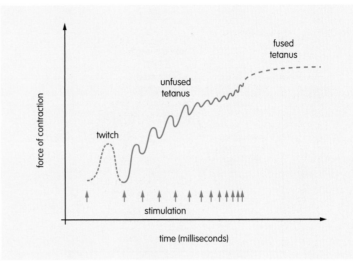

Fig. 2.29 Summation of twitches. As the time between each twitch decreases, the force of the contraction increases, showing the modulating effect of stimulation frequency. (Adapted with permission from *Physiology Colouring Book* by W. Kapit, Harper Collins, 1987.)

Modulation of force of skeletal muscle contraction

Force of muscle contraction is modulated by orderly recruitment and increasing frequency of stimulation. Other important factors include the length of the muscle and influence of the antagonistic muscle groups.

Force–velocity relationship

The force–velocity relationship is found by stimulating a muscle under isotonic conditions and measuring the speed of shortening with different loads. The speed of shortening is decreased with increasing loads (Fig. 2.31A).

Speed of shortening varies with different fibre types. This occurs because of the existence of myosin isoforms. In fast fibres, myosin ATPase activity is rapid and therefore cross-bridge cycling and shortening of muscle fibres is more rapid (Fig. 2.31B). The speed of shortening is inversely related to the load.

Power curves

Power = velocity × load (Fig. 2.32). The power of muscle contraction is influenced by the speed of shortening (velocity) and the load. Although increasing the load would seem to favour the equation this is not the case, because increasing the load would decrease the speed of shortening. Hence maximal power is actually achieved by a balance between the load and the speed of shortening.

Muscle plasticity

Muscle plasticity refers to changes in the characteristics of a muscle to match function. Factors that may be altered include muscle fibre diameter, length, strength and vascular supply.

The fibre types may also be altered, but to a lesser extent as these are determined by the motor neuron by which they are innervated.

Fast fibres are interconvertible, i.e. fast glycolytic fibres may be converted to fast oxidative and vice versa. Slow and fast fibres are not interconvertible.

Effect of exercise on muscle

An increase in muscle mass occurs owing to hypertrophy or hyperplasia.

Hypertrophy of muscle is an increase in the size of individual muscle fibres, resulting in an increase in the force of contraction. This is caused by regular contraction of the muscle at maximal force.

Hyperplasia of muscle occurs to a lesser extent than hypertrophy. Hyperplasia involves an increase in the number of muscle cells. This is not due to mitosis but rather to a splitting lengthwise of large fibres.

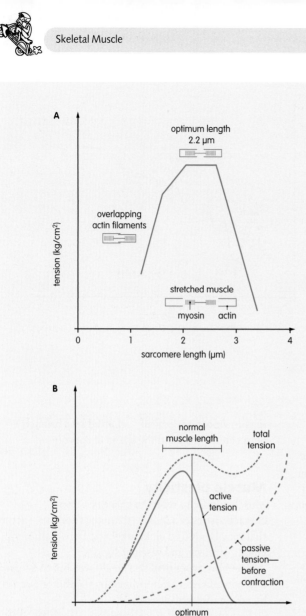

Fig. 2.30 (A) Effect of sarcomere length on the active tension developed by an individual muscle fibre upon contraction. (B) Effect of muscle length on tension. Increasing the passive tension initially increases the total tension. Further increases in passive tension lead to a decrease in active tension.

A lack of exercise causes muscle atrophy. This is a decrease in muscle fibre size resulting from lack of stimulation.

Relationship of muscle characteristics to function

Sprinters have a greater number of fast fibres, as they require rapid contractions of large force, while marathon runners have a greater number of slow muscle fibres as they require sustained low-force contractions. The number of slow muscle fibres is largely genetically determined. By training, the effect of these muscle fibres may be enhanced by increasing their size and vascular supply.

Clinical relevance of muscle plasticity

Cardiomyoplasty involves the training of a skeletal muscle near to the heart, usually latissimus dorsi. The skeletal muscle can then be wrapped around the heart to replace diseased or congenitally missing myocardium.

Fig. 2.31 Graphs showing that (A) speed of contraction decreases with increasing load, with maximum velocity occurring with zero load, and (B) maximum speed of contraction in fast fibres is greater than that in slow fibres.

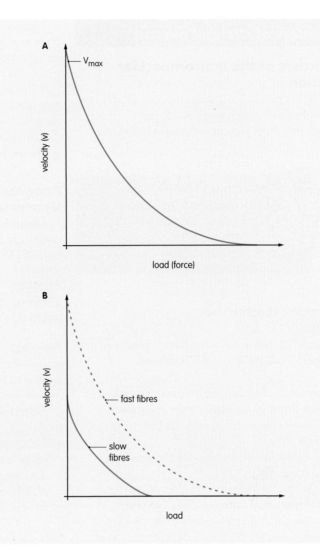

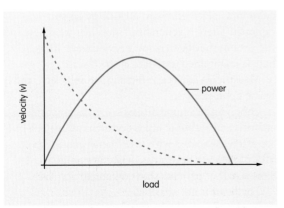

Fig. 2.32 Maximal power results from a balance between speed of shortening and load.

 Individual skeletal muscle fibres may be regarded as a syncytium as each fibre is made up of a number of myoblasts which have fused. However, skeletal muscle fibres contract independently of each other and therefore skeletal muscle is not referred to as a syncytium.

Disorders of skeletal muscle

Disorders of the neuromuscular junction

Disorders of the neuromuscular junction (NMJ) can be classified into two types: presynaptic or postsynaptic. Both present with muscle weakness.

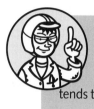

Disorders of the NMJ are not diseases of the muscle but rather disorders of function—hence atrophy tends to be a late feature.

Presynaptic abnormalities
Botulism
Aetiology   Botulinum is an endotoxin produced by an organism called *Clostridium botulinum*.

Pathogenesis   Poisoning by botulinum is called botulism. Botulism is caused by the ingestion of canned meat contaminated with the endotoxin of C. *botulinum*.

The endotoxin acts by blocking the uptake of choline at the NMJ.

Clinical features   Botulism causes symmetrical descending paralysis, particularly of the face and respiratory muscles. Signs include diplopia, loss of pupillary reflex and laryngeal palsy.

Diagnosis   The diagnosis of botulism is clinical and is confirmed by detection of the endotoxin in food or faeces.

Management   Management of botulism is by supportive care and antitoxin. Antibiotics may also be required.

Prognosis   There is an associated mortality of around 50% with botulism.

Lambert–Eaton myasthenic syndrome
The Lambert–Eaton myasthenic syndrome is a non-metastatic complication of malignancy that involves antibodies to voltage-gated Ca^{2+} channels in the presynaptic membrane.

Lambert–Eaton myasthenic syndrome is most often associated with small-cell lung carcinomas. The malignant cells express Ca^{2+} channels and may trigger the formation of the antibodies.

When nerves are stimulated at the NMJ, there is a decrease in Ca^{2+} influx. This leads to a decrease in the release of acetylcholine (ACh).

Patients with Lambert–Eaton myasthenic syndrome present with abnormal fatiguability.

Postsynaptic abnormalities
Myasthenia gravis
Epidemiology   Myasthenia gravis occurs most commonly in the third decade and has a male: female ratio of 1:2.

Aetiology   The cause of myasthenia gravis is unknown. It may be due to recurrent viral illness resulting in the formation of antibodies.

Pathology   Myasthenia gravis is an autoimmune disease (Fig. 2.33). In 90% of patients there are IgG antibodies to the ACh receptor in the postsynaptic membrane.

A decrease in functional ACh receptors results from:
- Stearic prevention of ACh binding to receptors because of the presence of antibody. The antibody does not itself bind to the ACh site, but prevents ACh from binding.
- Increased breakdown of receptors.

Clinical features   The main symptoms of myasthenia gravis are muscle weakness and fatiguability.

The ocular, bulbar and cranial muscles are most commonly affected. Signs include ptosis and diplopia. There is generalized muscular weakness and the patient may be in respiratory distress. Muscle bulk is maintained until late in the disease.

Myasthenia gravis is remitting and relapsing, and is worse upon exercise.

Other autoimmune diseases, e.g. rheumatoid arthritis and systemic lupus erythematosus (SLE), are often associated with myasthenia gravis. About 10% of patients have an associated thymoma and almost half of patients show thymic hyperplasia.

The heart is not affected.

Neonatal myasthenia may be seen in the newborn babies of mothers with the disease. The babies present with poor limb movements and poor feeding.

Fig. 2.33 Features of the neuromuscular junction in myasthenia gravis.

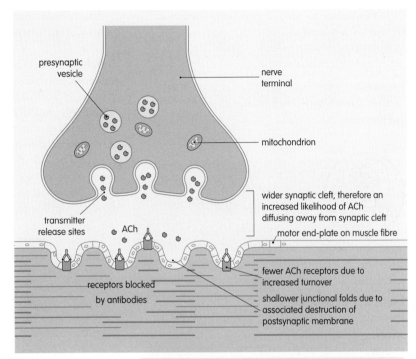

presynaptic vesicle

nerve terminal

mitochondrion

wider synaptic cleft, therefore an increased likelihood of ACh diffusing away from synaptic cleft

motor end-plate on muscle fibre

transmitter release sites

ACh

fewer ACh receptors due to increased turnover

receptors blocked by antibodies

shallower junctional folds due to associated destruction of postsynaptic membrane

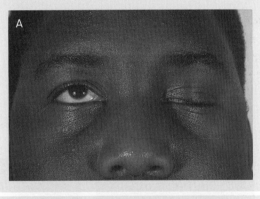

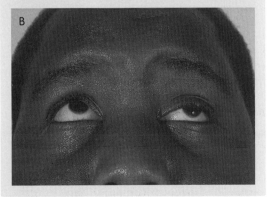

These symptoms last a few weeks until the maternal antibodies decrease.

Diagnosis About 90% of patients with myasthenia gravis have circulating anti-ACh receptor antibodies.

Diagnosis is based on the Tensilon test (Fig. 2.34). This test involves giving an injection of a short-acting anticholinesterase drug called edrophonium to the suspected myasthenic patient. As anticholinesterase drugs inhibit the enzyme acetylcholinesterase (which hydrolyses ACh, thereby terminating the activation of ACh receptors on the muscle fibre), ACh is present in the synaptic cleft for longer and there is a greater probability that it will bind to the ACh receptor. In this way, muscle contraction can take place sufficiently for the patient to regain normal muscle strength temporarily.

An electromyogram (EMG) shows a decrease in response to stimulation.

Management Management of myasthenia gravis is by the administration of longlasting anticholinesterases, the dose varying according to the patient's response. Longlasting anticholinesterases prolong the presence of ACh in the synaptic cleft, thereby increasing the likelihood of ACh binding to a receptor.

Fig. 2.34 The Tensilon test. (A) Muscle weakness caused by repeated facial movements. (B) There is rapid improvement after administration of edrophonium, a short-acting anticholinesterase. (Courtesy of Dr G.D. Perkin.)

In those patients with an associated thymoma, thymectomy is needed.

Immunosuppressives such as prednisolone or azathioprine are also useful.

Prognosis   The course of myasthenia gravis is variable. Death may result from aspiration pneumonia.

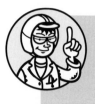
Understand myasthenia gravis because it is a common exam question.

Inherited myopathies
Muscular dystrophies

The muscular dystrophies are a group of disorders involving a progressive degeneration of skeletal muscle.

X-linked dystrophies
Duchenne muscular dystrophy

Epidemiology   Duchenne muscular dystrophy occurs in 1 in 4000 live male births. One-third of the cases have no family history.

Spontaneous mutations are likely because the gene involved is large.

Aetiology   Duchenne muscular dystrophy is an X-linked recessive disorder.

Pathology   In Duchenne muscular dystrophy, a mutation occurs on the short arm of the X chromosome, the site (Xp21) coding for dystrophin protein. The lack of dystrophin protein results in impaired anchorage of muscle fibres to the extracellular matrix. This makes the muscle fibres more susceptible to tearing upon repeated contraction.

Damaged fibres allow an influx of calcium ions, leading to irreversible cell death.

Clinical features   Children with Duchenne muscular dystrophy usually present at 2 years of age.

Symptoms include weakness of the pelvic and shoulder girdle muscles, and signs include selective atrophy, waddling gait, pseudohypertrophy of the calves and Gower's sign (Fig. 2.35).

Diagnosis   The average age of diagnosis of Duchenne muscular dystrophy is 5 years.

Diagnosis is based on a raised serum creatinine phosphokinase concentration. Muscle biopsy also

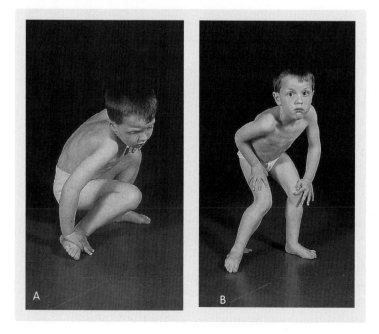

Fig. 2.35 Gower's sign showing the difficulty encountered in standing from the prone position in patients with Duchenne muscular dystrophy. (A) This child needs to turn prone to rise, then uses his hands to climb up on his knees. (B) Once at knee level the hands are released and the arms and trunk are swung sideways and upwards to reach an upright position. Note the hypertrophied calves (due to deposition of fat and fibrous tissue). (Courtesy of Dr T. Lissauer and Dr G. Clayden.)

Fig. 2.36 Histological changes in Duchenne muscular dystrophy showing variation in fibre diameter, increased fibrous and fatty connective tissue, and fibre generation.

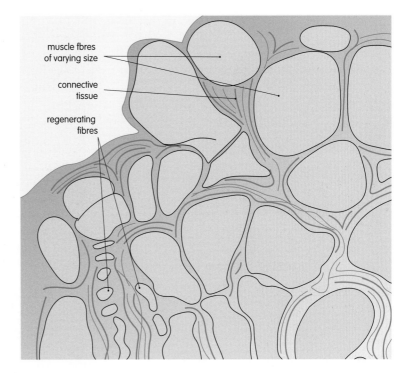

muscle fbres of varying size

connective tissue

regenerating fibres

reveals necrosed muscle fibres surrounded by fibrous tissue and fat (Fig. 2.36). The muscle fibres are of variable diameters, owing to the body's attempt at regeneration.

Complications Complications of Duchenne muscular dystrophy include marked scoliosis, impaired learning (30%), contractures and cardiomyopathy.

Management There is no treatment that will halt Duchenne muscular dystrophy; management is supportive and is aimed at maintaining the use of the muscles and decreasing respiratory symptoms.
Identification of female carriers is possible and genetic counselling may be offered.

Prognosis Most people with Duchenne muscular dystrophy are wheelchair-bound by their teens. Death occurs in the late teens or the early twenties, and is due to cardiac failure or failure of the respiratory muscles.

Becker muscular dystrophy
Becker muscular dystrophy is a less common X-linked variant of Duchenne muscular dystrophy. It shows similar clinical features to Duchenne muscular dystrophy, although the progression of the disease is slower. The average age of onset is 11 years with death occurring in the 40s.

Of the inherited myopathies, Duchenne muscular dystrophy is a common topic in exams.

Autosomal dystrophies
Limb girdle dystrophy
Limb girdle dystrophy, one of the autosomal recessive dystrophies, presents in childhood or adult life with pelvic and shoulder girdle weakness (Fig. 2.37).
Pseudohypertrophy of the calves is less common than in Duchenne muscular dystrophy.
Muscle biopsy shows findings similar to those of Duchenne muscular dystrophy.
Prognosis involves a variable degree of disability.

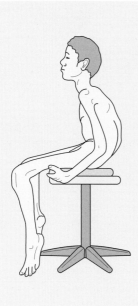

Fig. 2.37 Severe limb girdle dystrophy demonstrating proximal muscle wasting and kyphosis.

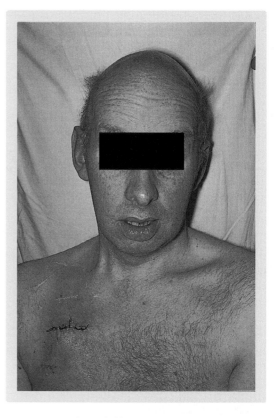

Fig. 2.38 Typical 'monk-like' appearance seen in an adult with myotonic dystrophy. Note the facial weakness, atrophy of temporal and sternocleidomastoid muscles, and frontal baldness. (Courtesy of Dr G.D. Perkin.)

Facioscapulohumeral dystrophy

Facioscapulohumeral dystrophy is an autosomal dominant disorder. The condition presents in childhood or adult life with face and shoulder girdle weakness. Winging of the scapulae is characteristic.

Pseudohypertrophy is rare.

Muscle biopsy shows findings similar to those of Duchenne muscular dystrophy.

Individuals show a mild degree of disability.

Myotonic disorders

Myotonic disorders are a group of conditions in which there is a delay in muscle relaxation after voluntary contraction. Administration of general anaesthetics is more likely to cause complications in patients with muscle disorders of this sort.

Myotonic dystrophy

Epidemiology   Myotonic dystrophy occurs in 1 in 8000 people.

Aetiology   Myotonic dystrophy is an autosomal dominant disorder.

Pathology   The condition is caused by a mutation on chromosome 19, the site coding for a cAMP-dependent kinase.

In affected families the disease is more severe in later generations. This is known as anticipation.

Clinical features   Myotonic dystrophy may occur in the newborn period, with hypotonia. More commonly, it presents in the early 20s with limb weakness, distal wasting, characteristic facies and cranial muscle involvement (Fig. 2.38). Learning difficulties may also be present.

Other associated findings include cataracts, baldness, gonadal atrophy and glucose intolerance.

Diagnosis   Diagnosis of myotonic dystrophy is mainly clinical, although an EMG is characteristic.

A muscle biopsy shows dystrophic changes.

Management The management of myotonic dystrophy involves treating the myotonia, although this does not influence the course of the disease.

Prognosis Death from myotonic dystrophy is usually due to cardiomyopathy or involvement of the respiratory muscles.

Congenital myotonia
Congenital myotonia, or Thomsen's disease, is a rare disorder that may be dominant or recessive. Symptoms include myotonia—this is worse in cold temperatures and with rest.

Generalized muscle hypertrophy is prominent.

Paramyotonia congenita
Paramyotonia congenita is an autosomal dominant condition. The mutation occurs on chromosome 17, the site coding for the sodium channel.

Paramyotonia congenita is a non-progressive muscle weakness that is worse in cold temperatures.

Metabolic myopathies
The metabolic myopathies are a heterogeneous group of conditions in which there are abnormalities in muscle energy metabolism.

Primary metabolic myopathies
Glycogen storage disorders Glycogen storage disorders are caused by enzyme anomalies inherited in a recessive manner.

The degree of muscle involvement is variable between the major types of primary metabolic myopathies.

Symptoms arise as a result of the decreased availability of energy from glycolysis. This is because of an impaired ability to mobilize glucose from glycogen.

Glycogen storage disorder type V (McArdle's syndrome) is an autosomal recessive disorder in which there is a deficiency of skeletal muscle myophosphorylase. Symptoms include temporary weakness and muscle cramps on exercise. There is an associated myoglobinuria. There is no rise in venous lactate during exercise, which aids diagnosis by enzyme analysis of muscle tissue. Life expectancy is not affected. Patients are advised to avoid exercise.

Lipid disorders In the lipid disorders, there is a decreased availability of energy to muscle due to abnormalities in fatty acid metabolism.

Patients usually present with hypotonia in infancy or muscle weakness and cramps later.

Symptoms are worse with prolonged exercise or fasting.

Mitochondrial disorders The mitochondrial disorders are inherited. These are abnormalities of either the mitochondrial genome (more commonly) or the nuclear genome.

The age of onset is variable. The muscle weakness (particularly of the extraocular muscles) may be isolated or associated with neurological and metabolic disturbances.

Muscle biopsy shows abnormal mitochondria with crystalline inclusions.

Mitochondrial myopathy may develop in patients on long-term zidovudine therapy, i.e. patients infected with HIV.

Secondary metabolic myopathies
Myopathic symptoms can occur as a result of a whole range of electrolyte disturbances, e.g. Ca^{2+}, Mg^{2+}, K^+, etc.

Endocrine disorders are examples of secondary metabolic myopathies which are acquired.

Periodic paralyses
The periodic paralyses are a rare group of disorders characterized by repeated attacks of muscle weakness.

There are three types: hypokalaemic, hyperkalaemic and normokalaemic.

Hypokalaemic periodic paralysis Hypokalaemic periodic paralysis is an autosomal dominant condition. It presents in adolescence and is remitting in the late 30s.

Attacks often occur after strenuous exercise or a heavy carbohydrate meal. During an attack, the serum potassium concentration is low (2.5–3.5 mmol/l): attacks are terminated by the administration of intravenous potassium chloride.

Diuretic therapy and thyrotoxicosis must be excluded as possible causes of the myopathy.

Hyperkalaemic periodic paralysis
Hyperkalaemic periodic paralysis is an autosomal dominant condition. It presents in childhood and is remitting in the 20s.

Attacks may occur after strenuous exercise and are terminated by intravenous calcium gluconate. During an attack the serum potassium concentration is high (6–7 mmol/l).

Attacks last for a shorter period than those associated with hypokalaemia.

Normokalaemic periodic paralysis
Normokalaemic periodic paralysis is a very rare condition. The attacks respond to sodium.

Acquired myopathies
Idiopathic inflammatory myopathies
The idiopathic inflammatory myopathies are uncommon disorders and have a male: female ratio of 1:2.

Most people with idiopathic inflammatory myopathy present in middle age.

Polymyositis
Polymyositis is the most common inflammatory myopathy.

Aetiology   The cause of polymyositis is not known, although it may be autoimmune in origin. A viral cause (Coxsackie virus) has been suggested.

Polymyositis is a non-metastatic complication of malignancy, as more than 10% of patients have an underlying malignancy that presents later, e.g. carcinoma of the breast, bronchus or gastrointestinal tract. In this instance the male: female ratio is reversed.

Pathology   In polymyositis there is inflammation and destruction of both type I and type II muscle fibres because of the action of cytotoxic T lymphocytes. Histologically there is fibre necrosis, muscle atrophy and evidence of fibre regeneration.

Clinical features   There is progressive, symmetrical, proximal muscle weakness in polymyositis. The respiratory and heart muscles may also be affected. Dysphagia and dysarthria are other features.

Polymyositis is associated with other connective tissue diseases such as SLE and rheumatoid disease. Features typical of connective tissue diseases may be present, e.g. Raynaud's phenomenon, in which there is intermittent vasospasm of arterioles in the hands and feet in response to cold and emotional stimuli. It is usually painful and the affected part of the body goes through the following colour changes: pale–blue–red.

Diagnosis   The diagnosis of polymyositis involves two of three findings:
- Raised serum creatine phosphokinase concentrations.
- A characteristic EMG.
- A muscle biopsy.

Antinuclear antibodies (Jo-1) and rheumatoid factor may also be present.

Management   The management of polymyositis includes immunosuppressive drugs (causing remission), and physiotherapy to prevent disuse atrophy of muscles.

Underlying malignancy must be excluded.

Prognosis   The course of polymyositis is variable.
Death results from aspiration pneumonia and respiratory or heart failure.

Dermatomyositis
Dermatomyositis is closely related to polymyositis, sharing features previously described.

In addition to muscular symptoms there are associated skin changes:
- A characteristic purple heliotrope rash, usually on the eyelids, although it may spread to other sites.
- An erythematous rash on the face, scalp, shoulders and hands.

Inclusion body myositis
Inclusion body myositis affects mainly the elderly and is clinically similar to polymyositis.

Electron microscopy demonstrates the presence of filamentous inclusions in the muscle fibres.

It is a progressive disorder and immunosuppressive therapy is not as effective.

Endocrine myopathies (or secondary metabolic myopathies)
Corticosteroid-induced myopathy
Corticosteroid-induced myopathy is caused by an excess of corticosteroid, e.g. Cushing's syndrome or people on steroid therapy.

The myopathy is proximal, i.e. it affects the upper parts of the arms and legs.

There is a raised creatine kinase concentration, and muscle biopsy reveals selective atrophy of type II muscle fibres.

Myopathy of thyroid dysfunction

Thyrotoxicosis may be associated with a proximal myopathy.

Hypothyroidism may result in symptoms of muscle stiffness and a proximal myopathy.

Myopathy of osteomalacia

All causes of osteomalacia (e.g. vitamin D deficiency, liver failure, liver enzyme-inducing drugs) may result in a proximal myopathy.

 It is useful to remember endocrine and toxic causes of myopathy as they can be easily included on a list of differential diagnosis for myopathy.

Toxic myopathies

Toxic myopathies are caused by excess alcohol or drugs.

Excess alcohol

In toxic myopathy caused by excess alcohol, two patterns of myopathy are seen:

- Subacute proximal myopathy (which may be reversed in the early stages); this is seen in chronic alcoholics. Selective atrophy of type II muscle fibres occurs.
- Acute myopathy associated with severe muscle pain due to acute alcohol excess—myoglobinuria may also occur.

Drug-induced myopathies

Agents that may cause a subacute proximal myopathy include cholesterol-lowering agents (e.g. benzofibrate), as well as chloroquine, penicillamine and lithium. Patients respond to removal of the drug.

Viral myalgias

The viral myalgias are muscle weaknesses associated with a viral illness, usually respiratory.

Myalgic encephalomyelitis (ME; also known as postviral/chronic fatigue syndrome or 'yuppie flu') is a disorder in which the patient presents with muscular fatigue and pain on movement. The cause is unknown and other associated symptoms include poor concentration and depression. The disorder tends to affect women and opinions differ as to whether this is a psychological or a skeletal muscle disorder.

- Outline the differences between the three types of muscle found in the body.
- What are the sites at which the three types of muscle are found?
- Distinguish between neurogenic and myogenic contraction.
- Describe how muscle is arranged and how shape can alter the characteristics of contraction.
- Explain the terms origin, insertion, tendon, aponeurosis and sesamoid bone.
- Demonstrate diagrammatically the organization of skeletal muscle into fasciculi and muscle fibres.
- What is the difference between a myofibre, myofibril and myofilament.
- Explain the term sarcomere.
- Explain the term triad in describing the cellular structure of skeletal muscle.
- Describe the role of satellite cells in adult skeletal muscle.
- Describe the ionic composition of the ICF and ECF in muscle fibres.
- What is the difference between the RMP and the equilibrium potential?
- What is the ionic basis of an AP (demonstrate on a diagram)? Describe its initiation and propagation.
- Explain the following terms: all-or-none law, local circuit theory, and safety factor associated with saltatory conduction.
- With regard to the NMJ, describe the events that occur upon arrival of an AP at the nerve terminal to initiation of an AP in the muscle fibre.
- Describe the synthesis, storage and breakdown of ACh.
- What are the types of drugs acting at the NMJ?
- Describe Huxley's cross-bridge cycle and the role of ATP.
- Describe the role of dystrophin protein.
- Explain the terms motor unit, innervation ratio and size principle.
- Discuss the different types of motor units and relate these to the different muscle fibre types.
- Explain the effects of denervation and reinnervation on motor units.
- Explain the terms isometric and isotonic contraction.
- Describe how summation occurs.
- What is the difference between tetanus and tetany?
- Draw graphs to demonstrate length–tension and force–velocity relationships.
- Define plasticity.
- Give examples of presynaptic and postsynaptic disorders of the NMJ.
- What is myasthenia gravis?
- Describe a simple classification of the inherited myopathies.
- Describe Duchenne muscular dystrophy and give a differential diagnosis.
- Describe the clinical features of myotonic dystrophy.
- Give examples of metabolic myopathies.
- List the three types of periodic paralyses.
- Give a simple classification of the main acquired myopathies.

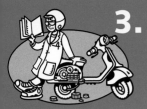

3. Cardiac and Smooth Muscle

Cardiac muscle

Structural organization of cardiac muscle

The heart consists of three layers: the inner layer (endocardium), middle layer (myocardium) and outer layer (pericardium) (Fig. 3.1).

Inner layer

The inner layer, or endocardium, is made up of endothelial cells that respond to pressure changes, stretch and a variety of circulatory substances.

Middle layer

The middle layer, or myocardium, is thickest in the ventricles.

Outer layer

The outer layer, or pericardium, consists of the epicardium (visceral pericardium), which is intimately related to the myocardium, and the pericardium (parietal pericardium), which forms the outermost layer of the heart. The two layers are separated by the pericardial cavity.

Microstructure of cardiac muscle

Intercalated discs are low-resistance junctions between myocytes (Fig. 3.2). These allow rapid propagation of action potentials (APs) from cell to cell, hence the term 'cardiac syncytium'.

Individual skeletal muscle fibres may be regarded as a syncytium as each fibre is made up of a number of myoblasts which have fused. However, skeletal muscle fibres contract independently of each other and therefore skeletal muscle is not referred to as a syncytium.

Types of cardiac myocytes

There are two types of cardiac myocytes: atrial and ventricular. The APs associated with these myocytes vary (Fig. 3.3).

Cellular physiology of cardiac muscle
Initiation of cardiac AP

Under normal circumstances the AP is initiated in the sinoatrial node (SA node). APs occur at the greatest rate in the SA node; hence, it acts as the pacemaker, setting the rate in other myocytes.

Propagation of cardiac AP

Propagation occurs rapidly owing to the presence of gap junctions. The AP is propagated from the SA node to the atrioventricular node (AV node), before propagation to the bundle of His into the left and right bundle branches and Purkinje fibres to the ventricular myocytes.

Conduction is slow in the AV node, resulting in a delay of 0.1 s before excitation of the ventricles. This is important as it results in contraction of the atria before the ventricles, thereby allowing greater emptying of the atria.

Ionic basis

There are two types of AP in cardiac muscle.

AP in SA node and AV node: SA node and AV node cells have the property of automatic rhythmicity, owing to the leakiness of the membrane to Na^+ in the absence of an AP and a decrease in K^+ conductance. This results in a resting membrane potential (RMP) that drifts from a threshold of -55 mV (lower than the RMP of ventricular and atrial myocytes) to -40 mV.

Ca^{2+} influx is responsible for the rising phase of the AP (Fig. 3.4).

AP in Purkinje cells and *atrial and ventricular myocytes:* Three types of channel are involved in the AP: fast Na^+ channels, slow Ca^{2+}/Na^+ channels (which are not found in skeletal muscle and are responsible for the plateau phase), and K^+ channels (Fig. 3.5).

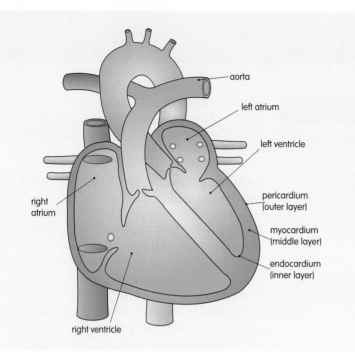

Fig. 3.1 Macroscopic organization of the heart.

The AP in ventricular cells differs from Purkinje cells in that the RMP is level in ventricular myocytes, whereas in Purkinje cells the RMP slowly rises to threshold, i.e. the cells are self-excitable.

Pacemaker tissue

Under normal conditions the SA node functions as the heart's pacemaker. In SA node pacemaker cells, APs are generated at a greater rate than in pacemaker tissue elsewhere in the heart. Hence the SA node sets the rhythm for the heart overall.

Pacemaker tissue is also found in the AV node, bundle of His and Purkinje fibres. These are often referred to as latent pacemakers as they can take over if the normal pacemaker fails.

Excitation–contraction coupling

Excitation–contraction coupling of cardiac muscle is essentially the same as skeletal muscle. This involves:
- Spread of the AP over the myocyte membrane.
- Influx of Ca^{2+}.
- Contraction due to formation of cross-bridges and sliding of filaments.

Bioenergetics of cardiac contraction

Cardiac muscle is mainly dependent on oxidative phosphorylation for contraction, as totally anaerobic conditions would not provide sufficient energy to sustain ventricular contraction.

Energy substrates vary according to dietary intake, e.g. during starvation, fat is the main substrate.

Cardiac muscle has a rich blood supply derived from the coronary arteries during diastole.

Cardiac muscle differs from skeletal muscle in that:
- The cardiac AP is 100 times longer.
- There is a long refractory period and therefore tetanus does not occur. However, upon increasing the frequency of APs there is an increase in intracellular Ca^{2+} levels. This results in an increase in the force of successive contractions and is known as the treppe or staircase effect.
- It is self-excitatory.
- The sarcoplasmic reticulum and T-tubules are organized in dyads (at the Z lines), not in triads. The sarcoplasmic reticulum is not as well developed and therefore stores less Ca^{2+}. Additionally, extracellular Ca^{2+} enters the cell directly through the T-tubules via slow Ca^{2+} channels. Hence, the force of contraction in cardiac muscle is largely dependent on the extracellular Ca^{2+} concentration.

Inotropes

Inotropes are agents that increase the force of cardiac contraction (Fig. 3.6).

Fig. 3.2 (A) Microscopic structure of cardiac muscle. Note that there are far fewer mitochondria in cardiac muscle than in skeletal muscle. (B) Components of the intercalated disc.

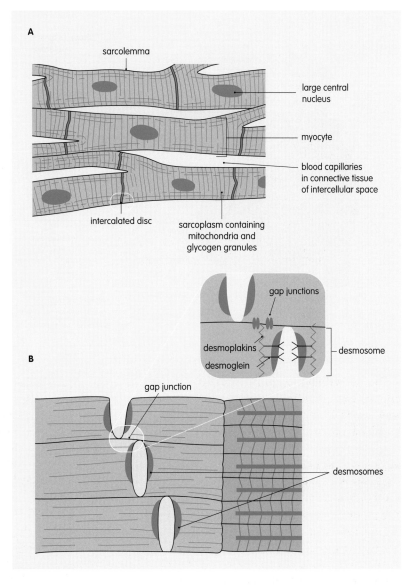

Mechanism of action: Inotropes increase the intracellular Ca^{2+} concentration. Digitalis glycosides, e.g. digoxin, inhibit the Na^+/K^+ ATPase pump. This results in an increase in intracellular Na^+ and therefore an increase in intracellular Ca^{2+} caused by the action of the Ca^{2+}/Na^+ exchanger.

Sympathomimetics, e.g. dobutamine, act on β_1 receptors, which increase intracellular Ca^{2+} via a rise in cyclic adenosine-5-monophosphate C (cAMP).

Phosphodiesterase (PDE) inhibitors, e.g. milrinone, also increase cAMP.

Function of cardiac muscle
Control of heart rate

Heart rate is affected by the autonomic nervous system.

Activation of the parasympathetic (vagal) nerves

Activation of the parasympathetic (vagal) nerves has the effect of decreasing heart rate, decreasing contractility and slowing transmission of the cardiac impulse. These nerves mainly innervate the SA and AV nodes.

51

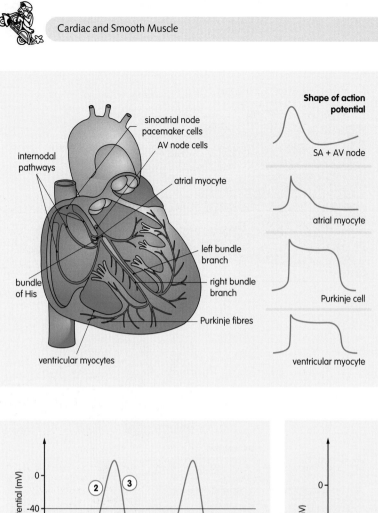

Shape of action potential

SA + AV node

atrial myocyte

Purkinje cell

ventricular myocyte

Fig. 3.3 Conducting system of the heart showing the location of the different types of myocytes and the action potentials associated with them. (AV, atrioventricular; SA, sinoatrial.)

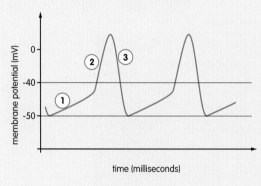

Fig. 3.4 Characteristics of the action potential seen in sinoatrial and atrioventricular node cells. (1) Drifting resting membrane potential caused by slow Na⁺ influx, or 'pacemaker potential'; (2) influx of Ca²⁺; (3) repolarization because of K⁺ efflux.

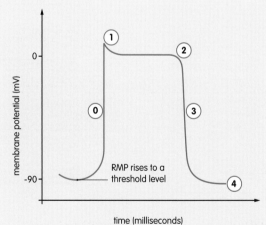

Fig. 3.5 Phases of the cardiac action potential in Purkinje cells. (0) Depolarization because of rapid Na⁺ influx; (1) initial rapid repolarization due to inactivation of Na⁺ channels and a passive influx of Cl⁻; (2) prolonged plateau phase with opening of slow Ca²⁺/Na⁺ channels. This prolongs depolarization owing to Ca²⁺ influx and results in contraction of the myocyte; (3) late repolarization caused by closure of Ca²⁺–Na⁺ channels and K⁺ efflux owing to opening of K⁺ channels; (4) restoration of RMP. (RMP, resting membrane potential.)

Mechanism of action: Activation of the parasympathetic (vagal) nerves causes hyperpolarization of the myocytic membrane via muscarinic acetylcholine (ACh) receptors. Anticholinergic drugs antagonize this effect.

Activation of the sympathetic system

Activation of the sympathetic system has the effect of increasing heart rate and force of contractility; β-adrenoceptor antagonists inhibit this effect.

Fig. 3.6 Inotropic drugs and their sites of action in the cardiac cell. (PDE, phosphodiesterase; ECF, extracellular fluid; ICF, intracellular fluid.)

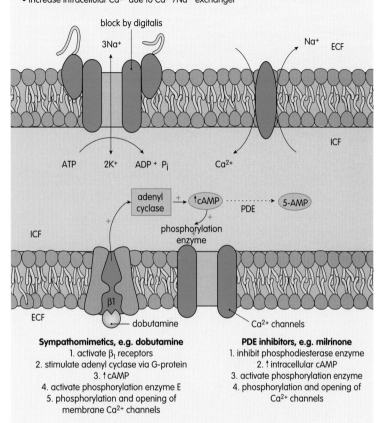

Digitalis glycosides, e.g. digoxin
- inhibit Na$^+$/K$^+$ ATPase pump
- increase intracellular Na$^+$
- increase intracellular Ca^{2+} due to Ca^{2+}/Na$^+$ exchanger

block by digitalis

3Na$^+$

Na$^+$ ECF

ICF

ATP   2K$^+$ ADP + P$_i$ Ca^{2+}

adenyl cyclase   +   ↑cAMP   PDE   5-AMP
+
phosphorylation enzyme

ICF

ECF   β1   dobutamine   Ca^{2+} channels

Sympathomimetics, e.g. dobutamine
1. activate β$_1$ receptors
2. stimulate adenyl cyclase via G-protein
3. ↑cAMP
4. activate phosphorylation enzyme E
5. phosphorylation and opening of membrane Ca^{2+} channels

PDE inhibitors, e.g. milrinone
1. inhibit phosphodiesterase enzyme
2. ↑ intracellular cAMP
3. activate phosphorylation enzyme
4. phosphorylation and opening of Ca^{2+} channels

Length–tension relationship in cardiac muscle

As with skeletal muscle, force of contraction increases with muscle fibre length (p. 13).

Starling's law

Starling's law states that the force of contraction is proportional to the initial length of the cardiac muscle fibre.

Muscle fibre length increases as the volume of blood in the heart chamber increases. Within physiological limits, the heart is able to pump out all the blood entering it.

Starling's law does not hold in situations where excessive stretching of cardiac muscle fibres is caused by a decrease in actin–myosin interaction.

Smooth muscle

The majority of smooth muscle found within the body is of the single-unit type (Fig. 3.7).

Organization of smooth muscle
Microstructure of smooth muscle

Smooth muscle cells are organized into small groups or bunches within the muscle (Fig. 3.8). These are surrounded by connective tissue containing the nerves and blood vessels.

The cells within a bunch are:
- Surrounded by an external lamina.
- Arranged in parallel to one another.

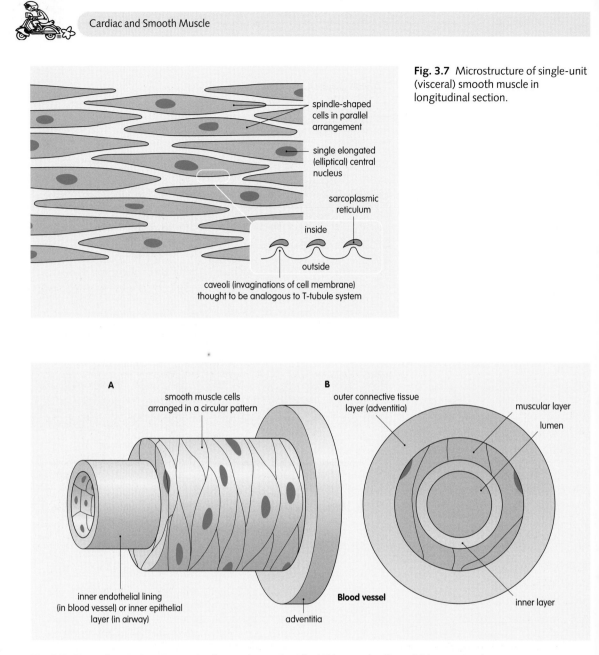

Fig. 3.7 Microstructure of single-unit (visceral) smooth muscle in longitudinal section.

spindle-shaped cells in parallel arrangement

single elongated (elliptical) central nucleus

sarcoplasmic reticulum

inside

outside

caveoli (invaginations of cell membrane) thought to be analogous to T-tubule system

A

smooth muscle cells arranged in a circular pattern

B

outer connective tissue layer (adventitia)

muscular layer

lumen

inner endothelial lining (in blood vessel) or inner epithelial layer (in airway)

Blood vessel

adventitia

inner layer

Fig. 3.8 Circumferential arrangement of smooth muscle cells, (A) longitudinally and (B) transversely.

- Adherent at multiple sites.
- Able to communicate with each other via gap junctions (nexus junctions), which are present at sites where the external lamina is deficient.
- Able to contract together as a functional single unit.

Arrangement of smooth muscle in different tissues

Smooth muscle cells are arranged circumferentially in blood vessels and airways (see Fig. 3.8).

In the intestines and lower two-thirds of the oesophagus (the upper third comprises skeletal muscle), smooth muscle is arranged in two layers (Fig. 3.9). In the inner layer, cells are arranged circumferentially and alter the diameter of the lumen, while in the outer layer cells are arranged longitudinally and influence the length. In this way both the diameter and length of the tract can be altered, causing movement of contents by peristalsis.

In the stomach, smooth muscle cells are arranged in three layers. These are the:

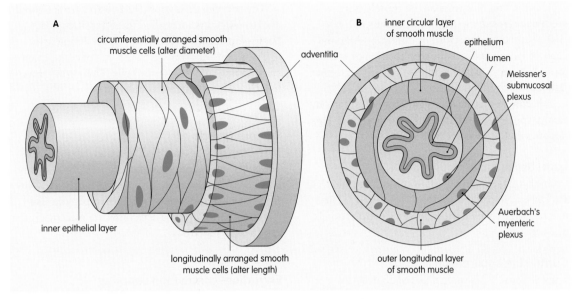

Fig. 3.9 Arrangement of smooth muscle cells in the intestine, (A) longitudinally and (B) transversely.

- Inner oblique layer.
- Middle circular layer.
- Outer longitudinal layer.

In the bladder, smooth muscle cells are arranged in three layers. These are the:
- Inner longitudinal layer.
- Middle circular layer.
- Outer longitudinal layer.

Cellular physiology of smooth muscle

Initiation of contraction of smooth muscle may result from several mechanisms.

Autonomic nervous system stimulation

In smooth muscle, branching nerve fibres contain neurotransmitter within swellings called varicosities. Released neurotransmitter diffuses to receptors on smooth muscle fibre, so there is usually no direct contact between nerve fibres and muscle cells (Fig. 3.10).

According to the type of receptor activated, the effect will be either excitatory or inhibitory.

The neurotransmitter released by a parasympathetic nerve may be ACh or, if released by a sympathetic nerve, noradrenaline. The two types of neurotransmitter have opposite effects in any one tissue.

If a section of smooth muscle has many layers, usually only the outer one is innervated. The

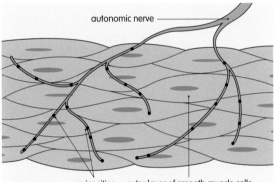

Fig. 3.10 Arrangement of autonomic nerve fibres in smooth muscle.

resulting AP is conducted to other layers via gap junctions. In the intestinal tract, peristalsis is coordinated by the Auerbach's (myenteric) and Meissner's (submucosal) plexuses, which lie on either side of the inner circular layer of smooth muscle; closest to the epithelium.

Action of circulating hormones

The most common hormones influencing smooth muscle contraction are ACh, adrenaline, noradrenaline, angiotensin and vasopressin; others include serotonin and histamine.

These act on receptors on the muscle fibre membrane, resulting in opening/closing of ion channels, thereby initiating or inhibiting APs, and changes within the cell due to activation of second-messenger pathways, e.g. release of Ca^{2+} from the sarcoplasmic reticulum.

A hormone may have an excitatory effect in one tissue type yet an inhibitory effect in another. This depends on the receptor activated.

Local tissue factors
Local tissue factors involved in smooth muscle tone are carbon dioxide, H^+ and Ca^{2+} (Fig. 3.11). The mechanism by which these produce contraction is unclear.

Contractile apparatus (Fig. 3.12)
Smooth muscle has three types of contractile protein: actin, myosin and desmin. Desmin is an intermediate filament.

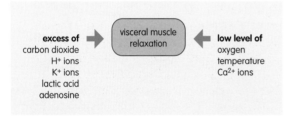

Fig. 3.11 Effect of local tissue factors on the tone of smooth muscle.

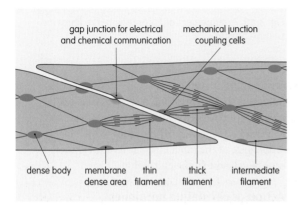

Fig. 3.12 Organization of contractile proteins in smooth muscle. (Adapted with permission from *Physiology* 3rd edn, by R.M. Berne and M.N. Levy, Mosby Year Book, 1993.)

The proteins criss-cross the cell and are anchored at cytoskeletal points called focal densities or dense bodies (analogous to Z discs in skeletal muscle).

Focal densities transmit the force of contraction to surrounding smooth muscle cells. This allows smooth muscle cells to contract as one unit.

Smooth muscle AP
In smooth muscle, the RMP is usually about −50 to −60 mV (i.e. less negative than skeletal muscle), and Ca^{2+}, not Na^+, is usually responsible for the AP. The AP can be spike- (skeletal muscle) or plateau-like.

Smooth muscle cells communicate electrically via gap (nexus) junctions.

Excitation–contraction coupling
During excitation–contraction coupling of smooth muscle, there is a rise in intracellular Ca^{2+}. Four Ca^{2+} bind to calmodulin protein present in the cytoplasm. This results in the formation of a myosin kinase–calmodulin–Ca^{2+} complex.

Myosin kinase phosphorylates a site on the myosin light chain. The phosphorylated myosin is then able to interact with actin to form cross-bridges.

A decrease in myoplasmic Ca^{2+} concentration inactivates myosin kinase—the enzyme is only active when it is part of the calmodulin complex.

The dephosphorylation of myosin takes place by myosin phosphatase.

Regulation of intracellular Ca^{2+} concentration
In smooth muscle intracellular Ca^{2+} is elevated by:
- Mobilization of intracellular stores: Ca^{2+} is rapidly released from the sarcoplasmic reticulum upon activation of the cell.
- Voltage-activated Ca^{2+} channels in the sarcolemma.
- Receptor-activated Ca^{2+} channels in the sarcolemma.
- Caveolae—these are invaginations in the sarcolemma and are believed to be analogous to T-tubules in skeletal muscle. The exact mechanism by which they control the entry of Ca^{2+} into the cell is unknown.

Intracellular Ca^{2+} concentration is restored by:
- Active pumping back into the sarcoplasmic reticulum.

- Active pumping of Ca^{2+} out of the cell.
- Na^+/Ca^{2+} exchange across the sarcolemma.

Smooth muscle contraction differs from skeletal muscle in that troponin is not a component of the thin filament and Ca^{2+} binds to the cytoplasmic protein calmodulin.

Disadvantages of smooth muscle contraction are that:

- Phosphorylation is a relatively slow process, therefore cross-bridge turnover and hence contraction velocities are low.
- ATP is required for both phosphorylation and powering of cross-bridges. Therefore, smooth muscle contraction is less efficient.

Advantages of slow cross-bridge turnover are that:

- The lower ATP consumption is adequately provided by oxidative phosphorylation hence no fatigue is shown.
- There is prolonged contraction.

Organic nitrates

Examples of organic nitrates include glyceryl trinitrate and isosorbide dinitrate.

Mechanism of action: Organic nitrates relax smooth muscle by increasing intracellular nitric oxide (NO) which interferes with contractile proteins and Ca^{2+} regulation.

Indications: Organic nitrates are drugs used in the treatment of angina and hypertension.

Adverse effects: There are no serious side effects from organic nitrates, although headache and postural hypotension may occur.

The organic nitrates act in the same way as the vasodilator NO produced by endothelial cells. Prostacyclin is also a vasodilator produced by endothelial cells. The vasoconstrictor released by endothelial cells is endothelin.

Functions of smooth muscle

The functions of smooth muscle depend on the site, such that:

- In blood vessels and airways it is important in maintaining tone and diameter.
- In the gastrointestinal tract it is important in mixing and propelling the contents along the tract via peristalsis.
- In the urinary system it is responsible for bladder emptying.

Myoepithelial cells

Myoepithelial cells are contractile cells found in mammary glands, sweat glands, salivary glands and the iris. They comprise a layer of flat cells arranged around acini and ducts. The arrangement of contractile proteins is similar to that in smooth muscle.

Upon stimulation, myoepithelial cells contract and cause expulsion of glandular secretions.

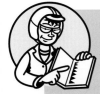

- Explain the term cardiac syncytium.
- Describe the initiation and propagation of the cardiac AP.
- Describe the ionic basis of the AP in the SA node compared to that in the Purkinje cells.
- Describe the differences in contraction of cardiac muscle to that in skeletal muscle.
- Explain the effect of the autonomic nervous system on heart rate.
- Describe how smooth muscle cells are arranged.
- Illustrate the arrangement of myofilaments in smooth muscle.
- Describe the mechanisms involved in changing intracellular calcium levels.
- Describe how smooth muscle contraction differs from skeletal muscle contraction and the effect of this.
- Outline the functions of smooth muscle in the body.
- What is the treppe or staircase effect?

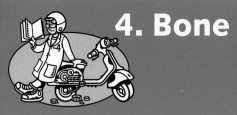

4. Bone

Overview of the skeleton

The skeletal system is composed of various types of connective tissue, including bone and cartilage.

Bone and cartilage comprise cells embedded in an extracellular matrix. This matrix consists of an amorphous ground substance permeated by a system of collagen and elastic fibres. These fibres differ from general connective tissue because their matrices are solid, although they do share the same origin from embryonic cellular connective tissue, the mesenchyme.

Components of the skeleton
Bone
Bone is rigid and forms most of the skeleton. It is the main supporting tissue of the body and provides a framework for most of the body's tissues.

Cartilage
Cartilage is a resilient tissue and provides a semi-rigid support for certain parts of the skeleton, e.g. the costal cartilages, respiratory airways and external ear.

Joints
Joints are composite structures that unite the bones of the skeleton. Depending on their form, joints allow for varying degrees of movement of the skeleton.

Ligaments and tendons
Ligaments and tendons are fibrous tissues that form part of the musculoskeletal system. Ligaments are flexible bands that connect bone or cartilage, stabilizing and strengthening joints. Tendons are the connections between muscles and their points of insertion into bones.

Functions of the skeleton
The skeleton performs the following functions:
- Support for the body, as it is a rigid frame work.
- Protection for organs, e.g. the cranium over the brain and the thoracic cage over the heart and lungs.
- A mechanical basis for locomotion.
- Mineral storage—the majority of calcium, phosphorus and magnesium salts are found in bone.
- Provides the site for bone marrow, where the development of blood cells, or haemopoiesis, occurs postnatally.

In newborn infants, red bone marrow produces red blood cells, some lymphocytes, granulocytic white blood cells and platelets. In adults, yellow bone marrow is mature bone marrow that has filled with adipocytes.

Organization of bone and cartilage

Distribution of bone and cartilage
The human skeleton is bilaterally symmetrical. It comprises the axial and appendicular skeleton (Fig. 4.1).

The axial skeleton consists of the bones of the head (skull), neck (hyoid bone and cervical vertebrae) and trunk (ribs, sternum, thoracic and lumbar vertebrae, and sacrum).

The appendicular skeleton consists of the bones of the upper and lower limbs and includes those forming the pectoral and pelvic girdles.

With age, the proportion of bone and cartilage in the skeleton changes. In the fetus, most long bones are initially represented by cartilage that resembles the shape of adult bone. In the adult, the only remnants of hyaline cartilage are the articular cartilages of joints, the tracheal ring cartilages.

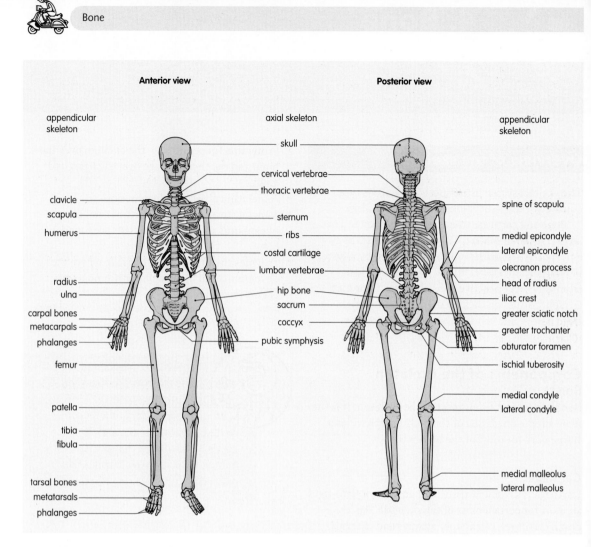

Fig. 4.1 Anterior and posterior views of the adult axial and appendicular skeleton.

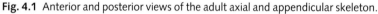

Cartilage
Cartilage microstructure
Cartilage consists of cells called chondroblasts and chondrocytes, which are laid in an extensive matrix. This matrix is composed of fibrous elements and a ground substance.

The chondroblasts and chondrocytes produce and maintain the matrix.

Cartilage formation and cell types
Cartilage derives from mesenchyme, embryonic cellular connective tissue. During development, the primitive mesenchymal cells become round, retract their extensions, and undergo rapid mitotic divisions. This process forms mesenchymal condensations.

Chondroblasts
Chondroblasts are the precursors of cartilage and arise from the differentiation of mesenchyme. They secrete cartilage matrix. The synthesis and deposition of this matrix separates the chondroblasts from each other and traps them within the matrix. Each chondroblast then undergoes up to eight further mitotic divisions to form groups of isogenous cells (i.e. developed from the same cell) surrounded by a smaller amount of condensed matrix.

Chondrocytes
Chondrocytes are mature cartilage cells occupying small cavities, or lacunae, within the matrix. Chondrocytes maintain the integrity of the matrix. Chondrocytes that are active have a basophilic

cytoplasm (indicating protein synthesis), plenty of rough endoplasmic reticulum, and a large Golgi complex. Older, less active, cells are smaller and have a pale cytoplasm and reduced Golgi complex.

The sequence of differentiation and maturation of cartilage cells is most developed in the centre of growing cartilage. Towards the periphery of the cartilage, chondroblasts at earlier stages of maturation merge with the surrounding perichondrium (Fig. 4.2).

Perichondrial cells differentiate into chondroblasts, then chondrocytes, growing inwards from the periphery. Cartilage matrix, rich in collagen, lies between the cells. The lacunae are rich in glycosaminoglycans.

Matrix

Cartilage matrix is firm and solid, but pliable, causing it to be resilient. The matrix contains varying types and amounts of fibres and ground substance.

The fibres are made up of either collagen—type II (hyaline) and type I (fibrocartilage)—or elastin.

The ground substance is rich in glycosaminoglycans. Chondroitin and keratin sulphates are joined to a core protein to form a proteoglycan monomer. A hyaluronic acid molecule is associated with about 80 proteoglycan units; these are joined by link proteins to form a large hyaluronate proteoglycan aggregate. Cross-linking glycoproteins bind these aggregates to collagen fibrils in the tissue (Fig. 4.3).

Perichondrium

All hyaline cartilage, apart from articular cartilage, is covered by a layer of perichondrium. This is a dense connective tissue. Perichondrium is rich in type I collagen fibres. The outer layer contains fibroblasts and the inner layer chondroblasts.

Growth

Cartilage can increase in size by either interstitial growth or appositional growth.

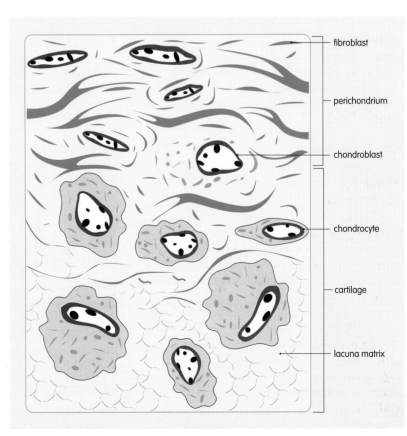

Fig. 4.2 Diagram of an area of perichondrium overlying hyaline cartilage. Perichondrial cells differentiate into chondroblasts, then chondrocytes, growing in from the periphery. Cartilage matrix lies between the cells; it is rich in collagen, apart from the lacunae which are rich in glycosaminoglycans. (Adapted with permission from *Basic Histology*, 8th edn, by L.C. Junqueira, Appleton & Lange, 1995.)

fibroblast

perichondrium

chondroblast

chondrocyte

cartilage

lacuna matrix

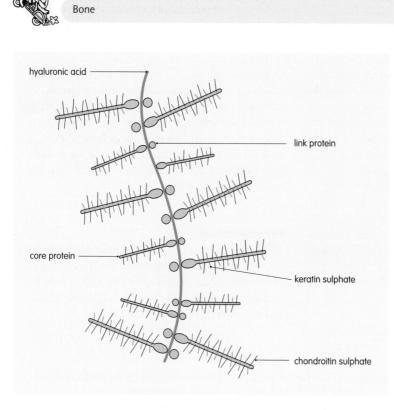

Fig. 4.3 Proteoglycan macromolecule, formed from chondroitin and keratin sulphates joined to a core protein.

Labels in figure: hyaluronic acid, link protein, core protein, keratin sulphate, chondroitin sulphate

Interstitial growth

Interstitial growth takes place in the middle of cartilage by the mitotic division of mature chondrocytes. This occurs in relatively young cartilage, which is malleable enough to allow for internal expansion.

Appositional growth

Appositional growth occurs on the periphery of cartilage from the differentiation of perichondrial cells.

Blood supply

As mature cartilage is an avascular tissue, the exchange of metabolites between chondrocytes and surrounding tissue relies on diffusion through the matrix.

In sites where cartilage is particularly thick, e.g. costal cartilage, small blood vessels are carried into the centre of the tissue by cartilage canals.

Poor blood supply to cartilage:
- Limits the extent of its thickness, as the innermost cells need to be maintained.
- Makes repair after injury difficult. Injured areas are usually replaced by fibrous tissue.

Cartilage types

Cartilage type depends on the composition of its matrix components. Three types of cartilage occur: hyaline cartilage, elastic cartilage and fibrocartilage.

Hyaline cartilage

Hyaline cartilage is the most common type of cartilage. It is characterized by a uniformly amorphous matrix and contains type II collagen fibres orientated along lines of stress.

Throughout childhood and adolescence, hyaline cartilage is present in the epiphyseal plates of long bones. It has a great resistance to wear and covers the surface of nearly all synovial joints, areas that are subjected to much stress.

Elastic cartilage

Elastic cartilage is composed of large numbers of elastic fibres and elastic lamellae embedded in matrix, making it flexible. It is found in the auricle of the ear, the external auditory meatus, the auditory tube and the epiglottis.

Fibrocartilage

Fibrocartilage comprises a large number of type I collagen fibres embedded in a small amount of matrix. It is found in discs within joints, e.g. the temporomandibular, sternoclavicular and knee joints, and also on the articular surfaces of the clavicle and the mandible.

Bone
Bone shape
Bone is defined according to its shape, i.e. long, short, flat, irregular or sesamoid.

Long bone
Long bone is longer than its width; most bone in the appendicular skeleton is of this type. The ends of long bones are composed of cancellous (spongy) bone surrounded by a thin layer of compact bone. Their shafts contain a bony network along stress-bearing lines and surround cavities filled with bone marrow. The articular surfaces are covered by hyaline (articular) cartilage.

Short bone
Short bone has a similar-sized length and width, and is roughly cuboidal or round in shape. Such bones are found in the wrist and ankle. Short bone is composed of cancellous bone surrounded by a thin layer of compact bone and is covered by periosteum. Hyaline cartilage covers the articulating surfaces.

Flat bone
Flat bone is usually thin, flat and curved. It is found in the vault of the skull, ribs, sternum and scapula. It consists of thin inner and outer layers of compact bone separated by a layer of cancellous bone called the diploë.

Irregular bone
Irregular bone does not fit into any of the previous groups. Vertebrae and sphenoid bone are examples of this type. Irregular bone is composed of cancellous bone with a covering of thin compact bone.

Sesamoid bone
Sesamoid bone is a small bone found in some tendons where they rub over bony surfaces. Tendons such as quadriceps femoris and flexor pollicis brevis contain the patella and the sesamoid bones, respectively. Most of a sesamoid bone is buried in the tendon; the free surface is covered with cartilage. Sesamoid bone reduces friction on the tendon and may also alter its direction of pull.

Bone anatomy
Long bone
Long bone comprises a shaft called the diaphysis; each end is expanded into an epiphysis (Fig. 4.4).

The diaphysis contains a large central medullary cavity surrounded by a thick-walled tube of compact bone. A small amount of cancellous bone lines the

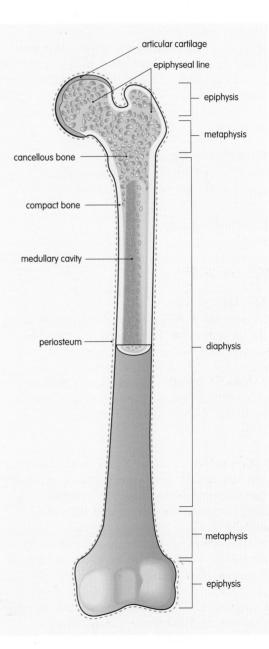

Fig. 4.4 Features of long bone.

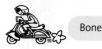

inner surface of the compact bone, forming a network of trabeculae.

In adults, the medullary cavity is filled with yellow (inactive) marrow, which is mostly adipose tissue; red (active) marrow is confined to the proximal epiphyses of larger adult long bone.

The epiphyses consist mainly of cancellous bone and have a thin outer shell of compact bone. Their articular surfaces are covered with a layer of hyaline cartilage.

In growing bone, the site of elongation of the bone is known as the epiphyseal cartilage (growth plate). When bone stops growing, the epiphyseal growth plate becomes ossified and forms the epiphyseal line.

The metaphysis, the flared epiphyseal end of the diaphyses, is very vascular.

Long bone is covered by periosteum and lined by endosteum.

Short, flat and irregular bone

Short, flat and irregular bone is composed of compact bone surrounding cancellous bone.

Bone microstructure

Bone is composed of cells called osteoblasts, osteocytes and osteoclasts, which are embedded in an extracellular matrix.

Bone cells

Osteoblasts: Osteoblasts lie on the inner periosteum and the endosteum. They secrete an organic bone matrix in which they become entrapped, forming osteocytes. Active osteoblasts have a large Golgi complex, plenty of rough endoplasmic reticulum and a basophilic cytoplasm. Resting (inactive) osteoblasts are smaller, flattened cells and have a paler cytoplasm.

Osteocytes: Osteocytes are found in small cavities called lacunae. Each cell has many processes, which run along canaliculi to connect with other cells via gap junctions. Osteocytes maintain the matrix, although they have less rough endoplasmic reticulum and a smaller Golgi complex than osteoblasts. When the cells die, the lacunae remain empty and there is resorption of the matrix.

Osteoclasts: Osteoclasts are large multinucleated cells with many branched processes. They are derived from the fusion of monocytes in blood and are therefore phagocytic. The cells resorb bone and

are found in troughs, called Howship's lacunae, on surfaces where bone is being removed. Cells in the process of actively resorbing have a pale acidophilic cytoplasm, and many vacuoles and lysosomes for enzymatic digestion. They also have a ruffled border facing the bone matrix; an adjacent clear zone is responsible for adhesion to the matrix and provides a suitable environment of low pH for the lysosomal enzymes.

Bone matrix

Bone matrix has an organic component, responsible for flexible strength, and an inorganic component, responsible for rigidity and mechanical strength.

The organic matrix (osteoid) is composed of type I collagen embedded in a ground substance of proteoglycan aggregates. Also present are specific glycoproteins such as bone sialoprotein (rich in sialic acid) and osteocalcin (binds calcium).

The inorganic matrix is composed of deposited mineral salts, which make up more than half the weight of dried matrix. The most abundant minerals in the inorganic matrix are calcium and phosphate. These form hydroxyapatite crystals $[Ca_{10}(PO_4)_6(OH)_2]$, the surface ions of which are hydrated to facilitate the exchange of water between the mineral crystals and body fluids. Bicarbonate, citrate, potassium and sodium are also found but in smaller quantities.

Periosteum

Periosteum covers the outer surface of bone. Its outer layer contains blood vessels, nerves and lymphatics, and its inner layer a few osteoblasts and osteoclasts.

Sharpey's fibres penetrate into the outer layer of bone to hold the periosteum, ligaments and tendons in place.

The enthesis is the site of insertion of ligaments and tendons, and the articular capsule. Rheumatoid arthritis (enthesitis) commonly begins at the enthesis.

Endosteum

Endosteum is a single layer of tissue containing osteoblasts and osteoclasts. It lines inner bone surfaces.

Blood supply and lymph drainage of bone

Several arteries supply blood to bone, which they enter from the periosteum (Fig.4.5). These blood vessels include:
- The periosteal arteries, which enter the bone shaft at many points and supply the compact bone. At the midshaft of the bone, a nutrient artery

Fig. 4.5 Blood supply of bone. The periosteal, epiphyseal and nutrient arteries supply the bone.

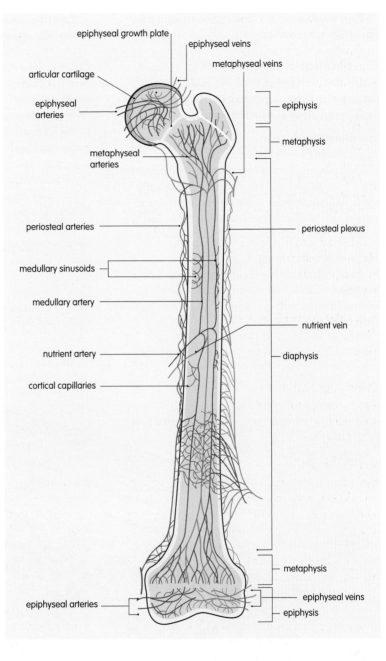

epiphyseal growth plate

epiphyseal veins

metaphyseal veins

articular cartilage

epiphysis

epiphyseal arteries

metaphysis

metaphyseal arteries

periosteal arteries

periosteal plexus

medullary sinusoids

medullary artery

nutrient vein

nutrient artery

diaphysis

cortical capillaries

metaphysis

epiphyseal veins

epiphyseal arteries

epiphysis

passes through the compact bone to supply the cancellous bone and bone marrow.
- The metaphyseal and epiphyseal arteries, which supply the ends of the bone.

The arteries are accompanied by veins. They are large and numerous in long bone and in areas of red bone marrow. The veins exit through vascular foramina near the articular ends of bones.

Lymph vessels are most abundant in the periosteum. They drain into the regional lymph nodes.

Nerve supply of bone

Many nerve fibres travel with the blood vessels to bone. They are mostly vasomotor, i.e. cause constriction or dilatation of blood vessels.

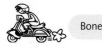

Periosteal nerves are sensory and contain pain fibres. They are sensitive to tearing or tension.

Classification of bone

There are two types of bone, depending on the pattern of collagen deposited: immature or woven bone, and mature or lamellar bone.

Immature (woven) bone

In immature (woven) bone, an irregular array of coarse collagen fibres, a large number of osteocytes and a low mineral content make it mechanically weak. Immature bone is the first type of bone to develop in the embryo and after fractures, and is gradually remodelled and replaced by lamellar bone.

Mature (lamellar) bone

In mature (lamellar) bone, collagen fibres appear in a regular parallel arrangement and have a highly organized infrastructure, which make it mechanically strong (Fig. 4.6).

Lamellar bone may be formed either as compact or cancellous bone.

Compact bone: Compact bone is composed of parallel columns along the long axis of a bone. Each column is made of concentric osteocyte layers fixed in the matrix in cavities called lacunae. The lacunae surround central neurovascular channels called Haversian canals. The units of lamellae and canals are known as Haversian systems or osteons. The vertical Haversian canals are linked with each other and with the endosteum and periosteum via transverse Volkmann's canals. Circumferential lamellae cover the outer surface of compact bone. Interstitial lamellae, which are remnants following bone remodelling, are also present.

Cancellous bone: Cancellous bone contains lamellae that form lattices called trabeculae. They are orientated along lines of stress and provide structural

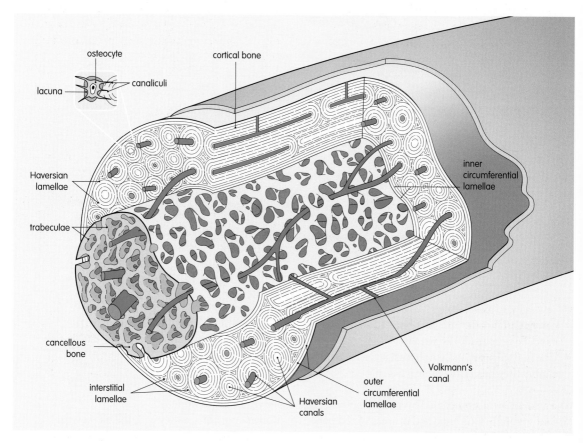

Fig. 4.6 Arrangement of mature bone.

strength. Cancellous bone has greater metabolic activity, hence it is more affected in conditions such as osteoporosis.

Bone formation, growth and remodelling

Types of ossification

Although all bones are derived from mesenchyme, the type of process they undergo for their formation, or ossification, can be either intramembranous or endochondral.

In intramembranous ossification, bone develops directly from primitive mesenchyme tissue, e.g. the skull bones and clavicle.

In endochondral ossification, bone develops indirectly from mesenchyme through an initial cartilage model, i.e. most bones.

The two processes result in an identical bone microstructure—both compact and cancellous bone can develop from either method.

After ossification, immature bone grows and is continuously remodelled by osteoclasts and osteoblasts until it is mature. This process continues throughout life.

The development of bone is controlled by hormones—growth hormone, thyroid hormones and sex hormones.

Intramembranous ossification

Intramembranous ossification occurs within 'membranes' of condensed mesenchyme tissue. Ossification takes place from the centre outwards (Fig. 4.7).

Some mesenchymal cells differentiate into osteoblasts at primary ossification centres. Osteoblasts secrete new bone matrix, which calcifies and encapsulates the cells in lacunae. These cells then become known as osteocytes.

Osteoprogenitor cells beneath the periosteum divide mitotically to produce further osteoblasts, which lay down more bone. This process forms the outer surface of bone.

Islands of new bone tissue within the mesenchyme are known as spicules. Spicules are penetrated by blood vessels and haematopoietic precursor cells, which will become bone marrow.

As bone formation progresses, there is fusion of adjacent centres of ossification to form immature bone with a woven appearance.

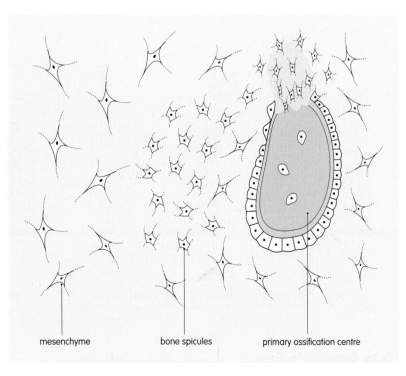

Fig. 4.7 Intramembranous ossification. Some mesenchymal cells differentiate into osteoblast within the primary ossification centre. The islands of bone formed within the mesenchyme which will eventually become bone marrow are known as spicules. (Adapted with permission from *Basic Histology*, 8th edn, by L.C. Junqueira, Appleton & Lange, 1995.)

mesenchyme   bone spicules   primary ossification centre

Endochondral ossification

Endochondral ossification refers to new bone formation occurring from established cartilage. Chondroblasts develop in the primitive mesenchyme (Fig. 4.8A), forming a hyaline cartilage and perichondrium model (Fig. 4.8B).

Osteoprogenitor cells and osteoblasts are formed at the midshaft of the diaphysis, creating periosteum and a collar of bone by intramembranous ossification. Calcium is deposited in the cartilage matrix (Fig. 4.8C).

Blood vessels grow from the periosteum and bone collar. They transport osteoprogenitor cells which differentiate to create a primary ossification centre in the middle of the diaphysis (Fig. 4.8D).

Osteoblasts form lamellae on the calcified cartilage to make lamellar bone. This growth spreads from the centre outwards. The outer bone collar makes cortical bone. This happens prenatally, when the epiphyses are still made of cartilage (Fig. 4.8E).

Secondary ossification centres form in the epiphyses at different times, mostly after birth. There is endochondral growth until fusion of the epiphyses occurs at around 25 years of age (Fig. 4.8F).

Bone growth
Appositional growth

Appositional growth involves bone formation on the outer surface of bone contributed to by the periosteum. In long bone this results in an increase in width while in short, flat and irregular bone, there is an increase in general size.

Endochondral growth

Endochondral growth involves interstitial growth of a cartilage model and then replacement with bone (Fig. 4.9). Overall this results in an increase in bone length.

At the epiphyseal plate, the diaphysis lengthens until the plate becomes fused, forming the epiphyseal line at puberty.

At articular cartilage, endochondral growth results in enlargement of the epiphyses.

Factors affecting growth

Factors that have an influence on bone growth include:

- Genetic influences, which determine bone shape and size.
- Dietary factors, such as vitamins D and C, which affect the formation of the organic and inorganic components of bone matrix.

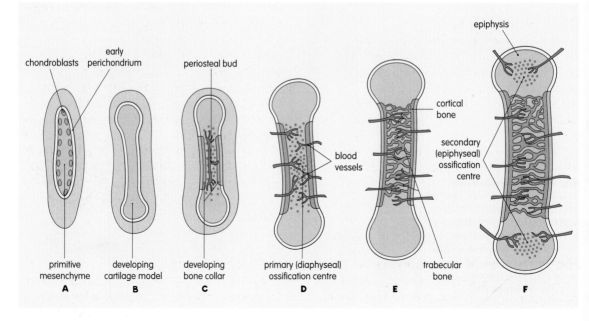

Fig. 4.8 Endochondral ossification. Parts A–F are explained in the text.

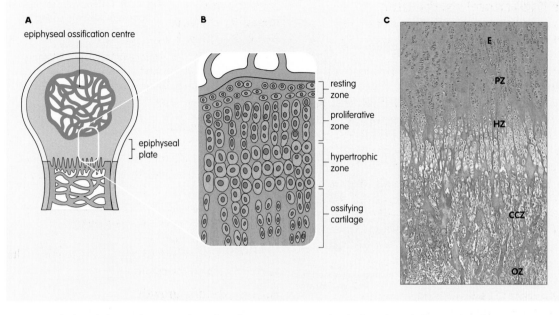

Fig. 4.9 Endochondral growth. (A) Epiphyseal ossification centre; (B) detail of epiphyseal plate; and (C) low-power electron micrograph. E, resting zone of the epiphyseal plate cartilage; PZ, proliferative zone; HZ, hypertrophic zone; CCZ, calcified cartilage zone; OZ, beginning of the ossification zone. (Courtesy of Dr A. Stevens and Prof. J. Lowe.)

• Hormones: growth hormone, thyroid hormones and sex hormones usually stimulate bone growth, and also cause fusion of the epiphyseal plates to stop bone growth.

Bone remodelling

Immature woven bone undergoes progressive remodelling by osteoclastic resorption and osteoblastic deposition to form mature compact or cancellous bone (Fig. 4.10).

Cancellous bone is laid along fibres of the mesenchyme, and compact bone is laid beneath the periosteum.

The primitive mesenchyme that remains in the network of developing bone differentiates into bone marrow.

Functions of bone

Maintenance of calcium levels

The skeleton contains 99% of the body's calcium. It maintains the levels of calcium in the blood within narrow limits so that muscle contraction and membrane potential activity can occur.

Normally, calcium levels in blood and tissues are stable and there is a continuous interchange of calcium between the blood and bone (Fig. 4.11).

When levels of calcium in the blood decrease, calcium is mobilized from bones. Conversely, excess levels of calcium in the blood can be removed and stored in bone.

One method for regulating blood calcium levels involves the transfer of calcium ions, firstly from hydroxyapatite crystals to interstitial fluid and then into blood. This takes place in cancellous bone and is a rapid mechanism helped by the large surface area of the hydroxyapatite crystals.

Other ways of regulating blood calcium levels are through parathyroid hormone and calcitonin release (Fig. 4.12). (Refer to *Crash Course: Endocrine and Reproductive Systems* for more details of hormones.)

Parathyroid hormone

Parathyroid hormone (PTH) is the main regulator of calcium levels in blood. It is responsible for raising low blood calcium levels to normal. When blood calcium levels are high, less PTH is secreted.

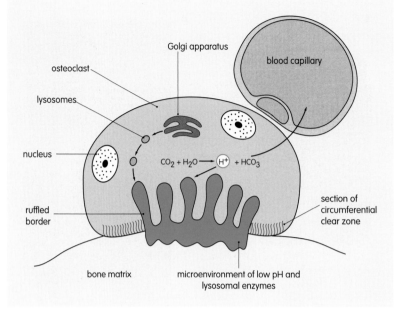

Fig. 4.10 Osteoclastic resorption in bone remodelling. (Adapted with permission from *Basic Histology*, 8th edn, by L.C. Junqueira, Appleton & Lange, 1995.)

osteoclast

Golgi apparatus

blood capillary

lysosomes

nucleus

$CO_2 + H_2O \longrightarrow H^+ + HCO_3$

ruffled border

section of circumferential clear zone

bone matrix

microenvironment of low pH and lysosomal enzymes

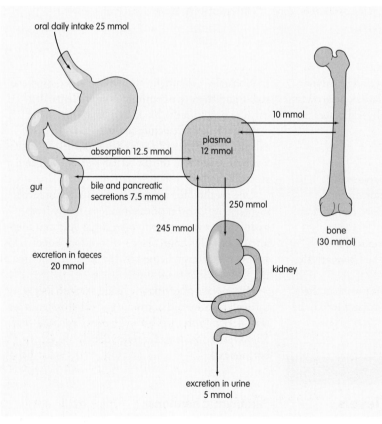

oral daily intake 25 mmol

10 mmol

plasma 12 mmol

absorption 12.5 mmol

gut

bile and pancreatic secretions 7.5 mmol

250 mmol

245 mmol

bone (30 mmol)

excretion in faeces 20 mmol

kidney

excretion in urine 5 mmol

Fig. 4.11 Daily calcium exchange in the body tissues. A continuous exchange of calcium between blood and bone takes place to keep calcium levels stable.

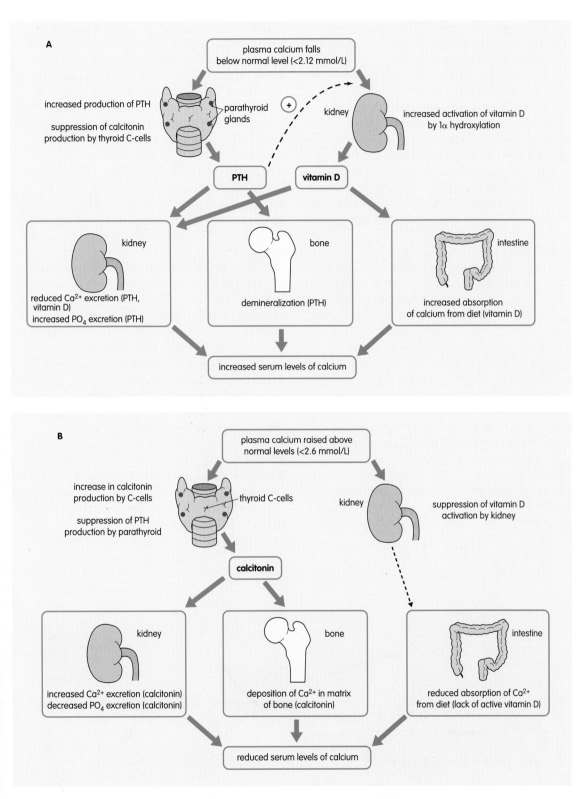

Fig. 4.12 Control of serum calcium levels by parathyroid hormone (PTH), calcitonin and vitamin D where (A) serum calcium falls below normal levels; and (B) where serum calcium rises above normal levels. (Adapted with permission from *Colour Atlas of Physiology*, by Depopoulous, Thieme, 1991.)

PTH is a peptide made of 84 amino acids. It is secreted from the parathyroid glands in response to low blood calcium levels.

PTH stimulates osteoclast activity and results in bone resorption and calcium release into blood. It also increases renal reabsorption so that less calcium is lost in the urine. PTH also promotes the formation of vitamin D in the kidneys. Vitamin D increases the absorption of calcium from the small intestine.

Hyperparathyroidism, the excessive production of PTH, leads to demineralized bone and elevated blood calcium levels. The excess calcium is deposited at other sites, such as arterial walls and kidney.

Calcitonin

Calcitonin is responsible for reducing high blood calcium levels to normal. It is a peptide made of 32 amino acids, and is secreted from the parafollicular cells of the thyroid gland in response to high blood calcium levels.

Calcitonin inhibits osteoclast activity and so opposes the action of PTH. It also decreases calcium and phosphate reabsorption in the kidney.

Excessive calcitonin production has no effect on calcium balance, so people with no calcitonin, e.g. thyroidectomy patients, do not need hormone replacement. The reasons for this are unknown.

Nutrition

During growth, bone is sensitive to nutritional factors. For bone and matrix formation to occur, the diet needs to contain proteins, calcium, and vitamins D and C.

Vitamin D

Vitamin D is required for the absorption of calcium and phosphate from the small intestine and, to a lesser extent, kidney (see Fig. 4.12). It also stimulates calcium reabsorption from bone.

Small amounts of vitamin D occur in foods such as fish liver oil and egg yolks. Most vitamin D, however, is produced in the epidermis from 7-dehydrocholesterol by a photolytic reaction mediated by ultraviolet light (Fig. 4.13).

Hydroxylation occurs in the endoplasmic reticulum of the hepatocytes of the liver to form 25-hydroxyvitamin D_3, which enters the circulation and is transported to the kidney by vitamin D-binding protein.

Further hydroxylation to 1,25-dihydroxyvitamin D_3 takes place in the mitochondria of the proximal tubules of the kidney. This most active form of vitamin D is called calcitriol. Its synthesis is promoted by PTH, and it has similar actions to PTH.

A decrease in vitamin D can lead to demineralization and poor calcification of bone. In adults this is called osteomalacia, while in children whose epiphyseal lines have yet to fuse it is known as rickets. Both conditions involve a loss of bone density, large epiphyses and bowing of the legs.

Vitamin C

Vitamin C is essential for the synthesis of collagen in the bone matrix by osteoblasts. It is a reducing agent, required for the hydroxylation of collagen residues, to allow calcification to occur.

Vitamin C is found in fresh fruit and vegetables.

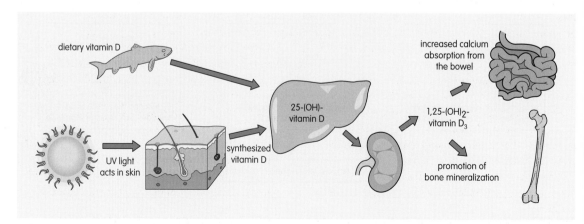

Fig. 4.13 Formation and actions of vitamin D.

A deficiency of vitamin C results in scurvy. The defective connective tissue leads to sore, spongy gums, loose teeth, fragile blood vessels, swollen joints and anaemia. There is also interference with bone growth and slowed tissue repair.

Hormonal influences
Sex hormones
Sex hormones influence the time of the appearance of the ossification centres and stimulate closure of the epiphyses.

Sex hormones initially stimulate bone growth during puberty, when their production is increased. This accounts for the growth spurts seen at this time. However, they also stimulate closure of the epiphyseal plates so that growth stops. Oestrogens cause quicker ossification of the epiphyseal plates than does testosterone, which is why girls stop growing earlier than boys and are normally shorter than boys.

Precocious sexual development caused by hormone-secreting tumours or administration of sex hormones tends to retard growth by causing early epiphyseal closure, whereas deficiencies of sex hormones caused by abnormal gonadal development tend to delay epiphyseal closure, prolonging the growth phase and resulting in tall stature.

Low oestrogen levels, common in immobilized patients and postmenopausal women, give rise to osteoporosis. In osteoporosis, although bone morphology is normal, there is a net decrease in bone mass caused by less bone formation and more bone resorption.

Growth hormone
Growth hormone increases general tissue growth. It is a peptide hormone released from the anterior pituitary gland, and is regulated by growth hormone-releasing hormone and the inhibiting hormone, somatostatin.

Growth hormone stimulates interstitial cartilage growth and appositional bone growth.

During the growing years, too much growth hormone abnormally increases the length of long bone, resulting in gigantism. Adults with elevated growth hormone levels have acromegaly. In acromegaly, the epiphyseal plates have closed so the bones cannot grow in length and instead become wider.

A lack of growth hormone gives rise to pituitary dwarfism.

Thyroid hormones
Thyroid hormones regulate gene expression, metabolism and the general development of all tissues.

Triiodothyronine (T_3) and tetraiodothyronine (T_4) are peptide hormones released by the follicular cells of the thyroid gland. They are regulated by thyroid-stimulating hormone (TSH), which is released from the anterior pituitary.

Thyroid hormone deficiency in neonates leads to cretinism and associated dwarfism.

Haemopoiesis in bone
Haemopoiesis is the formation of mature blood cells from precursors. In humans, haemopoiesis occurs in the medullary cavities of bone.

Red bone marrow is actively haematopoietic while yellow bone marrow, former red marrow, has become filled with adipocytes and is therefore inactive. When stress is applied to the haematopoietic system, yellow bone marrow can revert to red marrow.

Although the number of active sites of blood production in bone marrow lessens from birth to maturity, all bone marrow retains some haematopoietic potential. Haematopoietic activity can reappear in anaemia and extramedullary haemopoiesis.

Location of haemopoiesis
In humans, haemopoiesis takes place in various sites according to the stage of development.

In the embryo, primitive blood cells arise in the yolk sac within 4 weeks of conception.

At 6 weeks' gestation, the embryonic liver becomes the major site of haemopoiesis. The spleen and lymph nodes also show some activity.

Bone marrow starts to produce blood cells when bones form medullary cavities after 20 weeks' gestation; it is the only site to do so by birth, when all marrow is red.

In children, the diaphyses of long bone, but not the epiphyses, show replacement of red marrow by yellow marrow.

In adults, haemopoiesis occurs only in some bones, e.g. the vertebrae, sternum, ribs, clavicles, hip bones and upper femora, i.e. the axial skeleton (Fig. 4.14).

The bone marrow receives its blood supply from vessels that supply cancellous bone. Nutrient arteries

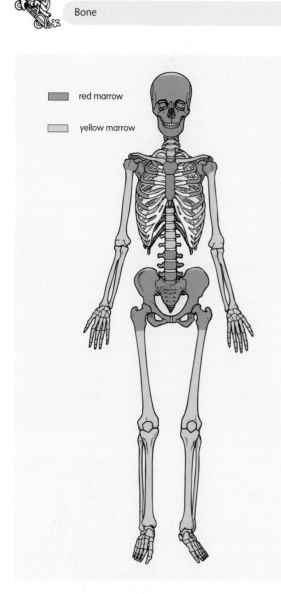

red marrow

yellow marrow

Fig. 4.14 Sites of haemopoiesis in an adult. (Adapted with permission from *Anatomy and Physiology*, 3rd edn, by R.R. Seeley, T.D. Stephens and P. Tate, Mosby Year Book, 1995.)

enter the midshaft of bone through the periosteum and pass through compact bone to reach the medullary space.

Response of bone to stress

Within limits, bone is a labile tissue that is capable of remodelling its internal structure according to different stresses (Fig. 4.15).

The two main mechanical stresses on bone are those from:

- The pull of skeletal muscles.
- The pull of gravity.

In response to mechanical stress, the increased deposition of mineral salts and production of collagen fibres make the bone stronger. In sites that are stressed frequently, bone is thicker, develops heavier prominences, and the trabeculae are rearranged (Fig. 4.16). Stress also increases the production of calcitonin, which inhibits bone resorption.

The bones of athletes, which are repeatedly subjected to high stresses, are notably thicker than those of non-athletes. Weightbearing activities, such as walking, help build and retain bone mass.

The removal of mechanical stress weakens bone through demineralization and collagen reduction. Bone is unable to remodel normally since resorption outstrips bone formation.

People who are bedridden or wear a cast lose strength in their unstressed bones. Astronauts subjected to the weightlessness of space also lose bone mass. In these situations bone loss can be as much as 1% per week.

Disorders of bone

Hereditary abnormalities of bone
Osteogenesis imperfecta

Osteogenesis imperfecta, or brittle bone disease, is a group of disorders that may be inherited in several ways and which have varying degrees of severity (Fig. 4.17). The genes responsible for osteogenesis imperfecta are found on chromosomes 7 and 17. The incidence of osteogenesis imperfecta is 1 in 20 000.

Pathology

In osteogenesis imperfecta, there is an abnormal synthesis of type I collagen that makes up 90% of bone matrix. Some forms of the disorder are fatal in the perinatal period; others predispose to fractures but there is overall survival.

Morphology

Osteopenia (decreased bone) occurs in osteogenesis imperfecta. This involves thinning of the cortex and trabeculae.

Fig. 4.15 Factors affecting bone remodelling in response to stress. (1,25(OH)$_2$D$_3$, 1,25-dihydroxyvitamin D$_3$; PGE$_2$, prostaglandin E$_2$; PTH, parathyroid hormone.) (Adapted with permission from *Essential Endocrinology*, by J. Laycock and P. Wise, Oxford University Press, 1996.)

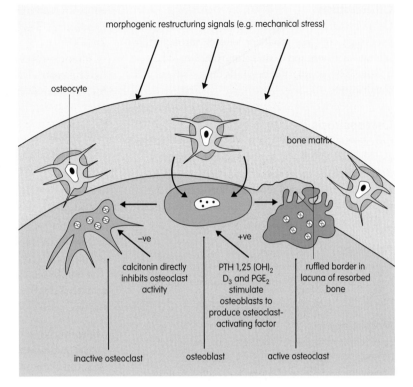

Fig. 4.16 Orientation of trabeculae along lines of stress. (Adapted with permission from *Anatomy and Physiology*, 3rd edn, by R.R. Seeley, T.D. Stephens and P. Tate, Mosby Year Book, 1995.)

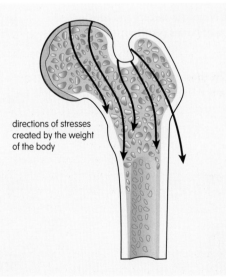

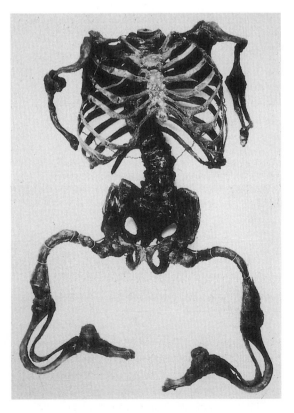

Fig. 4.17 Skeleton of a child with osteogenesis imperfecta congenita. Note the deformed limbs, scoliosis, and chest and pelvic deformities. (Courtesy of Dr P.G. Bullough and Dr V.J. Vigorita.)

Other features

Other features of osteogenesis imperfecta include uveal pigment (blue) that can be seen through thin sclerae, deafness and dental abnormalities. The prognosis is variable and depends on the severity of the disease.

Osteopetrosis

Osteopetrosis, also known as Albers–Schöenberg or marble bone disease, is a group of rare inherited disorders of different severities (Fig. 4.18). If the condition is autosomal recessive it presents from birth as anaemia and leucocytopenia. Adult types predispose to fractures and infection.

Pathology

Osteopetrosis is a defect in osteoclast function leading to decreased bone resorption and net bone overgrowth.

Morphology

In osteopetrosis there is overgrowth and sclerosis of bone, marked thickening of cortex, and narrowing and filling of medullary cavity (inhibits haemopoiesis). Treatment is with marrow transplant. In the severe form there is mental retardation and early death; in the mild form, there may only be changes in radiography detectable.

Achondroplasia

Achondroplasia is also known as dwarfism. It is a disorder caused by a single gene inherited in an autosomal dominant manner with complete penetrance. The incidence of achondroplasia is 1 in 25 000.

Homozygotes die soon after birth, whereas heterozygotes have a normal lifespan and normal mental, sexual and reproductive development.

Pathology

In achondroplasia there is derangement of endochondral ossification.

Morphology

Achondroplastic heterozygotes have short limbs and a normal-sized trunk. The skull is enlarged and there is a big forehead and depression of the nasal bridge. The epiphyses are abnormally wide (appositional growth is unaffected).

Malformations

Occasionally, malformations of the bones in the skeleton occur in achondroplasia. These result from either:

- Failure of formation.
- Extra bones (in fingers and toes).
- Fusion of bones (skull sutures).

Generally, these malformations are of no consequence. However, correction is possible for cosmetic reasons.

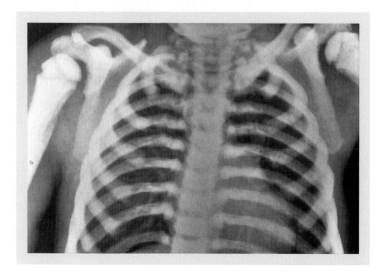

Fig. 4.18 Radiograph of the upper body of a child with osteopetrosis, showing a marked increase in density of all the bones. (Courtesy of Dr P.G. Bullough and Dr V.J. Vigorita.)

Infections and trauma

Osteomyelitis

Osteomyelitis, or infection of bone, can be caused by any bacterial agent, especially in people who are immunosuppressed (Fig. 4.19).

Pyogenic osteomyelitis
Causes

In immunocompromised people, pyogenic osteomyelitis can be caused by *Staphylococcus aureus, Escherichia coli, Klebsiella* spp., *Pseudomonas* spp., *Salmonellae* spp., *Haemophilus influenzae* and *Streptococcus* spp.

Spread

Spread of infection into bone can be by blood, local tissues, open fracture or surgery. In developing countries, spread is usually haematogenous, whereas in developed countries it is due to trauma.

Histology

Infection of bone leads to ischaemic necrosis, fibrosis and bony repair. The focus of infection starts initially around small vessels in the metaphysis. Necrosis of a bone segment is known as a sequestrum. This is surrounded by a sheath of subperiosteal new bone called the involucrum. Very sclerotic new bone forms a pattern called Garré's sclerosing osteomyelitis. There may be formation of sinus tracts or abscesses called Brodie's abscesses (these are sometimes sterile).

Clinical features

Infection of bone causes acute bone pain and fever. The infection usually starts in the metaphysis, where the good blood supply encourages bacterial growth and enables spread to other areas. A lytic area surrounded by a zone of reactive new bone can be seen on radiographs.

Complications

Complications of bone infection include sinus tracts to the skin surface (called cloacae), fracture, septicaemia, endocarditis, pyogenic arthritis and an alteration in growth rate.

Management

Antibiotic treatment is critical to the management of pyogenic osteomyelitis. If a diagnosis is suspected, intravenous antibiotics against the most likely causative organisms should be started immediately. Once the culture is identified from appropriate tissue or pus samples, the antibiotics can be adjusted accordingly. The course should include 2 weeks of intravenous antibiotics and 4 weeks of an oral dose.

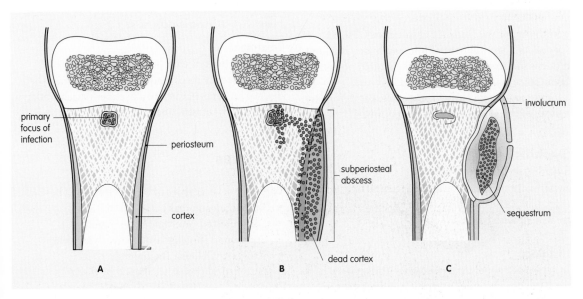

Fig. 4.19 Sequence of osteomyelitis. The primary focus of infection (A) has spread through bone, causing the death of cortical bone, and formation of a subperiosteal abcess (B). Death of a segment of bone (sequestrum) occurs (C), and the area is surrounded by new subperiosteal bone (involucrum).

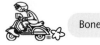

Surgery should only be undertaken if there is dead bone present, which acts as a nidus of infection and may lead to recurrence.

Tuberculous osteomyelitis
Tuberculous osteomyelitis is relatively uncommon in people who are immunocompetent. About 2% of all cases of tuberculosis have bone involvement.

Spread
Tuberculous osteomyelitis is spread haematogenously. It is more destructive and resistant to control than the pyogenic form.

Clinical features
Tuberculous osteomyelitis is usually a chronic condition with involvement of a single bone (except in patients with AIDS). It occurs in long bones, and in the thoracic and lumbar vertebrae, where it is called Pott's disease.

Complications
Tuberculous osteomyelitis causes fractures, nerve compression and tuberculous arthritis.

Management
The management of tuberculous osteomyelitis is both medical and surgical. Combination chemotherapy with rifampicin, isoniazid and para-aminosalicylic acid is administered over several months under the guidance of infectious disease specialists. Debridement of infected bones and joints reduces the amount of infectious material present. If the spine is involved, prolonged bed rest, administration of a plaster cast to prevent deformity and surgical stabilization may be required.

Syphilis
Syphilis in the skeleton
Syphilis of bone can be either congenital or acquired (Fig. 4.20). The condition is rare because of its early treatment with penicillin.

Histology
In syphilis of bone, local periostitis leads to new bone formation on the outer cortex. Gummata are the characteristic lesions of syphilis. They have a centre of rubbery, grey–white coagulation necrosis surrounded by epithelioid or fibroblastic cells.

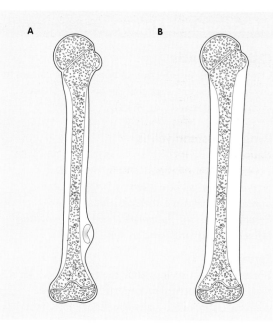

Fig. 4.20 Syphilis in bone showing (A) localized and (B) diffuse bone thickening.

Clinical features
On radiographs of affected skulls, the effects of syphilis are seen as a 'crew-cut' outline. When the tibia is involved there is a 'sabre shin' appearance. The destruction and collapse of nasal and parietal bones can create a 'saddle nose'.

Treatment
Syphilis is treated with penicillin, usually for 2 weeks, but may be extended to 3 weeks when the disease presents in the late stage. For patients allergic to penicillin, tetracycline or erythromycin is also effective.

Fractures
Types
There are several types of bone fractures. These are:
- Simple (clean break).
- Comminuted (multiple bone fragments).
- Compound (breaks through overlying skin).
- Stress (small linear fragments).
- Pathological (bones weakened by disease).

Causes
Fractures are usually caused by trauma, which is either substantial or minor and repeated.

Pathological fractures arise from diseases, e.g. tumours, osteoporosis, Paget's disease, osteomalacia.

Healing
Healing of fractures requires immobilization of approximated bone ends and good alignment.

Delayed or imperfect healing
The delayed or imperfect healing of bone fractures can be caused by malalignment, movement during healing, poor blood supply and soft tissue interposition in the fracture gap. These can occur in the elderly, those in poor general health and in people who are immunosuppressed.

Histology of healing
Healing of a fracture follows a sequence (Fig. 4.21). The histological changes that take place during healing include:

- Development of a haematoma, which forms a soft procallus (Fig. 4.21A).

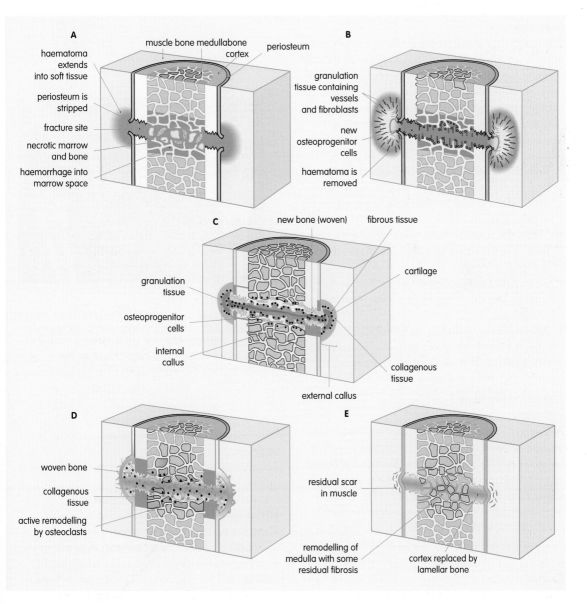

Fig. 4.21 Sequence of fracture repair. See text for explanation.

- Conversion of the procallus to a fibrocartilaginous callus (Fig. 4.21B).
- Replacement of fibrocartilaginous callus to an osseous callus—trabecular lamellar bone (Figs 4.21C and D).
- Remodelling along weightbearing lines by osteoclasts (Fig. 4.21E).

Complications

Complications of fractures can include malunion of bones, avascular necrosis, shock, osteoarthritis, infection and deep vein thrombosis.

Management

The immediate management involves immobilization of the fracture, coverage of the wound with a sterile dressing and pain relief. Individual management of fractures depends on the age and expectation of the patient, the pathology present and the patient's personal requirements in terms of occupation, etc. The basic principles of fracture management are as follows:

- Reduction of the deformity, replacing the bone fragments in their previous anatomical position—external or internal fixation may be necessary to achieve this.
- Maintenance of the reduction until the fractured bone reunites either by a plaster cast, brace and/or traction.
- Encouraging the healing of the fracture and surrounding structures by providing optimum conditions.
- Rehabilitation, including early mobilization of adjacent joints to prevent stiffness and wasting.
- Minimization of complications (see above).

Avascular necrosis
Pathology

Avascular necrosis involves the death of bone and marrow without infection, and is caused by a poor blood supply. It is mostly seen in the head of femur and scaphoid, occurring when fractures deprive adjacent areas of their blood supply (Fig. 4.22). Medullary infarctions affect cancellous bone and bone marrow, with cortical sparing. Subchondral infarctions lead to wedge-shaped areas of damage.

Causes

Avascular necrosis can be idiopathic or caused by trauma, thromboembolism, sickle-cell

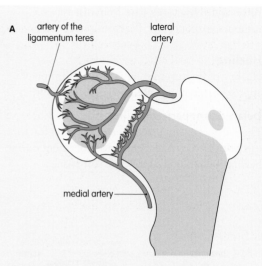

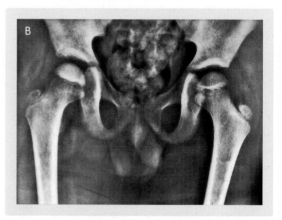

Fig. 4.22 Avascular necrosis of the femoral head (Perthe's disease). (A) Normal blood supply; and (B) radiograph showing widened joint space, cessation of growth of the bony epiphyses and increased growth of cartilage. (Courtesy of Dr P.G. Bullough and Dr V.J. Vigorita.)

disease, polycythaemia, immunosuppression or decompression sickness (divers).

Histology

Dead bone is identified by empty lacunae surrounded by necrotic adipocytes. The adipocytes may rupture to release fatty acids, which bind calcium and form deposits. There is osteoclastic resorption of trabeculae and the articular cartilage is distorted.

Clinical features

There is pain and immobility in avascular necrosis—the patient cannot walk, especially if the condition is a complication of fracture (elderly).

Metabolic diseases of bone

Osteoporosis

Osteoporosis is a very common disease of the elderly, especially postmenopausal women, resulting in abnormally decreased bone mass. Osteoporosis causes a major social and economic problem.

Classification

Osteoporosis can be localized or generalized, and can be classed as primary or secondary:

- Primary occurs in old age and postmenopausal women.
- Secondary is caused by endocrine abnormalities, gut malabsorption and neoplasia.

Histology

In osteoporosis the bone cortex has thinned, the trabeculae are attenuated, and there are wide Haversian canals (Fig. 4.23). Increased osteoclastic resorption with slowed bone formation occurs. The main sites affected are the vertebrae, femoral necks, wrists and pelvis. In the spine there may be disc herniation and nerve root compression.

Aetiology

Possible causes of osteoporosis include decreased exercise, oestrogen deficiency, lack of calcium, vitamin D or fluoride, hyperadrenocorticism, hypogonadism, thyrotoxicosis, hypopituitarism, pregnancy, immobilization, diabetes and long-term heparin administration.

Clinical features

Osteoporosis causes bone pain, loss of height, fractures and deformities such as lumbar lordosis and kyphoscoliosis. Diagnosis is by bone density scans or biopsy. A 30% loss of bone mass is required before radiographs show translucency.

Clinical consequences:

- Increased mortality (especially in the first year following hip fractures).
- Pain.
- Deformity (loss of height, kyphosis).
- Loss of independence.

Treatment for osteoporosis includes hormone replacement to increase oestrogen levels and exercise to strengthen weightbearing joints.

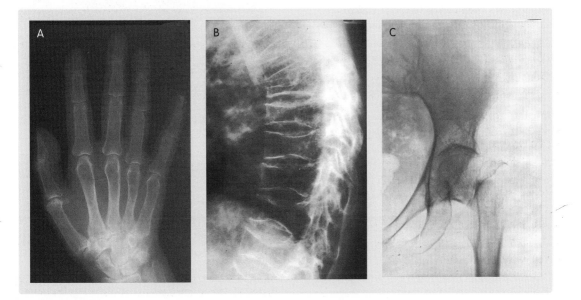

Fig. 4.23 Features of osteoporosis. (A) Loss of cortical thickening and reduction of trabeculae in the hand; (B) wedge-shaped flattening of vertebral bodies leading to loss of height; and (C) fracture of the neck of the femur in an elderly person. (Courtesy of Dr P.G. Bullough and Dr V.J. Vigorita.)

Management

The rapid bone loss in postmenopausal women may be countered to some extent by hormone replacement therapy (HRT); it is recommended that HRT is maintained for a minimum of 5 years to be useful in preventing osteoporosis. Bisphosphonates inhibit osteoclast action and increase bone density. They may be given orally or intravenously. Protracted treatment with calcium and vitamin D has also been proven to reduce the risk of fracture.

Rickets and osteomalacia

Rickets occurs in growing children and osteomalacia in adults. These are caused by either vitamin D deficiency or phosphate depletion—the latter is less common.

Aetiology

Vitamin D deficiency can be caused by low quantities in the diet, insufficient exposure to sunlight, malabsorption, or deranged liver or kidney metabolism. Phosphate depletion can be caused by X-linked phosphataemia, neoplasia or poisoning from heavy metals.

Pathology

Rickets and osteomalacia arise from a failure of bone mineralization, which leads to softer and wider channels of matrix. Excess unmineralized matrix and underdeveloped epiphyseal cartilage calcification leads to endochondral bone that is deranged and overgrown.

Clinical features

Rickets presents with bowing of the legs, overgrowth of costochondral junctions (forming a 'rachitic rosary'), widened epiphyses and either a flattened ('bossed') square skull or craniotabes (the skull snaps back into shape after being pressed in) (Fig. 4.24).

Osteomalacia presents with spontaneous incomplete fractures ('Looser's zones') in long bones and the pelvis, bone pain, weakened proximal limb muscles and a decreased serum calcium.

Bone biopsy is needed to confirm the diagnosis of rickets or osteomalacia. Treatment involves oral or intravenous administration of vitamin D, and an improved diet.

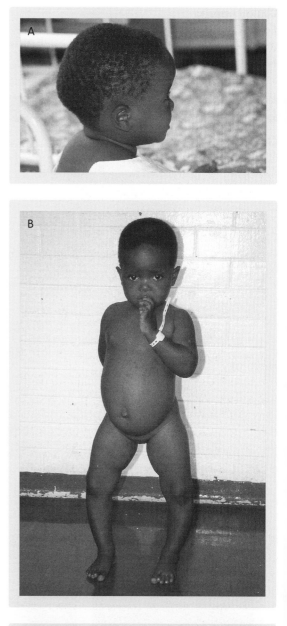

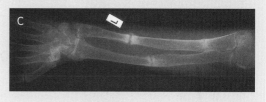

Fig. 4.24 Rickets and osteomalacia. (A) Skull 'bossing' in rickets; (B) lateral and forward bowing of legs in rickets; and (C) radiograph showing pseudofractures (Looser's zones) in the forearm in osteomalacia. (A and B courtesy of Dr S. Taylor and Dr A. Raffles; C courtesy of Dr P.G. Bullough and Dr V.J. Vigorita.)

Management

Treatment involving vitamin D and calcium regulates bone formation, and is used in the management of osteomalacia. Corrective osteotomies may also be required if the deformities are severe and established.

Hypercalcaemia, which leads to muscle weakness, lethargy, confusion, polyuria and dehydration, is caused by hyperparathyroidism or bone malignancy caused by metastatic bone disease or multiple myeloma. Less common causes include thyrotoxicosis, sarcoidosis and excess vitamin D. It is important to be aware of this condition, as severe hypercalcaemia leads to crisis, the main features of which are gross dehydration resulting from polyuria. It is treated by rehydration and intravenous bisphosphonate to reduce the loss of bone calcium.

Hyperparathyroidism

Classification

Hyperparathyroidism can be either:

- Primary—caused by a lesion of the parathyroid gland which increases PTH and thus raises calcium levels.
- Secondary—owing to bone metastases, inappropriate PTH secretion by tumours or renal failure (normal or lowered serum calcium).
- Tertiary—because of the development of an autonomous adenoma in the parathyroid glands, which occurs following the persistent hyperactivity of the glands as they secrete PTH.

Pathology

Increased PTH levels cause an increase in osteoclast activity that leads to increased bone resorption.

Histology

In hyperparathyroidism, demineralization leads to increased osteoclast activity and resorption. There is characteristic peritrabecular fibrosis, called osteitis fibrosa, and more marked fibrosis and cyst formation within the marrow (osteitis fibrosa cystica or von Recklinghausen's disease of the bone). 'Brown tumours' of osteoclasts, fibrosis and haemorrhage are also seen (Fig. 4.25). These resemble giant-cell granulomas.

Clinical features

In hyperparathyroidism, radiographs of the phalanges and clavicles show 'moth-eaten' erosions (see Fig. 4.25). This bone damage can be reversed by treating the cause of the excess PTH.

Management

Primary and tertiary hyperparathyroidism are treated by parathyroidectomy after the affected gland has been identified by biopsy. In secondary hyperparathyroidism, a subtotal parathyroidectomy is performed, which involves removal of three and a half of the four glands. Surgical risks include inducing hypocalcaemia if too much gland tissue is removed, and damaging the recurrent laryngeal nerve.

Renal osteodystrophy

Renal osteodystrophy is the collective term for all the skeletal changes occurring in chronic renal disease.

Pathology

Renal osteodystrophy is caused by:

- Inadequate renal tissue for making vitamin D— leads to osteomalacia.
- High serum phosphate—precipitates hyperparathyroidism.
- Prolonged haemodialysis—inhibits calcification of bone matrix and produces osteomalacia.
- Steroids—may induce osteoporosis or avascular necrosis.

Clinical features

The clinical features and management of renal osteodystrophy are similar to those of osteitis fibrosa cystica and osteomalacia. Osteosclerosis occurs and chronically there are metastatic calcifications in the skin, eyes, joints and arterial walls.

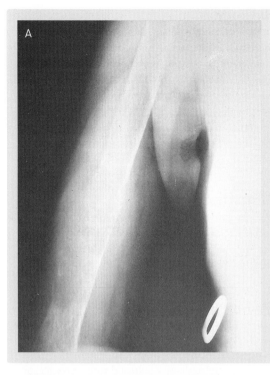

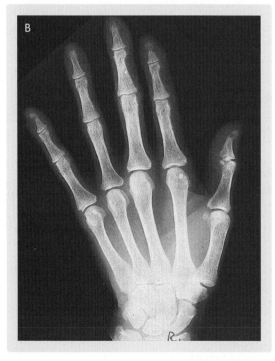

Fig. 4.25 Hyperparathyroidism. (A) Radiograph showing large destructive lesion (brown tumour) in the lower half of the humerus. (Courtesy of Dr P.G. Bullough.) (B) Radiograph showing subperiosteal erosion of the cortical surfaces of the phalanges. (Courtesy of Dr A. Norman.)

Tumours of the skeleton

Metastatic tumours of the skeleton
Metastatic tumours of the skeleton are much more common than primary bone tumours, particularly in adults.

Metastases arising from the breast, lung, kidney and thyroid are lytic, whereas those from the prostate are sclerotic.

Cartilage-forming tumours
Chondroma and endochondroma
Cartilage-forming tumours are benign tumours composed of mature hyaline cartilage. Those within bone are endochondromas and those on the surface are subperiosteal chondromas (Fig. 4.26).

Epidemiology
Males are more likely to develop cartilage-forming tumours than females—usually between 20 and 50 years of age.

Classification
There are two types of cartilage-forming tumours: solitary and multiple.

Multiple tumours involve non-familial types (endochromatosis or Ollier's disease) and familial types (Mafucci's syndrome). Familial types are associated with haemangiomas.

Clinical features
Features of cartilage-forming tumours include bone pain and fractures. The tumours consist of cartilage nests and arise at the epiphyses. There is a risk of chondrosarcoma in multiple lesions, especially if the condition is familial.

Management
Many of these lesions do not require treatment. When needed, treatment consists of curettage of the cartilage tissue and the grafting of bone onto the subsequent defect.

Chondrosarcoma
Chondrosarcomas are malignant tumours of cartilage. They grow slowly and occur half as frequently as osteosarcomas—75% are primary and the rest form endochondromas, osteochondromas and chondroblastomas.

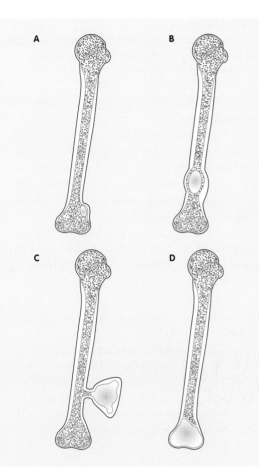

that are translucent when cut and show necrosis and spotty calcifications.

Chondroblastoma

Chondroblastomas, or Codman's tumours, are rare benign tumours that affect the epiphyses of young people. The tumours, which are composed of chondroblasts arranged in sheets, have a grooved nucleus and a surrounding calcified network; osteoclast-like cells may also be present.

Chondromyxoid fibroma

Chondromyxoid fibromas are rare benign tumours composed of cartilage matrix, and fibrous and myxoid tissue.

Epidemiology

Males are more likely to develop chondromyxoid fibromas than females—usually between 10 and 30 years of age.

Clinical features

Radiographs of chondromyxoid fibromas show circumscribed lucencies with scattered calcifications, usually in the metaphyses of the tibia, fibula and humerus.

Fig. 4.26 Benign bone tumours. (A) Osteoma; (B) endochondroma and chondroma; (C) osteochondroma; and (D) giant-cell tumour.

Bone-forming tumours
Osteochondroma

Osteochondromas, or exostoses, are benign mushroom-shaped outgrowths of bone capped with cartilage and attached to the skeleton by a bony stalk. Osteochondromas can grow up to 20 cm in diameter.

Epidemiology

Males are more likely to develop osteochondromas than females—usually under 20 years of age.

Epidemiology

Males are more likely to develop chondrosarcomas than are females—usually over 30 years of age.

Classification

Chondrosarcomas are graded from 1 to 3 according to nuclear atypia. Five-year survival rates range from 90% (low grade) to 40% (high grade).

Clinical features

Radiographs of chondrosarcomas show localized areas of bone destruction mottled with dense calcified spots. High-grade tumours spread haematogenously, notably to the lungs. Typical sites are central bones such as the pelvis, scapula and ribs. Histology shows large, gelatinous, lobulated tumours

Classification

There are two types of osteochondroma:
- Solitary, developing in young adults.
- Multiple, developing in children and inherited in an autosomal dominant pattern.

Clinical features

In osteochondroma, lesions are near the epiphyses of long bones. Malignant change is rare, but can occur in multiple lesions.

Management
Simple excision is the definitive treatment for osteochondromas.

Osteoma
Osteomas are slow-growing benign tumours composed of sclerotic bone that is well formed (see Fig. 4.26). Osteomas are unlikely to become malignant.

Epidemiology
Both young and middle-aged people can develop osteomas.

Classification
There are two types of osteoma. These are:
- Solitary, developing in middle age.
- Multiple, developing in young people and often associated with polyposis coli (Gardner's syndrome).

Common sites of bony metastases include the thoracic and lumbar spine, the proximal femur and the proximal humerus. Patients often present with pathological fractures — breaks in the bone caused by minimal stress. Patients may also present with hypercalcaemia.

Clinical features
Osteomas are likely to protrude from cortical surfaces, especially the skull and facial bones. They are usually harmless unless the location compromises organ function, e.g. growth on the inner skull.

Osteoid osteoma and osteoblastoma
Osteoid osteomas are small benign tumours surrounded by a dense sclerotic ring of new bone, and are usually less than 2 cm in diameter.

Osteoblastomas (also called giant osteoid osteomas) have a similar histology, without the sclerotic ring, and are usually more than 2 cm in diameter.

Epidemiology
Males are more likely to develop osteoid osteomas and osteoblastomas than are females—usually between 5 and 25 years of age.

Clinical features
Osteoid osteomas are located in the cortex of the tibia and femur, and are very painful. Radiographs show a small radiolucent 'nest' of trabecular bone surrounded by a ring of dense sclerotic bone. The nest consists of osteoid, osteoblasts and a vascular stroma.

Osteoblastomas are less painful than osteoid osteomas and are found in the vertebrae and long bones. They may become malignant and form osteosarcomas.

All patients with back pain, especially that which is unremitting and frequently severe at night, must have the most likely primary tumour sites — lung and breast — assessed.

Osteosarcoma
Osteosarcomas are the most common type of primary bone tumour (Fig. 4.27). They are composed of osteocytes and osteoid. Osteosarcomas are thought to be related to the retinoblastoma and p53 genes. They grow quickly and, with combination therapy, have a 60% 5-year survival rate. Some histological variants, such as juxtacortical and periosteal types, have a better prognosis.

Epidemiology
Males are more likely to develop osteosarcomas than females—usually up to 20 years of age, although the elderly with pre-existing bone tumours are also at risk.

Clinical features
Osteosarcomas are found in the medullary cavity of metaphyses of long bones (especially near the knee)

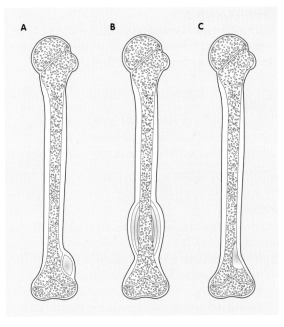

Fig. 4.27 Malignant bone tumours. (A) Osteosarcoma; (B) Ewing's sarcoma; and (C) metastatic bone tumours.

and, in the elderly, in flat bones. They produce bone pain, tenderness and swelling. Osteosarcomas are usually a complication of Paget's disease of bone. Radiographs show elevated periosteum (Codman's triangle) caused by new bone growth under the periosteum. There may be haematogenous spread to the lungs.

Management
Over the past 25 years, new multi-drug chemotherapy has been introduced which has led to a reduction in the mortality rate of patients with osteosarcomas. The adoption of aggressive surgical treatment has also led to an increase in patient survival; cure rates vary, but may reach up to 80%.

Fibrous and fibro-osseous tumours
Fibroma
Fibromas are benign, well-defined tumours composed of fibroblasts and collagenous tissue. They are usually found in the ovary, but may develop elsewhere.

Fibrous dysplasia
Fibrous dysplasia is a benign disorder in which there is progressive replacement of bone. This takes place

by fibroblasts that are arranged in a regular pattern with small spicules of immature bone. As a result, the bones become structurally weakened.

Epidemiology
Fibrous dysplasia affects children and young adults.

Classification
There are three types of fibrous dysplasia. These are:
- Monostotic (70%).
- Polyostotic (25%).
- Polyostotic and associated with endocrinopathies (5%).

Albright's syndrome is fibrous dysplasia with precocious sexual development and irregular skin pigmentation.

Clinical features
Fibrous dysplasia is found in the ribs, femur, tibia and skull. There is a 'ground glass' appearance on radiographs and *café-au-lait* spots over affected bones. Rarely, some can become osteosarcomas.

Miscellaneous tumours
Ewing's sarcoma
Ewing's sarcomas are aggressive malignant tumours of primitive neural differentiation (see Fig. 4.27). These grey tumours contain small round cells growing in sheets around blood vessels, and show focal necrosis and haemorrhage. However, they respond to drugs and have an overall 5-year survival of 60%. The tumour metastasizes to lungs and lymph nodes.

Epidemiology
Females are more likely to develop Ewing's sarcoma than males—usually under 25 years of age. Ewing's sarcoma is very rare in Afro-Caribbean children.

Clinical features
Ewing's sarcoma presents as a soft-tissue mass—periosteal 'onion-skinning' is seen on radiographs. This is often followed by a 'moth-eaten' or mottled appearance of the bone, accompanied by the extension of the lesion into soft tissue.

Management
Treatment for Ewing's sarcoma is medical and surgical. Preoperatively, chemotherapy with vincristine, dactinomycin and cyclophosphamide (VAC), and radiation are used. Following tumour resection, chemotherapy is used to reduce the chance of recurrence.

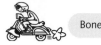

Giant-cell tumour

Giant-cell tumours, or osteoclastomas, are low-grade malignant tumours of giant multinucleate cells and stroma; 10% form metastases (see Fig. 4.26).

Epidemiology

Females are more likely to develop giant-cell tumours than males—usually between 20 and 40 years of age.

Clinical features

Radiographs of giant-cell tumours show large lytic 'soap-bubble' lesions with absent calcified spots. These can often be mistaken for 'brown tumours' that occur in hyperparathyroidism. Giant-cell tumours are found at the metaphyses and epiphyses of long bones, especially the knees.

Management

The treatment depends on the history and histological grading of the lesion. Recommended methods of removal include curettage and bone grafting, and cryosurgery involving the use of liquid nitrogen to destroy residual tumour cells.

 Treatment of bone pain caused by tumours is palliative. Bones which are at risk of fracture because of malignant pathology are often treated prophylactically by internal fixation, as the risk of fracture is substantial if more than one-third of the bone's width is destroyed by tumour lesions.

Other diseases of bone

Paget's disease of bone

Paget's disease of bone is also known as osteitis deformans. It is a disease of disordered bone formation and resorption. It commonly occurs in people over 40 years of age and affects males more than females. Paget's disease of bone usually occurs in white populations of the western world; it is rare in Asians and Africans.

Classification

Paget's disease of bone affects either one bone (15%) or several (85%). Bones affected are the tibia, femur, ileum, vertebrae, humerus and skull (Fig. 4.28).

Causes

The cause of Paget's disease of bone is unknown, but may be due to infection of osteoclasts by paramyxovirus, measles virus or respiratory syncytial virus.

Pathology

Paget's disease of bone occurs in three phases. These are the:
- Initial osteolytic phase, when there is a huge increase in osteoclastic activity.
- Mixed osteoclast/osteoblast phase, when there is disordered activity and a mosaic pattern of bone is produced.
- Quiescent osteosclerotic phase, when new sclerotic bone is produced after a period of years.

Histology

In Paget's disease of bone, the bone is thickened but weak, and there is intertrabecular fibrosis and a mosaic pattern of new bone as the osteoid is very bulky and porous.

Clinical features

Fractures and coarsened facial bones in Paget's disease of bone lead to a leonine facies, bone pain and fractures. There may be deafness because of nerve compression by the overgrown skull. Serum alkaline phosphatase and calcium levels are raised and hydroxyproline is present in the urine.

Complications

Complications of Paget's disease of bone include secondary osteoarthritis, high-output heart failure caused by new blood vessels forming shunts, and Paget's sarcoma.

Management

Management is both medical and surgical. Salmon calcitonin and biphosphates are used to inhibit osteoclast action and slow down the pathological remodelling of bone. Surgical correction of severe deformities is also sometimes performed; as bone heals poorly in this condition, intramedullary fixation devices are usually applied at the end of the operation.

Hypertrophic pulmonary osteoarthropathy

Hypertrophic pulmonary osteoarthropathy is an uncommon, idiopathic condition causing changes to bones and joints.

Pathology

In hypertrophic pulmonary osteoarthropathy there is:

- New periosteal bone formation in the distal long bones, wrists, ankles and proximal phalanges.
- Arthritis of adjacent joints.
- Clubbing of digits.

Clinical features

Hypertrophic pulmonary osteoarthropathy is associated with lung cancer or pleural mesothelioma, and there is usually an increased blood flow to the limbs.

Management

Resection of the tumours usually leads to regression of the condition.

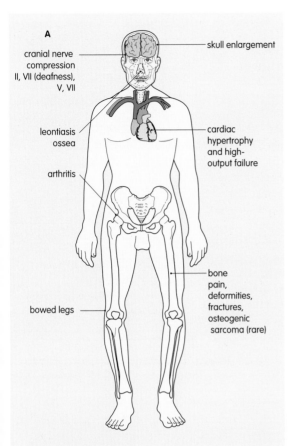

A

cranial nerve compression II, VII (deafness), V, VII

skull enlargement

leontiasis ossea

cardiac hypertrophy and high-output failure

arthritis

bone pain, deformities, fractures, osteogenic sarcoma (rare)

bowed legs

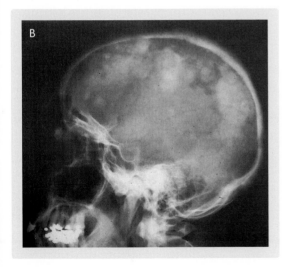

B

Fig. 4.28 Paget's disease of bone. (A) General features; and (B) radiograph of skull in late stage showing patchy sclerosis and loss of diploic architecture. (Courtesy of Dr P.G. Bullough.)

- List the functions of the skeleton.
- Describe the microstructure of the cartilage.
- Give a simple classification of cartilage type.
- Describe the microstructure of bone.
- Name two types of ossification.
- List the factors that affect bone growth.
- Describe remodelling of immature bone.
- Explain how calcium levels are maintained by PTH and calcium.
- List hormonal influences on bone.
- List the causes of hereditary abnormalities of bone.
- Describe the features of pyogenic osteomyelitis.
- List the different types of fracture and how they heal.
- Explain the causes and pathology of osteoporosis.
- What is the difference between osteoporosis and osteomalacia?
- Give a simple classification of hyperparathyroidism and its effects.
- Describe the effects of renal disease on bone.
- Describe the features of Paget's disease of bone.
- Give a simple classification of tumours of the skeleton.
- Distinguish between benign and malignant tumours.

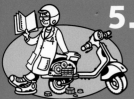

5. Joints and Related Structures

Classification of joints

Joints are the site at which two or more bones are united, regardless of whether there is movement between them. Joints are classified into fibrous, cartilaginous or synovial, according to the type of tissue between the bones (Figs 5.1–5.3).

Fibrous
Fibrous joints have fibrous tissue uniting the bones. This type of joint allows very little movement.

Cartilaginous
There are two types of cartilaginous joints—primary and secondary.

Primary cartilaginous
Primary cartilaginous joints unite two bones with a plate of hyaline cartilage. No movement is possible with this type of joint.

Secondary cartilaginous
Secondary cartilaginous joints unite two bones with a plate of fibrocartilage; there is also a thin layer of hyaline cartilage on the articular surfaces. A small amount of movement is possible with this type of joint.

Synovial
Synovial joints have a thin layer of hyaline cartilage on the articulating surfaces of the bones, which are separated by a joint cavity and covered by a joint capsule. The cells of the synovial membrane lining the capsule secrete a lubricating nutritive medium called synovial fluid. An extensive range of movement is possible with this type of joint.

There are several types of synovial joints, based on the shape of the articulating surfaces and the range of movements possible.

Structure and function of joints

The structure and function of joints are closely related. The range of movements available at a joint is related to its stability. This, in turn, depends on the shape, size and arrangement of the bones, and the flexibility of the ligaments and the tone of muscles around the joint.

Generally, the more stable a joint, the less movement it permits. If a joint is solid (no cavity), then it has limited mobility. If a cavity exists between the two ends of bone, movement can occur.

Fibrous and cartilaginous joints are both known as synarthroses, i.e. solid joints. Synovial joints are diarthroses, i.e. cavitated joints.

Fibrous joints
Fibrous joints consist of two bones united by fibrous tissue. These types of joints have no cavity, and little or no movement is exhibited.

Fibrous joints are further classified into sutures, syndesmoses and gomphoses.

Sutures
Sutures are interdigitating bones held together by dense fibrous connective tissue. This type of joint occurs in the skull. The inner and outer layers of periosteum of the adjacent bones are continuous over the joint; these two layers and the fibrous tissue form the sutural ligament.

 In newborn infants, the bone sutures are called fontanelles. The bones within the sutures undergo intramembranous ossification, forming a synostosis. This happens in normal adults between the frontal bones. However, in old age there can be fusion between the coronal, sagittal and lambdoid sutures, and also in the sternum.

Syndesmoses
Syndesmoses are where bones are separated by a larger distance than in sutures, and are joined by a

Fig. 5.1 Fibrous joint.

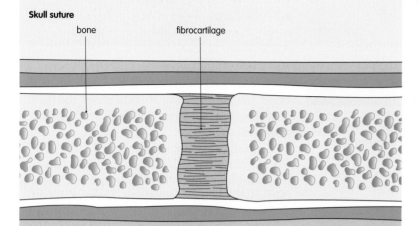

Skull suture

bone   fibrocartilage

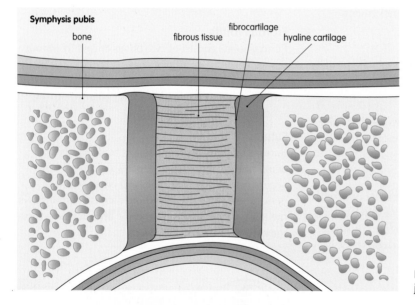

Symphysis pubis

bone   fibrous tissue   fibrocartilage   hyaline cartilage

Fig. 5.2 Secondary cartilaginous joint.

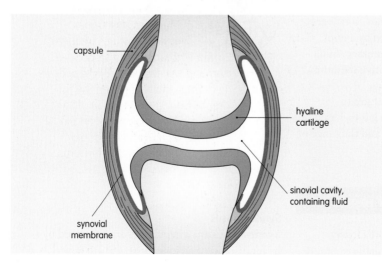

capsule

hyaline cartilage

sinovial cavity, containing fluid

synovial membrane

Fig. 5.3 Synovial joint.

sheet of fibrous tissue—either a ligament or a membrane. This type of joint occurs in the radioulnar interosseous membrane.

A small amount of movement may be achieved with syndesmoses. The degree of movement depends on the distance between the bones and the flexibility of the fibrous ligaments.

Gomphoses

Gomphoses are specialized joints that occur between teeth and their sockets, and the alveolar processes of the maxillae and mandible. Gomphoses are anchored by the fibrous tissue of the periodontal ligament.

Movement of a gomphosis usually suggests a pathological condition, e.g. disease loosening a tooth.

Primary cartilaginous joints

Primary cartilaginous joints are also known as synchondroses. The bones are united by hyaline cartilage. They are found in the epiphyseal growth plate and costosternal joints. Synchondroses appear in the normal development of long bones, so most are temporary unions.

This type of joint is slightly moveable.

Secondary cartilaginous joints

Secondary cartilaginous joints are also known as symphyses. The bone articulating surfaces are covered with hyaline cartilage and joined by fibrocartilage. They are found in the manubriosternal joint, symphysis pubis, intervertebral discs and the mandibular symphysis in the newborn.

This type of joint is slightly moveable and is strong.

Synovial joints

Synovial joints are the most common joint in the skeleton and also the most functionally important of joints (Fig. 5.4).

Fully formed synovial joints can be characterized by six features, namely:

- The articular surfaces of the bones involved are covered by a thin layer of hyaline cartilage.
- Lubrication is by a viscous synovial fluid.
- There is a joint cavity.
- The cavity is lined by synovial membrane.
- The joint is surrounded by a joint capsule.
- The capsule is reinforced externally or internally (or both) by fibrous ligaments.

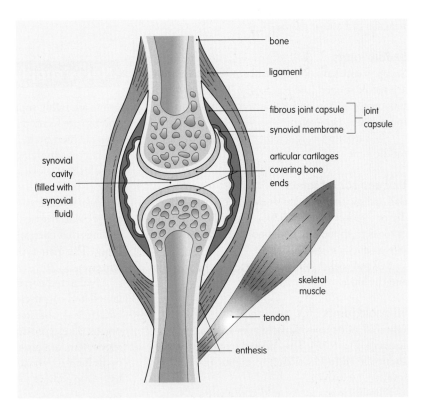

Fig. 5.4 Features of a synovial joint. The articular cartilages and fluid-filled synovial cavity prevent bone from rubbing against bone.

Synovial joints are classified according to the shape of the articular surfaces of the bones involved and the movements that are possible.

The movements at synovial joints can be described as:

- Monoaxial, i.e. occur in one direction or plane.
- Biaxial, i.e. occur in two directions or planes.
- Multiaxial, i.e. occur in many directions or planes.

Plane joints
Plane joints are shaped like two flat surfaces (Fig. 5.5A). They allow a sliding movement, i.e. monoaxial.

Plane joints are located in the sternoclavicular and acromioclavicular joints.

Hinge joints
Hinge joints have concave and convex-shaped surfaces (Fig. 5.5B). They allow flexion and extension movements, i.e. monoaxial.

Hinge joints are located in the elbow, knee and ankle.

Pivot joints
Pivot joints consist of a cylindrical projection inside a ring (Fig. 5.5C). They allow rotation movements, i.e. monoaxial.

Pivot joints are located in the atlantoaxial and superior radioulnar joints.

Saddle joints
Saddle joints have concave and convex surfaces that are saddle shaped (see Fig. 5.5D). They allow flexion, extension, abduction and rotation movements, i.e. biaxial.

The carpometacarpal joint of the thumb is a saddle joint.

Ball and socket joints
Ball and socket joints are shaped like a ball sitting in a dip or a socket (see Fig. 5.5E). They allow flexion, extension, abduction, and medial and lateral rotation movements, i.e. multiaxial.

Ball and socket joints are located at the shoulder and the hip.

Ellipsoid joints
Ellipsoid joints have ellipsoid concave and convex surfaces (Fig. 5.5F). They allow flexion, extension, abduction and adduction movements, but no rotation, i.e. biaxial.

Ellipsoid joints are located at the wrist.

Condyloid joints
Condyloid joints are shaped like two sets of concave and convex surfaces at right angles to each other (Fig. 5.5G). They allow flexion, extension, abduction, adduction and a small amount of rotation, i.e. biaxial movements.

Condyloid joints are located in the metacarpophalangeal (MCP) and metatarsophalangeal joints.

Blood supply and lymph drainage of joints

The periarticular arterial plexuses supply blood to the joints. These branch into articular arteries. They pierce the joint capsule to reach the synovium, and communicate with one another to create rich anastomoses around and inside the joint.

Articular veins accompany the arteries, so they too are present in the joint capsule and synovial membrane.

Lymphatic vessels are present in the synovial membrane and drain along the blood vessels to the regional deep lymph nodes.

Nerve supply of joints

Joints are richly supplied with articular nerves whose endings are located in both the fibrous capsule and synovial membrane. Articular nerves arise from the nerves supplying the overlying skin and the muscles that move a joint. This is known as Hilton's Law.

Both myelinated and non-myelinated nerve fibres are present in articular nerves. They have different endings that correspond to their roles in sensory input. The main types of input are proprioception and pain.

Myelinated nerves have Ruffini endings, lamellated corpuscles (rather like pacinian corpuscles), and some like Golgi neurotendinous organs. These provide information regarding the movement and position of the joint relative to the body. Non-myelinated and finely myelinated nerves have free endings, which are thought to mediate pain.

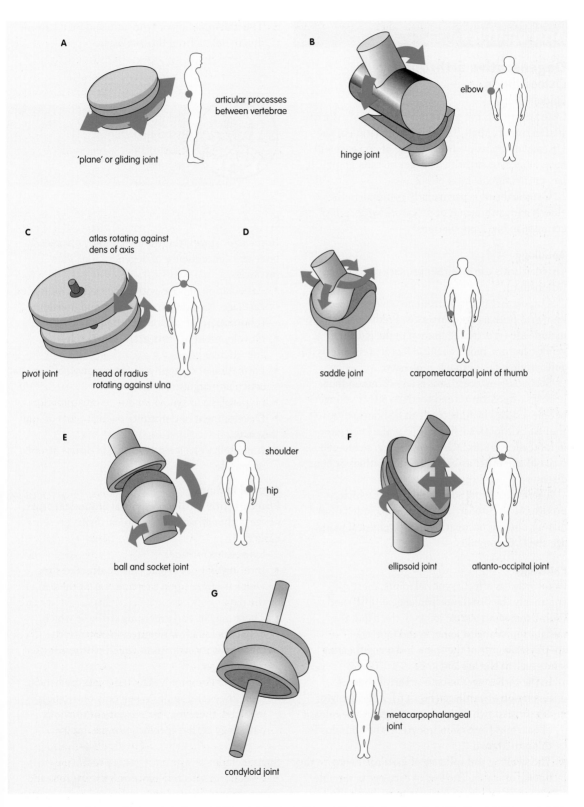

Fig. 5.5 Types of synovial joints: (A) plane; (B) hinge; (C) pivot; (D) saddle; (E) ball and socket; (F) ellipsoid; (G) condyloid.

Arthropathies

Degenerative arthropathy
Osteoarthritis
Epidemiology

Osteoarthritis is the most common type of arthritis. It affects more than 20% of the population of the UK, and most people over the age of 65 years will have some osteoarthritic changes on radiography. It has a male: female ratio of 1:2.

Osteoarthritis is particularly common in the elderly and, although it occurs worldwide, is less common in black populations.

Aetiology

Osteoarthritis can be either primary or secondary (idiopathic).

Osteoarthritis arising from no obvious cause is known as primary osteoarthritis. Predisposing factors include age (it is most common in the elderly), genetic factors, biomechanical factors (e.g. lifestyle) and systemic factors such as obesity.

Secondary osteoarthritis is less common than primary osteoarthritis and tends to affect younger people. Causes include congenital abnormalities, trauma, occupational hazards (e.g. the knee joint in footballers), avascular necrosis (e.g. sickle-cell disease) and other associated arthropathies or bone diseases.

There are several additional factors which predispose to osteoarthritis. These include family history, obesity, occupation (heavy physical work), age and hypermobility.

Pathology

Osteoarthritis affects synovial joints, most commonly the distal interphalangeal (DIP) and thumb carpometacarpal joints in the hand, the metatarsophalangeal joints in the foot, the apophyseal joints of the spine and weightbearing joints such as the hip and knee.

In the early stages of osteoarthritis there is degeneration of cartilage (Fig. 5.6). This involves:
- The breakdown of cartilage caused by the release of enzymes from chondrocytes—the stimulus for this is unknown.
- The swelling and splitting of cartilage owing to the uptake of water. The loss of cartilage is variable, ranging from irregularity of the surface to full-thickness loss. This destruction leads to loss of joint space.

- The inflammation of synovium and joint capsule due to debris from the cartilage.

The inflammation associated with osteoarthritis is secondary to degeneration.

In the later stages, there are secondary changes in bone as a consequence of degeneration. This involves:
- Articulation of bone with bone because of loss of cartilage, resulting in thickening and polishing (eburnation) of subarticular bone.
- Development of cysts in the newly sclerotic subarticular bone.
- Formation of osteophytes (overgrowth of bone) at articular margins.
- Hyperplasia of synovium due to inflammation.
- Development of deformity owing to loss of joint space.
- Immobility of a joint, resulting in disuse atrophy of muscle.

Clinical features

Osteoarthritis usually presents at around 50 years of age, although secondary osteoarthritis presents earlier.

Symptoms include:
- Intermittent or chronic pain at affected sites, which is worse upon exertion, e.g. at the end of the day.
- There may be early morning stiffness which only lasts for a few minutes, in contrast to inflammatory arthritis in which stiffness lasts much longer
- The most commonly affected joints are hands, hips, knees and spine. When only one joint is involved, there may be a history of previous pathology at that specific joint, i.e. injury.

Signs include:
- Swelling at affected joints due to effusions and osteophyte formation.
- Joint deformities with crepitus upon movement.
- Muscular wasting due to limited use of a joint.

Fig. 5.6 Pathological changes in osteoarthritis. Early changes and changes secondary to loss of cartilage.

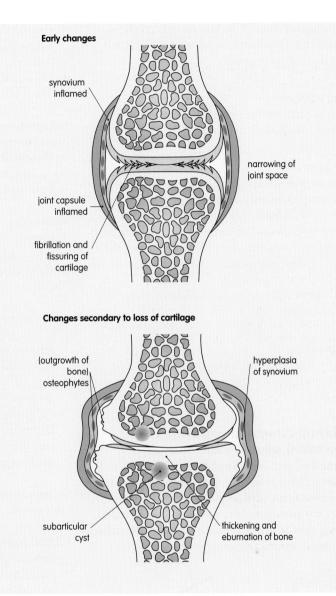

Early changes

synovium inflamed

narrowing of joint space

joint capsule inflamed

fibrillation and fissuring of cartilage

Changes secondary to loss of cartilage

(outgrowth of bone) osteophytes

hyperplasia of synovium

subarticular cyst

thickening and eburnation of bone

In the hands, the presence of Heberden's nodes (swellings at the DIP) and Bouchard's nodes [swellings at the proximal interphalangeal joints (PIP)] should be sought. There is also 'squaring' of the hand caused by changes at the thumb carpometacarpal joint.

At the hip, internal rotation is the first movement to be affected; passive movements also become painful at the end of the range of movement. There is also frequently a fixed flexion rotation (detected by Thomas' test).

Joints are usually affected bilaterally and symmetrically, although a unilateral pattern may be seen.

Diagnosis

Osteoarthritis is diagnosed clinically from the pattern of joints involved and the absence of systemic features.

A plain X-ray demonstrates narrowing of the joint space and the presence of osteophytes, subchondral cysts and osteosclerosis.

Blood tests are negative for rheumatoid factor and antinuclear antibodies (ANAs). As osteoarthritis is not a systemic disease, the erythrocyte sedimentation rate (ESR) is normal and there is no evidence of anaemia or abnormality of calcium metabolism.

Analysis of synovial fluid shows an increase in volume and the presence of white blood cells and crystals. Culture is negative.

Complications

Osteoarthritis has the potential to cause disability because of decreased mobility.

Management

Osteoarthritis is treated by non-steroidal anti-inflammatory drugs (NSAIDs) and analgesics to control pain, a balance between exercise and rest, and advising the patient on the progressive nature of the disease. Intra-articular steroids are occasionally used to reduce inflammation. Weight loss should be discussed if appropriate.

Surgery may be needed to replace severely diseased joints.

Prognosis

Osteoarthritis is a progressive disease—affected joints slowly get worse and other joints also become involved.

Inflammatory arthropathies
Rheumatoid arthritis: adult form

Rheumatoid arthritis is a systemic inflammatory disease which affects many parts of the body. It has a variable course, with periods of exacerbation and remission. Some patients have a self-limiting mild form of the condition, whilst the majority progress to a chronic destructive joint disease.

Epidemiology

Rheumatoid arthritis is polyarthritic, affecting at least 1% of Caucasians; the male: female ratio is 1:3. In adults, the peak of onset is between 35 and 45 years, although the disease can present at any age.

Aetiology

The cause of rheumatoid arthritis is unknown, although it is believed to involve an initiating factor that results in complex immunological changes. There is a number of possible hypotheses.

Evidence supporting autoimmune mechanisms in rheumatoid arthritis includes:
- The presence of rheumatoid factor (an autoantibody).

- Circulating immune complexes—these are believed to be responsible for the extra-articular features.
- Defective T cell-mediated immunity.
- The presence of other autoimmune diseases.

Genetic factors are due to an association between human leucocyte antigen (HLA) DR4 and DR1.

The initiating factor in rheumatoid arthritis has not been determined although possible candidates include the Epstein–Barr virus and parvoviruses.

Pathology

The most common sites affected in rheumatoid arthritis are the small joints of the hands (i.e. the PIP joints, as opposed to the DIP joints in osteoarthritis). The wrist, elbow, shoulder, cervical spine, hip and knee may also become involved.

The disease process can be split into three stages (Fig. 5.7). These include:
- Inflammation of the synovium—there is an infiltration of lymphocytes and macrophages.
- Destruction of cartilage—pannus (a layer of chronically inflamed fibrous tissue) extends across the cartilage, destroying it.
- Destruction of bone due to pannus—this results in joint deformities (e.g. ulnar deviation, swan neck and boutonnière deformities in the hand).

Secondary changes include muscle wasting and osteoporosis.

Clinical features

Symptoms include:
- Joint pain with prolonged early morning stiffness and 'gelling' of the joint after activity.
- Fatigue and general malaise.
- Weight loss during active disease.
- Anaemia.
- Extra-articular symptoms (Fig. 5.8).

Signs include:
- Warm and tender joints, with insidious onset, firstly affecting the small joints of the hands and then progressing to other joints.
- Swelling.
- Subcutaneous rheumatoid nodules.
- Decreased movement.

In the later stages the joint deformities mentioned above and muscle wasting may be seen.

Diagnosis

The diagnosis of rheumatoid arthritis is clinically from the pattern of joints involved, the presence of rheumatoid nodules and episodes of remission.

About 80% of patients have rheumatoid factor present and 30% have ANAs. The ESR and C-reactive protein levels are raised. There is an associated anaemia and thrombocytosis.

A plain X-ray will demonstrate narrowing of joint spaces with the presence of subchondral cysts. In addition, there may be osteoporosis in bone adjacent to the affected joint and focal erosions of bone.

Synovial fluid is usually turbid and green/yellow in colour. White blood cells are present and culture is negative.

Complications

Rheumatoid arthritis can cause secondary osteoarthritis and/or septic arthritis.

Rheumatoid arthritis can also be severely disabling.

Management

Rheumatoid arthritis is treated with NSAIDs to control pain, and immunosuppressive drugs such as penicillamine, gold and corticosteroids. Side effects of drug treatment include gastrointestinal bleeding and renal impairment. Patient education and physiotherapy are also important aspects of management.

Treatment is aimed at controlling the symptoms and at modifying disease activity rather than eradicating the cause.

Rheumatoid arthritis: juvenile form

The juvenile form of rheumatoid arthritis presents before the age of 16 years; the prognosis is worse than in adults.

Sjögren's syndrome

Affecting the exocrine glands, Sjögren's syndrome is a chronic inflammatory disease which is either primary or secondary to connective tissue diseases. The most common of these is rheumatoid arthritis, but the list also includes systemic lupus erythematosus, scleroderma, polymyositis and juvenile rheumatoid arthritis.

The lymphatic infiltration of exocrine glands leads to keratoconjunctivitis sicca (dry eyes) and xerostomia (dry mouth). It is treated symptomatically by artificial tears and pilocarpine

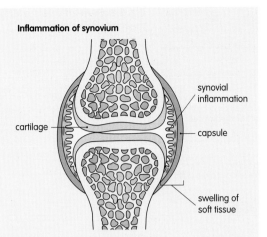

Inflammation of synovium

synovial inflammation

cartilage

capsule

swelling of soft tissue

Destruction of cartilage

pannus

Focal destruction of bone

oedematous and swollen synovium and capsule

osteoporotic lesions

erosion of the bone leading to joint deformity

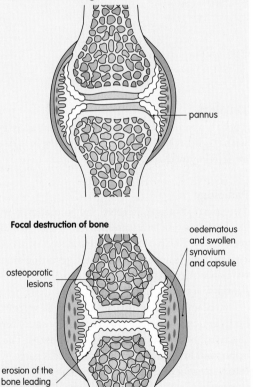

Fig. 5.7 Pathological changes in rheumatoid arthritis. Inflammation of synovium, destruction of cartilage and focal destruction of bone.

Splenomegaly and lymphadenopathy may be present.

The joints are affected symmetrically and the disease is progressive with remissions.

Extra-articular features of rheumatoid disease	
Site	**Manifestation**
nerves	carpal tunnel syndrome, peripheral neuropathy ('glove and stocking' sensory loss)
skin	subcutaneous nodules (particularly on extensor aspect of forearm near elbow), vasculitic lesions
blood vessels	vasculitis
eyes	episcleritis, scleritis, secondary Sjögren's syndrome (i.e. triad of dry mouth, dry eyes, and arthritis)
chest	intrapulmonary nodules, pleural effusions, fibrosing alveolitis, Caplan's syndrome
heart	myocarditis, pericarditis, pericardial effusion
kidney	amyloidosis, impaired renal function may be side effect of drug treatment
soft tissues around joints	bursitis, tenosynovitis

Fig. 5.8 Extra-articular features of rheumatoid disease.

hydrochloride tablets, which increase secretion from the salivary glands.

Seronegative arthritides

The seronegative arthritides are a group of related disorders. They are similar because they:

- Are often associated with HLA B27 (human leucocyte antigen B27).
- Are negative for rheumatoid factor and other autoantibodies.
- Have a familial tendency.
- Are more common in white people.

Patients may present with several different disorders, occurring either simultaneously or at different times.

Ankylosing spondylitis

Ankylosing spondylitis is the most common cause of inflammatory back pain in young adults (Fig. 5.9).

Epidemiology

The male: female ratio in ankylosing spondylitis is estimated to be of the order of 2–3:1. Women tend to show milder symptoms. Onset is usually in young adults.

Aetiology

There is a familial tendency in ankylosing spondylitis, with the HLA B27 association occurring in 90% of affected individuals.

Pathology

The spinal joints are affected. Inflammation starts in the lumbar spine and sacroiliac joints and extends proximally. The pathology begins at sites of ligamentous insertions (entheses), resulting in enthesiopathy—the hallmark of spondyloarthropathies.

There are initial erosive lesions on the vertebral body, which lead to the growth of bony spurs across the annulus fibrosis called syndesmophytes. The upper and lower syndesmophytes across each intervertebral disc fuse together, thus fusing the spine. On X-rays, there is 'squaring' of the vertebral bodies, and the appearance of the fused spine gives rise to the 'bamboo spine' tag.

Clinical features

Most patients with ankylosing spondylitis present in their late teens or early adulthood.

Symptoms include:

- Back pain, pelvic pain and joint pain in the lower limbs.

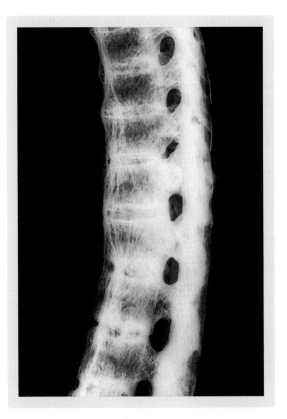

Fig. 5.9 Radiograph of a sagittal section through the vertebral column showing ankylosing spondylitis. There is complete fusion of the spine and apophyseal joints, and across the intervertebral disc. (Courtesy of Dr P.G. Bullough.)

- Systemic manifestations, including iritis and aortic valve incompetence.

Signs that may be present include:
- Kyphosis.
- Limited spinal flexion.
- Decreased chest expansion.

Diagnosis
Ankylosing spondylitis is diagnosed by the presence of HLA B27 (90%), although unaffected individuals may also carry this antigen (16%).

ESR and C-reactive protein levels are often raised.

A spinal radiograph may demonstrate calcification and ossification, the so-called tramline or bamboo spine appearance.

Management
Ankylosing spondylitis is usually treated with NSAIDs, immunosuppressive drugs such as sulphasalazine, regular exercise to maintain movement; hip replacement is occasionally required if the hip is ankylosed.

Prognosis
Although ankylosing spondylitis is progressive, most patients are able to lead a normal life.

Arthritis associated with gastrointestinal disease
Enteropathic arthritis
This is an arthritis associated with inflammatory bowel disease (IBD): ulcerative colitis or Crohn's disease. The severity of the arthritis, which affects the knees, ankles and elbows, reflects the activity of the IBD, with most episodes resolving within a few months. Successful treatment of the IBD usually leads to remission of enteropathic arthritis. The severity of the arthritis reflects the activity of the IBD. Most episodes resolve within a few months.

Arthritis associated with other systemic disease
Reactive arthritis
Reactive arthritis occurs in reponse to infection at a distant site, unlike septic arthritis where organisms can be isolated from the joint itself. The main causative organisms are:
- *Chlamydia*, causing genital infection.
- *Salmonella*, *Campylobacter* or *Shigella* causing gastrointestinal infection.

Reactive arthritis is more common in males and is the most common cause of arthritis in young males.

About 80% of patients show an association with HLA B27, suggesting an autoimmune process.

Reactive arthritis is often termed Reiter's syndrome when it follows a diarrhoeal or sexually transmitted infection and composes a triad of arthritis, urethritis/cervicitis and conjunctivitis. The arthritis usually affects the knees or ankles (asymmetrical oligoarthritis), although axial disease may occur.

The changes seen histologically are similar to those of rheumatoid arthritis, and diagnosis is clinical. Although symptoms may clear spontaneously, a large number of patients will suffer recurrences. In a minority, severe spondylitis may develop. In patients who are HIV-positive, a very severe form of reactive arthritis may result.

Psoriatic arthritis

Psoriatic arthritis occurs in 5–10% of psoriasis sufferers. It may also occur in individuals with a family history of psoriasis (p. 145).

HLA B27 association is often seen if spondylitis is also present.

Psoriatic arthritis may be clinically indistinguishable from rheumatoid arthritis, with the DIP joints most affected; axial involvement may also occur. Radiography may show bone erosion and periarticular osteoporosis.

Treatment is with NSAIDs and analgesics. Immunosuppressive drugs may also be used. In a minority of cases, severe destruction of bone may occur, i.e. 'arthritis mutilans'.

Behçet's syndrome

Behçet's syndrome is a rare condition of unknown aetiology. It is found most commonly in Japan and around the Mediterranean. The main features are polyarthritis, iritis and oral/genital ulceration. Less commonly there may be neurological, skin or gastrointestinal symptoms. It is characterized by exacerbations and remissions and is treated by oral steroids.

Still's disease

Still's disease is the most common cause of chronic juvenile arthritis, i.e. arthritis occurring in a person under 16 years of age.

Some forms of Still's disease are similar to rheumatoid arthritis.

Systemic symptoms include a salmon-coloured rash, spiking fever, lymphadenopathy, splenomegaly and pericarditis.

The number of joints affected is variable, depending on the subtype of Still's disease.

Most patients recover spontaneously before early adulthood.

Sarcoid arthritis

This is a transient polyarthritis or an acute monoarthritis which occurs in sarcoidosis. An acute arthritis is commonly a presenting feature of sarcoidosis, and is often accompanied by erythema nodosum and hilar lymphadenopathy. The sites affected are usually large joints such as ankles and knees. Sarcoidosis which presents with arthritis has a good prognosis and is usually self-remitting.

Neuropathic joint disease (Charcot's joint)

In neuropathic joint disease, or Charcot's joint, loss of sensation results in traumatic joint damage.

The conditions associated with Charcot's joint are:
- Diabetes mellitus, where joints in the feet are affected.
- Tabes dorsalis following syphilis, where the ankle and knee joints are affected.
- Leprosy, where the joint affected varies according to the site of sensory loss.

Arthritis associated with haemodialysis

Arthritis can arise as a result of haemodialysis, caused by the deposition of amyloid in the joints and pericortical tissues. Oxalate crystal deposition may occur in chronic renal disorders.

Systemic lupus erythematosus

Systemic lupus erythematosus (SLE) is a connective tissue disorder usually presenting with joint symptoms resembling rheumatoid arthritis.

Crystal arthropathies

The crystal arthropathies are a group of disorders in which the deposition of crystals in joints leads to inflammation.

Gout
Epidemiology

Gout is more common in men, although some postmenopausal women may be affected.

Aetiology

In gout, hyperuricaemia results in the deposition of monosodium urate crystals in the joint.

In primary gout, the causes of hyperuricaemia are commonly idiopathic, usually because of impaired excretion. There is a familial tendency.

Secondary gout may occur as a result of:

- Increased production of uric acid, e.g. increased cell turnover in carcinomas and leukaemia following chemotherapy, and in enzyme defects.
- Impaired excretion, e.g. renal failure, alcohol consumption, hyperlipidaemia and diuretics.
- High purine intake in the diet.

Pathology

Uric acid is a product of DNA (purine) breakdown and is normally excreted in the urine.

Excess uric acid results in the deposition of crystals in:

- Joints—the most commonly affected being the metatarsophalangeal (MTP) joint in the big toe. The ankle joint may also be affected.
- Soft tissues—this may lead to the formation of tophi (palpable masses).
- The urinary tract, in the form of urate stones.

The deposition of crystals in the synovium and periarticular soft tissues causes an acute inflammatory reaction. This may be precipitated by alcohol, diet, surgery or drugs.

Chronic gouty arthritis occurs following recurrent attacks. This is characterized by cartilage degeneration, synovial hyperplasia and secondary osteoarthritis.

Clinical features

Patients with gout present between the ages of 20 and 60 years, although most commonly in middle age.

An acute attack involves an extremely painful monoarthritis of sudden onset. The affected joint is oedematous and red; more than one joint may be affected in certain cases.

Diagnosis

The presence of tophi on the earlobes or around joints may aid in the diagnosis of gout.

Synovial fluid demonstrates the presence of needle-shaped crystals, which are diagnostic. These crystals are negatively birefringent. Neutrophils are also found.

Plasma uric acid levels are raised at >0.5 mmol/l, and there is also a raised ESR and white cell count.

Complications

Renal disease is a complication of gout.

Hyperuricaemia is genetically associated with an increased risk of hypertension and coronary artery disease.

Management

An acute attack of gout is treated with NSAIDs and aspiration of joint effusions.

Allopurinol, a drug that decreases uric acid synthesis, is used in the long term. The patient should be advised to maintain a good fluid intake and avoid precipitating factors.

Prognosis

Attacks of gout may be infrequent, and treatment can reduce the extent of joint damage. However, renal complications are frequent.

Pseudogout

Pseudogout is a condition that may mimic gout. It is more common in the elderly.

In pseudogout, calcium pyrophosphate crystals are deposited in the articular cartilage. Inflammation results if the crystals are shed into the joint space.

When pseudogout occurs in people younger than 60 years of age, it is often associated with hyperparathyroidism and haemochromatosis.

The joints most commonly affected are the knee, wrist, shoulder and ankle.

Pseudogout can be differentiated from gout by the presence of brick-shaped crystals in the synovial fluid which are positively birefringent.

Arthritis associated with infection
Septic arthritis
Epidemiology

Infectious (septic) arthritis is an uncommon condition, usually affecting children and young adults.

Aetiology

Infectious arthritis is usually caused by bacteria such as *Staphylococcus aureus*, *Streptococcus pyogenes*, *Neisseria gonorrhoea* and *Haemophilus influenzae*, and Gram-negative organisms. Tuberculous arthritis is now rare.

There are several predisposing factors. These include:

- Prosthetic joints.
- Drug addiction.
- Age between 5 and 15 years.
- Diabetes mellitus.
- Immunosuppressive drugs.
- Rheumatoid arthritis.

A viral cause, such as rubella or mumps, is less common.

Pathology

In infectious arthritis the infecting organism gains access to the joint:

- Haematogenously.
- As a result of local trauma.
- By direct spread from adjacent foci of infection.

Clinical features

Only one joint is usually affected in infectious arthritis, the patient presenting with a painful, swollen and erythematous joint and associated fever. Very little movement is possible at the joint, and there are systemic signs of sepsis present. The joint should be aspirated for culture if infection is suspected. Septic arthritis must be excluded in children who present with a painful joint, as the disease causes devastating damage to the joint if left undiagnosed.

Diagnosis

Synovial fluid is turbid in infectious arthritis, and white blood cells are present. Culture is positive. Patients need an X-ray to exclude trauma.

Management

Intravenous antibiotic treatment should be started immediately infectious arthritis is diagnosed. This is initially 'blind' until the culture results are available. Treatment with oral antibiotics is continued for 6 weeks.

Drainage of the joint is needed to remove debris. The joint should also be immobilized.

Prognosis

Infectious arthritis can be life-threatening, hence the importance of immediate treatment.

Recovery can take from a few days to a few weeks.

Disorders affecting specific joints

Disorders of the hand and wrist
Osteoarthritis of the wrist and hand

The joints of the hand are commonly affected by osteoarthritis. The carpometacarpal joint of the thumb feels tender and there is limited abduction.

Aetiology

In osteoarthritis of the wrist and hand, the interphalangeal joints become painful and stiff, with osteophytes creating swellings; these are called Heberden's nodes at the DIP and Bouchard's nodes at the PIP joints.

The wrists are usually affected at a later stage after trauma (lower radius or scaphoid fracture).

Rheumatoid arthritis of the wrist and hand
Complications

The wrists and hands usually suffer a major loss of function and deformities in rheumatoid arthritis. Progressively, there is synovitis of the proximal joints and tendon sheaths, then erosions, and finally joint derangement and tendon rupture leading to structural and functional loss.

The fingers have 'swan-neck' (hyperextended PIP joint and flexed DIP joint) or 'boutonnière' (flexed PIP joint, hyperextended DIP joint and extended MCP joint) deformities (Fig. 5.10).

The thumb acquires a Z deformity. The MCP joints and wrists undergo subluxation so that the fingers show ulnar deviation.

The ulnar styloid and radial head become prominent. There may also be firm rheumatoid nodules on the extensor surfaces and the flexor tendons.

De Quervain's tenosynovitis

De Quervain's tenosynovitis is inflammation of the fibrous sheath containing tendons of extensor pollicis brevis and abductor pollicis longus as it passes over the styloid process of the radius. Pain is felt at the styloid process of the radius, and there is tendon swelling and a palpable nodule proximal to the wrist joint on the radial aspect.

De Quervain's tenosynovitis may be caused by overuse of the tendons, e.g. wringing out washing. Treatment of De Quervain's tenosynovitis is by hydrocortisone injection or surgically splitting the tendon sheath.

Tendon lesions
'Trigger finger'

'Trigger finger' or digital stenosing synovitis is thickening of the tendon sheaths, constricting the flexor tendons (Fig. 5.11). It affects the ring and middle fingers in adults and the thumb in children. Extension of the finger has to be forced through a narrower space and elicits a snap noise. It is treated with steroid injections.

Fig. 5.10 Finger deformities in rheumatoid arthritis: normal finger, swan-neck and boutonnière deformities.

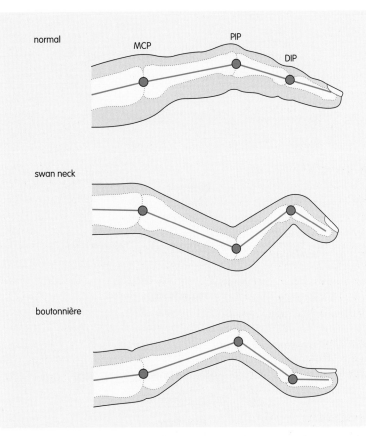

normal

MCP

PIP

DIP

swan neck

boutonnière

'Mallet finger'

'Mallet finger' is also called 'baseball finger' (see Fig. 5.11). The extensor tendon is damaged at its insertion into the distal phalanx so that the DIP joint cannot be fully extended. It is treated by splinting the finger with the DIP joint fully extended.

'Dropped finger'

'Dropped finger' is caused by tendon rupture at the wrist—either direct or as a complication of rheumatoid arthritis—resulting in loss of finger extension at the MCP joint.

Ganglia

Ganglia are smooth swellings containing clear viscous fluid which appear as painless lumps on the dorsum of the wrist (Fig. 5.12). They are mostly unilocular and have walls of fibrous tissue. Ganglia form around the joint capsule and tendon sheath but do not communicate with the joint space. Ganglia are treated by excision only if they press on the local ulnar or median nerves.

Dupuytren's contracture
Aetiology

In Dupuytren's contracture the palmar aponeurosis is thickened and contracted, and there is skin tethering (Fig. 5.13). Dupuytren's contracture is commonly bilateral, symmetrical and painless. The fingers become flexed at the MCP and PIP joints. There may be fibrous thickenings in the dorsal knuckle pads (Garod's pads) and on the soles of the feet.

Epidemiology

Dupuytren's contracture affects more men than women, may be familial, and has associations with alcoholism, antiepileptic drugs and Peyronie's disease (fibrosis of the corpus cavernosum).

Management

Dupuytren's contracture is treated by surgical excision of the thickened region, only when the deformity is progressive.

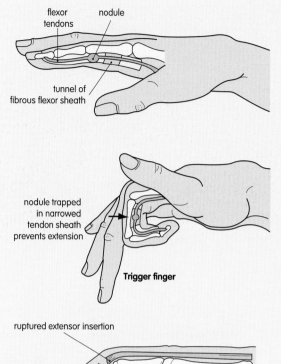

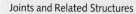

Fig. 5.11 'Trigger finger' and 'mallet finger' due to tendon injuries. See text for details.

flexor tendons

nodule

tunnel of fibrous flexor sheath

nodule trapped in narrowed tendon sheath prevents extension

Trigger finger

ruptured extensor insertion

Mallet finger

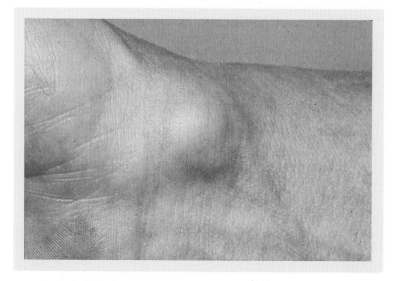

Fig. 5.12 Ganglion at the dorsal surface of the wrist. (Courtesy of Dr J.H. Klippel.)

Fig. 5.13 Dupuytren's contracture of the palmar fascia. (Courtesy of Dr J.H. Klippel.)

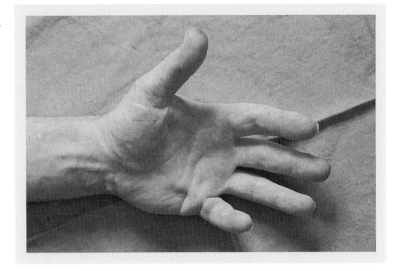

Carpal tunnel syndrome
Aetiology
Carpal tunnel syndrome is caused by median nerve compression as it passes under the flexor retinaculum. It occurs in premenstrual and pregnant women, and in cases of myxoedema and rheumatoid arthritis.

Clinical features
In carpal tunnel syndrome, there is paraesthesia and pain in the median nerve distribution in the hand (thumb, index, and middle and radial half of the ring finger). Pain is worse at night and after repetitive movements. Later, there is wasting and decreased sensation of the thenar eminence.

Management
Carpal tunnel syndrome is treated either conservatively with diuretics and hydrocortisone injections, or by surgical division of the flexor retinaculum.

Disorders of the elbow
Tennis elbow
Tennis elbow is inflammation of the common extensor attachment at the lateral epicondyle (lateral epicondylitis), causing pain.

Aetiology
Tennis elbow may be caused by hitting a tennis ball awkwardly during a backhand stroke.

Management
Tennis elbow is treated with steroid injections.

Golfer's elbow
Golfer's elbow is inflammation of the common flexor attachment at the medial epicondyle (medial epicondylitis).

Aetiology
Golfer's elbow may occur when a golfer hits the ground rather than the golf ball.

Management
Golfer's elbow is treated with steroid injections.

Olecranon bursitis
Olecranon bursitis occurs after trauma, sepsis, rheumatoid arthritis and gout. It involves a hot, painful swelling behind the olecranon.

Traumatic bursitis used to be called 'student's elbow'—caused by propping of the elbows on books for long periods. If infection is suspected, the joint must be aspirated.

Cubitus valgus and cubitus varus
Cubitus valgus is when the 'carrying angle' of the elbow joint is greater than the normal 10° in men and 15° in women (Fig. 5.14). It is caused by malunion of a previous lateral condylar fracture or retarded lateral epiphyseal growth. There may be an association with Turner's syndrome. Complications include ulnar neuritis and osteoarthritis.

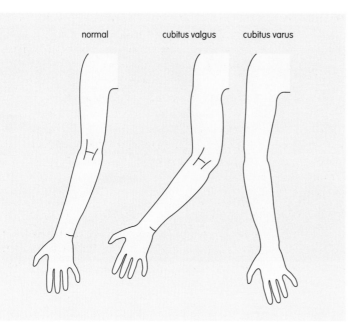

Fig. 5.14 Normal angle of the elbow, cubitus valgus and cubitus varus.

Cubitus varus is the opposite deformity, with a decreased carrying angle (see Fig. 5.14). Its most common cause is malunion of a supracondylar fracture. Cubitus valgus and cubitus varus may be corrected by osteotomy.

Ulnar neuritis
Aetiology
The ulnar nerve may be subjected to constriction (osteoarthritis, rheumatoid arthritis) or constant friction (cubitus valgus), as it lies in a groove behind the medial epicondyle. This can lead to nerve fibrosis and eventual ulnar neuropathy.

Complications
In ulnar neuritis there is hand clumsiness, reduced sensation over the little finger and the medial side of the ring finger, and weakened small muscles of the hand innervated by the nerve.

Management
Treatment of ulnar neuritis involves surgery for nerve release and transposition to the front of the elbow.

Loose bodies in the elbow joint
Loose bodies in the elbow joint may arise from osteochondral fractures, osteophytes of osteoarthritis, and other conditions such as synovial chondromatosis and osteochondritis dissecans. They cause locking of the elbow as the bodies become stuck between the bones, causing sharp pain and swelling, and are treated by surgical removal.

Rheumatoid arthritis of the elbow
The elbow joint is involved in over half of all patients with rheumatoid arthritis. There is pain and limitation of movement in both the elbow and superior radiohumeral joints.

The joint is treated conservatively; removal of the synovium or joint replacement may also be considered.

Disorders of the shoulder
Dislocation of the shoulder joint
A dislocated shoulder joint is a very common injury, usually caused by falling on to an outstretched arm, e.g. when playing rugby. The joint may be displaced in different directions, but anterior displacement of the humeral head to below the coracoid process is the most common occurrence.

Complications
Complications of a dislocated shoulder include neural (circumflex axillary nerve) and arterial

(axillary artery) damage, joint stiffness and recurrent dislocations.

Management
A dislocated shoulder is treated by reducing the joint and immobilizing it for about 3 weeks.

Painful arc syndrome
In painful arc syndrome, shoulder abduction causes pain in the mid-ranges but not extremes of movement, i.e. between 45 and 150°. Degeneration is the underlying defect and pain is caused by impingement of an inflamed structure between the greater tuberosity and the acromion (Fig. 5.15).

Aetiology
Painful arc syndrome is caused by incomplete tearing of the supraspinatus tendon, supraspinatus

tendonitis, subacromial bursitis and fracture of the greater tuberosity of the humerus.

The lesions may be associated with supraspinatus tendon calcification (perhaps a variation of crystal arthropathy), rheumatoid arthritis or acromioclavicular joint osteoarthritis.

Management
Painful arc syndrome is treated with hydrocortisone injections and surgery.

Rotator cuff tears
Rotator cuff tears are partial tears that often occur with supraspinatus tendonitis, leading to painful arc syndromes. Complete tears limit shoulder abduction, cause joint pain at the shoulder tip and upper arm,

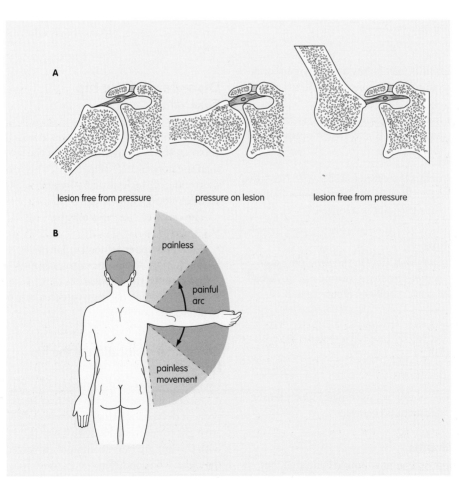

Fig. 5.15 Mechanism and aetiology of painful arc syndrome: (A) mechanical basis; and (B) areas of pain.

and tenderness under the acromion. The tears are usually in the supraspinatus tendon (although subscapularis and infraspinatus may be involved) and allow communication between the joint capsule and the subacromial bursa, seen by arthroscopy.

Aetiology
Rotator cuff tears may be caused by age-related degeneration or a fall, e.g. in epileptic subjects.

Management
Rotator cuff tears are treated by repairing the tendon; better results are obtained in young people with less degeneration.

Adhesive capsulitis (frozen shoulder)
Adhesive capsulitis or 'frozen shoulder' is a common but poorly understood condition affecting the glenohumeral joint. It causes pain and limitation of all movements (to about half the normal range) but no changes are seen on X-ray.

Aetiology
Adhesive capsulitis may follow a minor injury or be due to an autoimmune response to localized rotator cuff tissues.

Recovery follows the course of pain, stiffness, then recuperant phases. It may take months to heal.

Management
Adhesive capsulitis is treated initially with NSAIDs, analgesics and gentle exercise. Joint manipulation is undertaken when the joint is stronger.

Biceps rupture
In biceps rupture, an aching in the shoulder often occurs after 'something snaps' during lifting. A 'ball' appears in the muscle belly on elbow flexion.

Aetiology
Biceps rupture may be caused by degenerative changes or a fall.

Management
As the function of the biceps remains intact during rupture, no treatment is required.

Biceps tendonitis
Biceps tendonitis is an uncommon condition, but rotator cuff tears may involve the long head of biceps, giving pain in the anterior shoulder. This is made worse on forced muscle contraction.

Management
Biceps tendonitis is treated by hydrocortisone injection.

Rheumatoid arthritis and osteoarthritis in the shoulder
Rheumatoid arthritis and osteoarthritis are not as common in the shoulder as they are in weightbearing hip and knee joints. Pain and restricted movement are treated by joint replacement.

Pain referred to the shoulder
Pain referred to the shoulder may occur via C5 to the deltoid, C6, C7 and C8 to the superior border of the scapula, or C3 from the diaphragm to the shoulder tip.

The brachial plexus and roots (e.g. prolapsed cervical disc, herpes zoster, cervical rib), upper arm, abdomen (e.g. cholecystitis, subphrenic abscess) and thorax (e.g. angina, pleurisy) may contribute to referred pain.

Disorders of the hip
Coxa vara
Aetiology
Coxa vara includes any condition in which the angle between the neck and the shaft of the femur is less than the normal 125° (Fig. 5.16). This leads to true shortening of the limb and a limping walk due to a Trendelenburg 'dip'.

The cause of coxa vara may be:
- Congenital.
- A slipped upper femoral epiphysis.
- Fracture (trochanteric with malunion, non-united fractures of the femoral neck).
- Bone softening (rickets, osteomalacia or Paget's disease of bone).

Congenital dislocation of the hip
Epidemiology
Congenital dislocation of the hip (CDH) should be diagnosed and corrected in the first week of life to prevent delayed walking and abnormal gait. Girls are eight times more likely to have CDH than boys, with the left hip more commonly involved than the right. The condition occurs more frequently after a breech delivery and if a relative is affected. The acetabulum is abnormally shallow with a very upwardly sloping roof, the femoral head is displaced

Fig. 5.16 Normal femur and coxa vara.

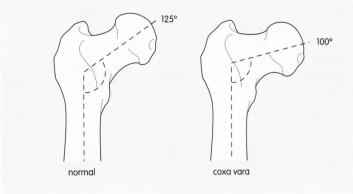

upwards and laterally, and the joint capsule may fold inwards.

Management
CDH is treated in various ways according to the age of the patient. Treatment may involve splints, joint reduction, osteotomy or hip displacement.

Perthes' disease
Perthes' disease occurs in children and involves osteochondritis of the epiphysis of the femoral head. There is avascular necrosis of unknown cause, resulting in bone fragmentation with concurrent revascularization and new bone formation. There is narrowing of the joint space and flattening of the femoral head, and these are risks for early arthritis. Surgical containment is necessary to treat severe cases of Perthes' disease.

Slipped upper femoral epiphysis
Aetiology
In adolescents, there may be a displacement of the upper epiphysis downward and backward from the femoral neck along the epiphyseal line (Fig. 5.17). This slipped upper femoral epiphysis affects overweight patients and males more than females. There is limping and pain in the groin, thigh, or knee, and limited abduction.

Complications include avascular necrosis and coxa vara.

Management
Slipped upper femoral epiphysis is treated by pinning the femur into position, and osteotomy.

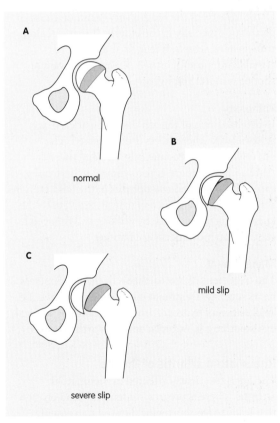

Fig. 5.17 (A) Normal femoral epiphysis; (B) mild; (C) severe slipped upper femoral epiphysis.

Transient synovitis
Transient synovitis is a short-lived condition of childhood, of unknown aetiology. It causes pain, limping and limited hip movements. X-rays are normal. No treatment is required for transient synovitis as it recovers spontaneously in about 4 weeks.

Tuberculous arthritis
Aetiology
Tuberculosis (TB) frequently affects the hip joint, causing pain, limping, limited movement and muscle spasm. X-rays show bone rarefaction (decreased density but normal volume) and subsequent articular cartilage and bony erosion.

Management
Tuberculous arthritis is treated with antituberculous drugs. If the joint has been destroyed, arthrodesis (joint fusion) is performed.

Osteoarthritis of the hip
Aetiology
Osteoarthritis of the hip is a very common cause of disability, especially in the elderly. It may develop from general wear and tear, or as a sequel to acetabular injuries, Perthe's disease, coxa vara or slipped femoral epiphysis.

Pathology
In osteoarthritis of the hip the articular cartilage is worn away where stress is transmitted. The underlying bone becomes sclerotic and there is cyst formation; there is also synovial hypertrophy, capsular fibrosis and osteophytes in the joint margins. Pain occurs in the groin and may also radiate to the knee; this is made worse by walking and relieved by rest. All hip movements are limited.

Management
The treatment of osteoarthritis of the hip depends on its severity. Treatment is either conservative, i.e. analgesics and hydrocortisone injections, or surgical, by osteotomy, joint replacement or arthrodesis.

Rheumatoid arthritis of the hip
The hip is frequently affected in rheumatoid arthritis. There is progressive femoral head erosion that leads to leg shortening, limited movement, gluteal and thigh muscle wasting, and gradual pain. Rheumatoid arthritis is treated conservatively with NSAIDs and immunosuppressants or by hip replacement.

Pain referred to the hip
Pain may be referred to the hip from the spine (prolapsed disc, sacroiliac arthritis), the pelvis and lower abdomen (appendicular abscess, pyosalpinx, irritation of the obturator nerve or muscle spasm), or from thrombosis of the lower abdominal aorta and its main branches.

Abnormal gait
Aetiology
Abnormal gait may arise when there is a loss of coordination in the movements of the spine, hip, knee, ankle and foot.

There are several types of abnormal gait, including:
- Osteogenic gait—bone shortening leads to limping.
- Arthrogenic gait—ankylosis; fixed flexion deformity making one or both buttocks prominent, and abduction deformity where a leg swings round during walking.
- Myogenic gait—weak gluteal muscles in muscular dystrophy giving a waddling gait.
- Neurogenic gait—disorders such as hemiparesis, cerebellar ataxia, parkinsonism, cerebral palsy, footdrop and bilateral leg spasticity all show characteristic gaits.

Disorders of the knee
Genu varum and genu valgum
Genu varum (bow legs) and genu valgum (knock knees) commonly occur in childhood, and usually correct spontaneously (Fig. 5.18). They may also occur secondary to injury or disease (fractures, rheumatoid arthritis or osteoarthritis, rickets, osteomalacia and Paget's disease of bone).

Meniscal tears
Epidemiology
Meniscal tears are common in young men. They are usually caused by a twisting injury, especially in sport.

Aetiology
The medial meniscus is torn more often than the lateral. When the meniscus splits longitudinally, a 'bucket-handle' tear occurs, where the meniscus remains attached at both ends; if either end becomes detached, 'anterior horn' or 'posterior horn' tears are produced (Fig. 5.19). The torn tags may either cause mechanical 'locking' of the knee by becoming jammed between the tibia and femur (preventing full extension) or predispose to secondary osteoarthritis because of the irritation to the joint.

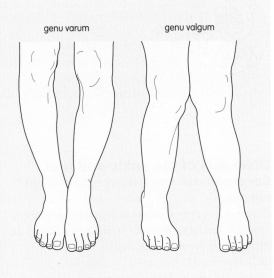

Fig. 5.18 Genu varum and genu valgum.

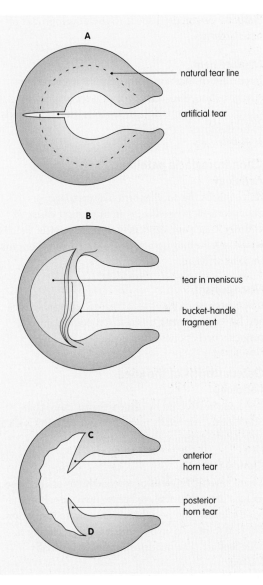

Fig. 5.19 Pattern of meniscal tears: (A) the natural tear line; (B) 'bucket-handle tear' (the most common type); (C) anterior horn tear; and (D) posterior horn tear.

Management
Meniscal tears are treated by arthroscopic excision of the displaced tag.

Meniscal cysts
Aetiology
Meniscal cysts are similar to ganglia and develop from the lateral joint line. They may either arise from a previous joint injury or occur spontaneously. The swelling is usually most painful at night.

Management
Meniscal cysts are treated by excision.

Osteochondritis dissecans
Osteochondritis dissecans is local ischaemic necrosis of bone and articular cartilage. It affects the knee more than any other joint. Osteochondral fragmentation produces loose bodies in the joint capsule.

    Other causes of loose bodies in the knee include osteoarthritis, fracture of the joint surface and synovial chondromatosis.

Recurrent dislocation of the patella
Aetiology
The patella is always displaced laterally when the knee is flexed. Predisposing factors for recurrent dislocation of the patella include generalized ligament laxity, anatomical abnormalities of the patella or lateral condyle of the femur, or a genu valgum deformity. Recurrent dislocation of the patella tends to affect adolescent girls, often bilaterally.

Clinical features
In recurrent dislocation of the patella there is severe pain in the front of the knee so that the patient cannot extend the joint and may collapse. Repeated

113

dislocations can predispose to the development of osteoarthritis.

Management
Recurrent dislocation of the patella is treated by strengthening the quadriceps muscle (especially vastus medialis muscle). If this fails, the joint needs to be stabilized surgically.

Chondromalacia patellae
Aetiology
Softening of the patellar articular cartilage, or chondromalacia patellae, is an important cause of anterior knee pain, especially in teenage girls. Pain is worse on climbing up and down stairs, and there may be joint effusion.

Management
Chondromalacia patellae is treated with analgesics and by strengthening the vastus medialis muscle; surgical correction is often unsuccessful.

Osteoarthritis of the knee
Aetiology
The knee is affected by osteoarthritis more than other joints, especially in overweight patients with a longstanding genu varum deformity.

Clinical features.
Characteristic features of osteoarthritis of the knee include articular cartilage breakdown, subchondral bone sclerosis and peripheral osteophyte formation. There is joint pain on use, and swelling, leading to knee locking. The quadriceps muscle is usually wasted.

Management
Treatment of osteoarthritis of the knee depends on the severity of the disease. It may be treated conservatively with analgesics and physiotherapy, or surgically by débridement, osteotomy or joint replacement.

Bursitis of the knee
Bursae can become inflamed because of infection, trauma, or repeated irritating friction giving rise to swelling and effusion.

The prepatellar bursa ('housemaid's knee'), infrapatellar bursa ('vicar's knee'), and semimembranosus bursa (popliteal cyst) are commonly affected.

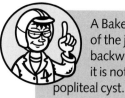

A Baker's cyst is a herniation of the joint synovium backwards and downwards; it is not the same as a popliteal cyst.

Disorders of the ankle and foot
Congenital club foot (talipes equinovarus)
Pathology
Congenital club foot shows as foot inversion, medial inversion (adduction), and plantarflexion (Fig. 5.20). The calf and peroneal muscles are also underdeveloped.

Boys are affected by congenital club foot more than girls. The condition may be associated with spina bifida.

Management
Congenital club foot is corrected by splinting and/or surgery.

Pes planus and pes cavus
Pes planus (flat foot) is a flattened longitudinal arch causing the medial border of the foot almost to touch the ground (Fig. 5.21). It can be caused by underlying general joint laxity. Often there are no symptoms, but there may be foot strain and osteoarthritis of the tarsal joints in later life.

Pes cavus (hollow foot) is a high longitudinal arch, which may be congenital or associated with neurological disorders, leading to weak intrinsic muscles (see Fig. 5.21). The toes may be clawed and the metatarsal heads prominent as they are weightbearing.

Hammer toes
In hammer toes, the toes are flexed at the PIP joint and extended at the MTP joint (Fig. 5.22). The second toes are most commonly affected. The disorder is treated by lengthening the tendons and excising the MTP joint (see Fig. 5.22).

Claw toes
In claw toes, the toes are flexed at both the PIP and DIP joints, and extended at the MTP joint (see

Fig. 5.20 Features of talipes equinovarus and talipes calcaneus.

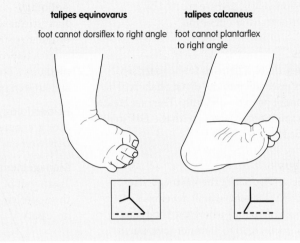

Fig. 5.21 Features of pes planus and pes cavus.

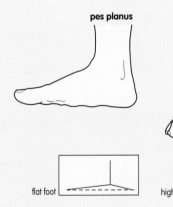

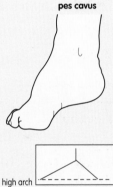

Fig. 5.22 Toe deformities: normal toe, 'claw toe', 'hammer toe' and 'mallet toe'.

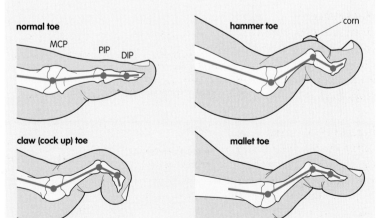

Fig. 5.22). Claw toes occur in rheumatoid arthritis and after poliomyelitis, and are treated by a flexor–extensor transfer operation.

Mallet toes

In mallet toes, there is damage to the extensor tendon at its insertion into the distal phalanx. The DIP joint cannot be extended fully. They are treated by placing a splint onto the toe, with the DIP joint fully extended.

Hallux valgus

In hallus valgus (Fig. 5.23), the big toe deviates laterally at the MTP joint, which develops a protective bursa (bunion) where the shoe rubs. This condition may lead to hammer toes, bursitis, metatarsalgia and secondary osteoarthritis of the MTP joint.

The wearing of high heels with pointed toes may contribute to this deformity; it is seen in elderly women.

Hallux rigidus

Aetiology

Joint stiffness in the big toe, or hallus rigidus, may be due to osteoarthritis of the MTP joint, trauma, osteochondritis dissecans in the head of the first metatarsal bone or gout. There is pain on walking and limited movement.

Epidemiology

Men are more commonly affected with hallus rigidus than women.

Management

Treatment of hallus rigidus involves dealing with the underlying cause, then replacing the joint if necessary.

Forefoot pain (metatarsalgia)

Forefoot pain may be caused by foot or toe deformities (pes planus, pes cavus, hallux valgus, claw toes); it also occurs in stress fractures and Morton's metatarsalgia (Fig. 5.24).

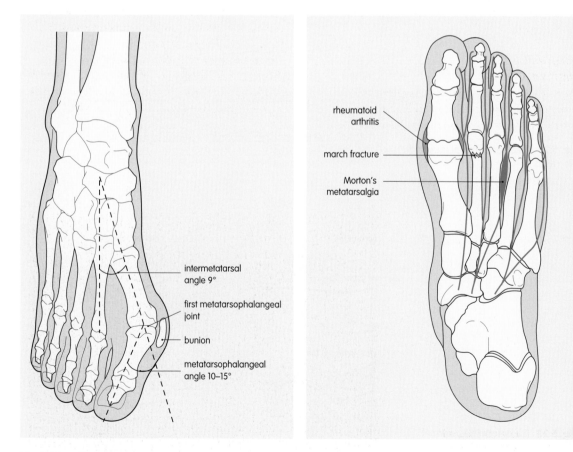

intermetatarsal angle 9°

first metatarsophalangeal joint

bunion

metatarsophalangeal angle 10–15°

rheumatoid arthritis

march fracture

Morton's metatarsalgia

Fig. 5.23 Hallux valgus.

Fig. 5.24 Causes of forefoot pain.

Stress fractures (march fractures)

Stress fractures occur in the shaft of the second or third metatarsals of young adults after excessive walking. The fractures are treated by rest and wearing a plaster during healing.

Morton's metatarsalgia (plantar digital neuritis)

Morton's metatarsalgia is a fibrous thickening of a digital nerve between the metatarsals. Wearing shoes causes compressional pain in this region, which then radiates to the third and fourth toes. Wearing rubber pads or excising the thickened nerve segment alleviates the pain.

Rheumatoid arthritis in the ankle and foot

Rheumatoid arthritis affects the ankle and foot joints in a similar way to the wrist and hands, with the added complication that the patient must walk on them.

There is subluxation of the metatarsal heads, with hallux valgus, clawed toes and prominent calluses causing pain.

Toenail lesions
Ingrown toenails

Ingrown toenails are nails that have become embedded in the lateral skin folds and formed inflamed (sometimes pus-filled) ulcerations.

Ingrown toenails can be prevented by the correct cutting of the nails, and are treated by inserting gauze under the ingrowing edges of the nail to separate them from the skin fold, or by removal of the nail and its germinal matrix.

Overgrowing toenails (onychogryphosis)

Overgrowing toenails are very thick, hard and curved laterally (Fig. 5.25). They are treated by excision.

Undergrowing toenails (subungual exostosis)

Undergrowing toenails have a bony outgrowth (exostosis) from the dorsal surface of the distal phalanx that pushes the nail upwards. They are treated by excision of the exostosis.

Disorders of the back
Congenital abnormalities

Lumbarization and sacralization are inconsequential anatomical anomalies. Lumbarization is when S1 remains as a vertebra, and sacralization is fusion of the body of L5 with the sacrum.

Hemivertebrae are congenital abnormalities where vertebrae are formed on one lateral side only (Fig. 5.26). The vertebral body is therefore wedge-shaped, causing the spine to angle laterally at this site.

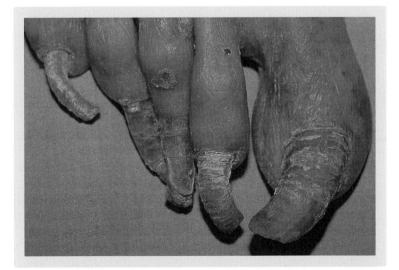

Fig. 5.25 Overgrown toenails. (Courtesy of Dr G. White, and the Department of Dermatology, UCSD.)

Torticollis

Torticollis is a contracted sternocleidomastoid muscle on one side of the body only. It is caused by poor blood supply during a birth injury. The head is tilted and rotated to one side and there is facial asymmetry (Fig. 5.27). Torticollis is corrected by surgery.

Scoliosis

Scoliosis is the lateral curvature of the spine (Fig. 5.28). The deformity may be mobile (reversible) or fixed (permanent).

Mobile scoliosis may be postural, compensatory (to a short leg or pelvic tilt), or sciatic (with disc prolapse and muscle spasm).

Aetiology

Fixed scoliosis can be caused by:
- Congenital vertebral abnormalities.
- Hemivertebrae.
- Asymmetrical muscle weakness.
- Muscular dystrophies.

Fixed scoliosis may be idiopathic in infants and adolescents.

Management

Fixed scoliosis can be treated either conservatively with exercise or by wearing supportive splints, or surgically.

Kyphosis

Kyphosis is excessive posterior curvature of the spine that is either gently rounded or sharply angled (Fig. 5.29). It can be a progressive deformity.

Kyphosis can be caused by tuberculosis of the spine, fractured vertebrae, ankylosing spondylitis and spinal tumours.

Lordosis

Lordosis is excessive anterior curvature of the spine, usually in the lumbar region (see Fig. 5.29). It may be caused by bad posture or be compensatory for hip deformities.

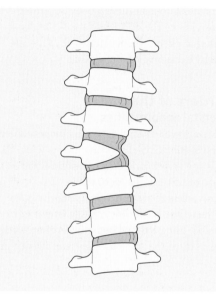

Fig. 5.26 Hemivertebra in the spine, producing scoliosis.

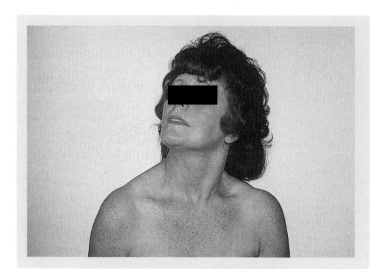

Fig. 5.27 Features of torticollis. (Courtesy of Dr G.D. Perkin.)

Fig. 5.28 Types of scoliosis. (A) Normal posture, and scoliosis due to (B) sciatica; (C) short leg; and (D) fixed deformity.

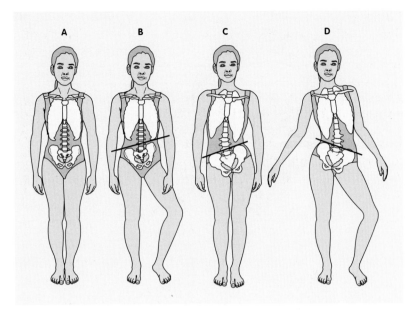

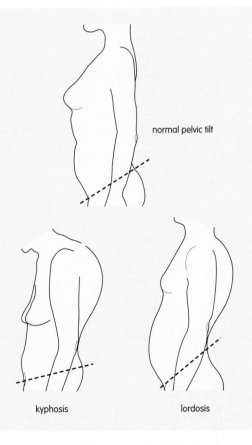

normal pelvic tilt

kyphosis

lordosis

Fig. 5.29 Features of kyphosis and lordosis. Normal posture, kyphosis and lordosis.

Disc prolapse

Disc prolapse usually occurs in the lumbar region—the nucleus pulposus herniates through a weak part of the annulus fibrosus (Fig. 5.30).

Sudden pain can be felt in the lumbar region (lumbago) or, if there is compression of a nerve root, may radiate to the buttocks and legs (sciatica). There is limited flexion and extension.

Management

Disc prolapse should be treated with analgesics, by injection of chymopapain (dissolves protruding disc), or disc excision.

Spondylolisthesis

In spondylolisthesis there is forward displacement of a lumbar vertebral body onto the one below. There may be pain and a 'step' can be palpated over the spine.

It can be treated conservatively by wearing a corset, or surgically by fusion of the vertebral joints.

Spinal stenosis

Spinal stenosis is narrowing of the spinal canal. It may be caused by long-term osteoarthritis and disc degeneration.

Standing and walking lead to severe pain in the buttocks and thighs, as nerves and blood vessels are cramped. The pain is relieved by rest.

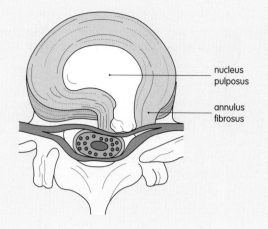

Fig. 5.30 Intervertebral disc prolapse.

nucleus
pulposus

annulus
fibrosus

Spinal stenosis is treated by the removal of osteophytes and part of the bony canal.

Back strain

Without an adequate warm-up, the muscles and ligaments of the lumbar spine can be strained during unaccustomed or sudden movements.

Back strain is treated by rest, analgesics, application of heat and gradual mobilization.

Tuberculosis in the back (Potts' disease)

Tuberculosis (TB) of the spine is called Pott's disease (Fig. 5.31). The spine is the most likely part of the skeleton to be affected by TB.

In Pott's disease, the vertebral bodies collapse onto each other, creating a sharply angled 'gibbus' deformity. There is also a risk of cord compression (Pott's paraplegia), chronic discharging sinus and the spread of TB to other organs.

Pott's disease is treated with antituberculous drugs. The pus is drained, any dead bone is removed, and the vertebrae are fused.

Arthritic disease in the back
Osteoarthritis

Osteoarthritis in the back tends to affect the thoracic or lumbar vertebrae (Fig. 5.32). It usually occurs in people who lift heavy objects or those with previous

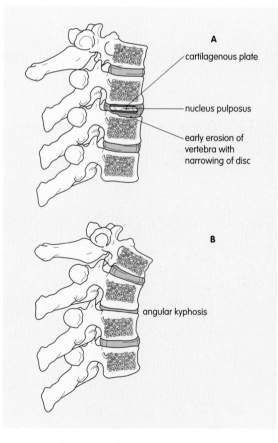

A

cartilagenous plate

nucleus pulposus

early erosion of vertebra with narrowing of disc

B

angular kyphosis

Fig. 5.31 Tuberculosis (Pott's disease) of the spine showing: (A) erosion of vertebra; and (B) subsequent collapse in front, resulting in angular curvature.

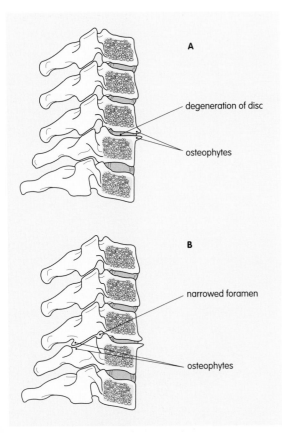

injuries, such as disc prolapse or degeneration. There is narrowing of the intervertebral discs and osteophyte formation in the lateral joint margins; these predispose to spinal stenosis and spondylolisthesis.

Rheumatoid arthritis

When rheumatoid arthritis occurs in the back, it often affects the cervical vertebrae. There is diffuse pain and impaired movement.

Ankylosing spondylitis

Ankylosing spondylitis affects the vertebral and sacroiliac joints before progressing to the limb joints. It occurs mostly in men.

There is erosion of the normal articular cartilage and underlying bone, then replacement with fibrous tissue, which also ossifies. This causes derangement of the normal structures.

Diffuse pain, a stiffened spine and marked restriction of chest expansion are the principal features of ankylosing spondylitis.

Pain referred to the back

Retroperitoneal disease in the abdomen (duodenal ulcer, pancreatic cancer, aneurysm) may give back pain.

Period pain and sciatic pain also radiate to the back.

Fig. 5.32 Osteoarthritis of the spine. (A) Degeneration and narrowing of intervertebral disc forming osteophytes anteriorly; (B) articular cartilage is worn away and marginal osteophytes surround the intervertebral foramen.

Labels in figure: A, degeneration of disc, osteophytes, B, narrowed foramen, osteophytes

- Give a simple classification of all joints.
- Describe the different types of joints with examples.
- Describe the structure and function of synovial joints.
- Describe the blood and nerve supply and lymph drainage of joints.
- Give a simple classification of the arthropathies.
- Differentiate the crystals found in gout and pseudogout.
- Describe the aetiology of De Quervain's tenosynovitis.
- Differentiate between tennis elbow and golfer's elbow.
- List the nerve roots which refer to the shoulder.
- Differentiate between osteoarthritis and rheumatoid arthritis.
- What is the difference between the pathology found in spinal stenosis and intermittent claudication?
- Describe the four different types of abnormal gait.
- Which bursae of the knee can be affected by bursitis and what are these lesions called?
- Differentiate between pes cavus and pes planus.
- What is the name of the lesions which cause the appearance of the 'bamboo spine', and how are they formed?

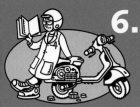

6. The Functioning Musculoskeletal System

Motor function and control

Central control of movement
Motor control
Motor systems responsible for movement have three levels of control, which are organized both hierarchically and in parallel (Fig. 6.1), namely:
- The cerebral cortex.
- The brainstem.
- The spinal cord.

Cerebral cortex
Three areas of the cerebral cortex are involved in motor control: the primary motor area, premotor area and supplementary motor area. The corticospinal tract originates from these areas and is the main descending tract involved in movement (Fig. 6.2).

Brainstem
The brainstem is the origin of other descending pathways, the extrapyramidal tracts. They play a role in posture, balance and hand–eye coordination, i.e. vestibulospinal, reticulospinal and tectospinal pathways.

Spinal cord
Spinal interneurons converge on spinal motor neurons, which innervate skeletal muscle. These interneurons act to inhibit certain muscle groups while activating others. In addition, movement can be modified by the basal ganglia and cerebellum.

Pyramidal tracts
Pyramidal tracts link the cerebral cortex, brainstem and spinal cord. They originate from pyramid-shaped cells in the motor cortex, descend into the brainstem, where 80% of fibres cross to the opposite side, and then terminate in the grey matter of the anterior horn of the spinal cord.

Coordination of movement
The coordination of movement involves the cerebellum and basal ganglia.

Cerebellum
The cerebellum improves the accuracy of movement by comparing actual movement (via feedback from the spinal cord) with intended movement (via input from the motor cortex). This information is passed forward to the brainstem, so that movement is modified as it occurs.

Basal ganglia
Basal ganglia play an important role in the planning and coordination of movement and posture. They have connections with the thalamus and cerebral cortex.

Peripheral control of movement
Peripheral control enables the monitoring of movement, while it is occurring, via sensory receptors in skeletal muscle.

Types of receptors
Two types of receptors are found in skeletal muscle: muscle spindles and Golgi tendon organs. They are important in both proprioception and spinal reflexes. The reflexes of muscle spindles and Golgi tendon organs exert opposite effects (Fig. 6.3).

Muscle spindles
Muscle spindles are spindle-shaped organs made up of modified muscle fibres, termed intrafusal fibres (Fig. 6.4). Intrafusal fibres are narrower than extrafusal fibres, and therefore do not contribute to muscle tension.

As muscle spindles lie parallel to muscle fibres they respond to changes in length.

Each spindle consists of several intrafusal fibres. These include:
- Two nuclear bag fibres, one for dynamic responses and the other for static responses.
- Five to six nuclear chain fibres for static responses.

Sensory innervation of muscle spindles is by group Ia afferent fibres, which supply both nuclear bag and nuclear chain fibres via primary endings. Group Ia

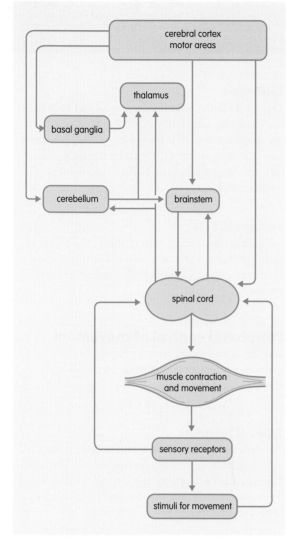

Fig. 6.1 Hierarchical organization of motor control in movement.

When the extrafusal fibres of muscle contract, the muscle spindle may no longer respond because its fibres are not being stretched. Activation of the γ-neurons causes shortening of the muscle spindles at the same time as the extrafusal fibres. During normal muscle contraction, descending pathways activate both the α-motor neurons, i.e. they stimulate extrafusal muscle contraction, and γ-motor neurons, i.e. they stimulate muscle spindle contraction, at the same time. This is known as α–γ coactivation.

Dynamic γ-motor axons supply the nuclear bag fibres. When activated, they enhance the dynamic response of group Ia fibres.

Static γ-motor axons supply the nuclear chain fibres. When activated, they enhance the static responses of both group Ia and II fibres.

Different descending pathways preferentially activate either dynamic or static motor neurons.

γ-Motor axons supply intrafusal muscle fibres while α-motor axons supply extrafusal, or 'regular', muscle fibres.

Golgi tendon organs

Golgi tendon organs consist of the terminals of a group Ib afferent fibre. These terminals are wrapped around bundles of collagen fibres in the tendon of a muscle. These lie in series with the extrafusal fibres, responding to changes in force.

There is no efferent innervation of Golgi tendon organs.

Posture and locomotion

Posture
Control of posture

Posture is the relative position of the trunk, head and limbs in space. To keep posture stable, the body's centre of gravity needs to be maintained in position over its support base.

Postural reflexes correct changes in posture caused by displacement of the centre of gravity—by either external forces or deliberate movement. Postural change is detected by musculoskeletal

afferent fibres show static and dynamic sensitivity, i.e. they respond to stretch and its rate.

One or more group II afferent fibres form secondary endings on nuclear chain fibres, although there may be occasional contact with a nuclear bag fibre. These fibres show static sensitivity only, i.e. they respond to change in muscle length.

Motor innervation of muscle spindles is important because it determines the sensitivity of muscle spindles to stretch (Fig. 6.5).

Fig. 6.2 Corticospinal tract.

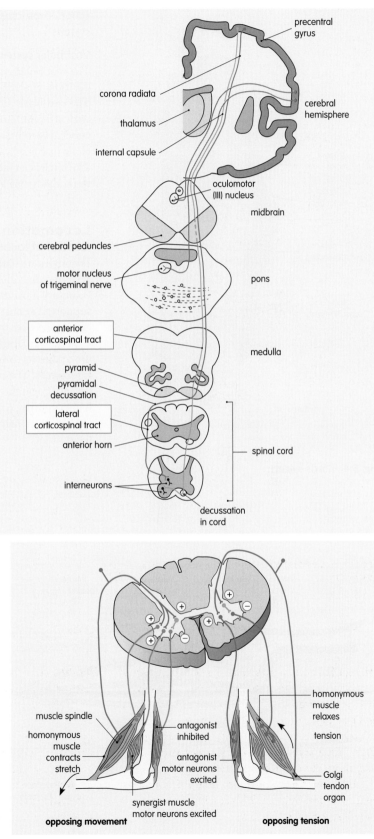

Fig. 6.3 Opposite effects of muscle spindle and Golgi tendon organ reflexes.

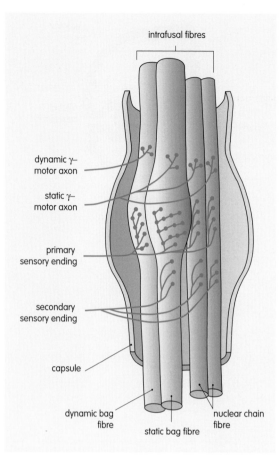

Fig. 6.4 Muscle spindle.

proprioceptors, the vestibular system and the visual system.

Vestibular system

The vestibular system detects changes in head position, linear acceleration and angular acceleration. The vestibular nuclei use this information, together with afferent nerves from the neck muscles and cervical vertebrae, to determine if the head is moving alone or if the head and the body are both moving. The nuclei can influence antigravity and axial musculature via a direct projection into the spinal cord.

Locomotion
Control of locomotion

Locomotion requires coordination between the systems controlling posture and those producing voluntary movement. This ensures that the body is supported against gravity and that the centre of gravity lies over the support base during propulsion.

A rhythm of muscle activity is needed, as each limb takes its turn in supporting the body and moving it forwards. The circuits that generate this pattern of activity are in the spinal cord and can be activated by higher centres, e.g. the brainstem. Sensory input is important in maintaining coordination of locomotion.

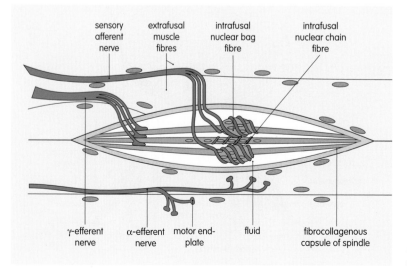

Fig. 6.5 Innervation of the muscle spindle.

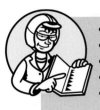

- Describe the hierarchical organization of the motor system.
- Locate the pyramidal tract.
- Describe the role of the cerebellum and the basal ganglia in coordination of movement.
- Describe the structure and innervation of muscle spindles.
- Describe the role of the central pattern generator in movement.

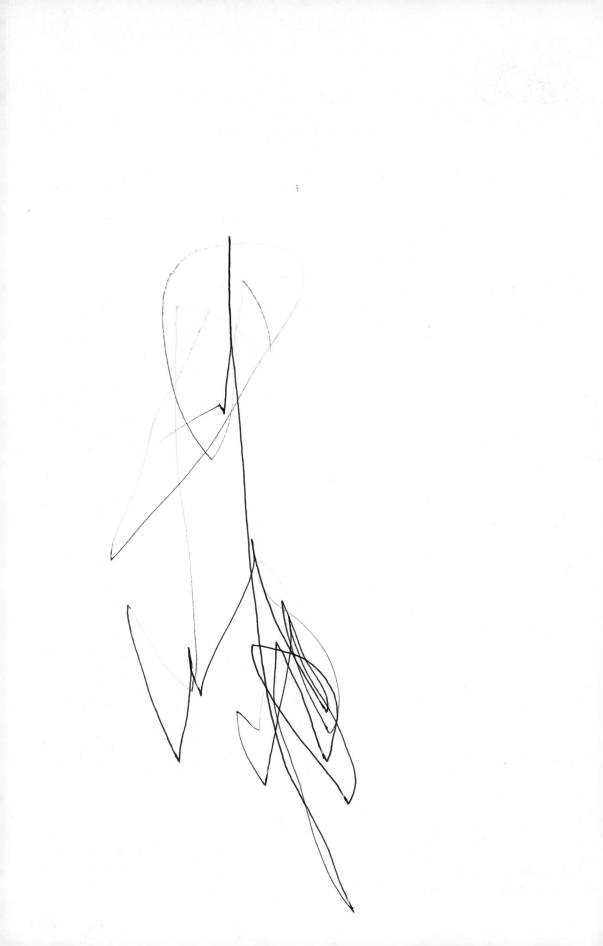

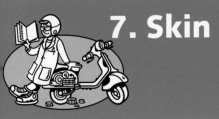

7. Skin

Organization of the skin

The skin is the largest organ in the body, making up 16% of the body's weight, and has a surface area of 1.8 m^2. It has an essential role in both homeostasis and protection of the body from external influences. The skin is composed of three layers:

- The epidermis—stratified squamous epithelium.
- The dermis—supportive connective tissue matrix.
- The subcutaneous layer—loose connective tissue and fat.

The epidermis (ectoderm) develops by the first month of gestation. The dermis (mesoderm) develops at a later stage, usually at around 11 weeks. By 17 weeks' gestation, the skin ridges which cause fingerprints have developed.

The composition of the three separate layers of the skin (see Fig. 1.2) is as follows:

Epidermis

The epidermis is generally around 0.1 mm thick, although it reaches depths of between 0.8 and 1.4mm on the palms of the hand and soles of the feet. The epidermis itself comprises four separate layers: the stratum corneum (horny layer), stratum granulosum (granular cell layer), stratum spinosum (prickle cell layer) and stratum basale (basal cell layer). These four layers are formed by the differing stages of maturation of keratin (Fig. 7.1), a protein produced by keratinocytes, the main cell of the epidermis.

Stratum basale

This layer is composed of keratinocytes (90%) which may be either dividing or non-dividing, melanocytes (5–10%) and infrequent Merkel cells. Keratinocytes are anchored to the basement membrane by hemidesmosomes; condensations of tonofibrils, which in turn are formed by synthesized keratin.

Melanocytes synthesize melanins, which absorb the energy of ultraviolet radiation and act as free radical scavengers. The cells originate from the neural crest and are most numerous on sites exposed to the sun.

Merkel cells appear to have a role in sensation and are found close to the terminal filament of cutaneous nerves.

Stratum spinosum

Here, the keratinocytes change from columnar to polyhedral. Desmosomes, again made of tonofibrils, connect the cells and help to distribute stress equally throughout the epidermis, as well as maintaining a distance of 20 nm between adjacent cells. When seen under a light microscope, these desmosomes form the 'prickles' that give the layer its name. Langerhans cells are also found in this layer: these are dendritic cells derived from the bone marrow and play an important role in the cellular immune system.

Stratum granulosum

As the keratinocytes mature, the cells flatten and lose their nuclei. The cytoplasm gains keratohyalin granules and membrane-coating granules which burst their contents into the intercellular spaces.

Stratum corneum

At the end of the maturation process, the keratocytes become overlapping, cornified cells which lack a nucleus—corneocytes. The cytoplasm is replaced by a matrix composed of keratin tonofibrils and keratohyalin granules, glued together by the contents of the membrane-coating granules. This horny layer forms the outermost layer of the skin. The keratin provides flexibility and strength, and the corneocyte layer can absorb three times its weight in water. If the layer becomes dehydrated, however, with the water content falling to below 10%, it is no longer pliable.

Dermis

The dermis varies greatly in thickness, ranging from 0.6 mm on the eyelids to 3 mm on the palms and soles. It is found below the epidermis and is composed of a tough, supportive cell matrix

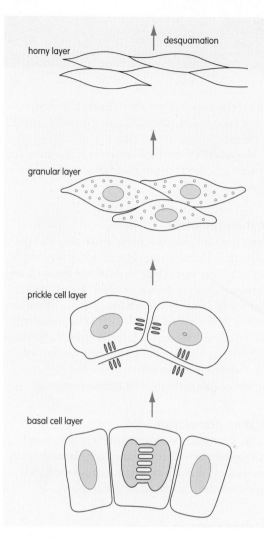

Fig. 7.1 The differing stages of keratinocyte maturation. (Adapted with permission from *Dermatology: an Illustrated Colour Text,* 2nd edn, by D.J. Gawkrodger, Churchill Livingstone, 1997.)

containing fibroblasts, dermal dendrocytes, mast cells, lymphocytes and macrophages.

Subcutaneous layer

Situated directly under the dermis, the subcutaneous layer is made up of loose connective tissue and fat. Most fat cells within the body are housed within this layer and these subcutaneous fat deposits are collectively referred to as adipose tissue.

Skin physiology

Keratinocytes, the basic building blocks of the skin, take around 14 days to mature fully as they travel

from the basal layer to the stratum corneum; the dividing cells in the stratum basale replicate every 200–400 h. The dead corneocytes are then shed from the horny layer of the skin in a process called desquamation within a further 14 days. This cell turnover rate of 28 days is dramatically shortened in keratinization disorders such as psoriasis.

Keratinocytes are also involved in the pathology of the blistering skin disorders. Circulating IgG autoantibodies, which are detectable in the serum by indirect immunofluorescence in 90% of affected patients, bind to components within the intercellular epidermal substance, and induce proteolytic enzyme release from the adjacent keratinocytes. These enzymes cause the loss of adhesion between cells and result in splits within the epidermis.

Derivative structures of the skin

Hair

In our now relatively bald state, humans no longer rely on hair to play a vital role in the conservation of heat. Although scalp hair still protects against the harmful effects of ultraviolet radiation and minor injuries, the main role of hair today is as an organ of sexual attraction.

Hair can be found in varying densities of growth over the entire surface of the body: exceptions are the vulval introitus, glans penis and the glabrous skin of the palms and soles of the feet. Follicles are most dense on the scalp and face. Follicles are derived from the epidermis (cells of the cortex matrix and the hair shaft) and the dermis (papilla).

Structure of hair

Each hair follicle is lined by germinative cells, which produce keratin and the other components of the hair shaft. The hair shaft itself consists of an outer cuticle, a cortex of keratinocytes and an inner medulla (Fig. 7.2). The root sheath that surrounds the hair bulb is composed of an inner and outer layer. An arrector pili muscle is associated with the hair shaft, which is the structure behind 'goose pimples'—it contracts with cold, fear and emotion to pull the hair erect.

Classification of hair types

There are three types of hair:

- Lanugo hairs—these are formed at 20 weeks' gestation and are usually shed before the fetus is

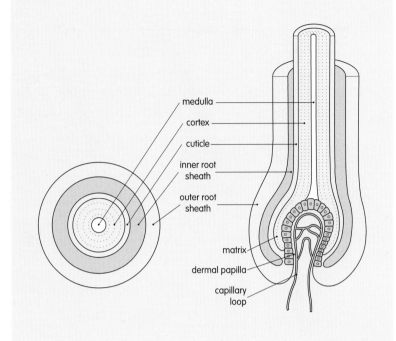

Fig 7.2 Structure of hair follicle. (Adapted with permission from *Dermatology: an Illustrated Colour Text,* 2nd edn, by D.J. Gawkrodger, Churchill Livingstone, 1997.)

born. They can be seen in premature babies, and are fine and long.

- Vellus hairs—this is the most common hair type; vellus hairs cover most of the surface of the body. They are short, fine and light in colour.
- Terminal hairs—there are around 100 000 terminal hairs on the scalp, and they are also found in the eyebrows, eyelashes, and the pubic and axilla regions. They are also the hairs which compose the beard.

Stages of hair development

Hair growth is cyclical, with the normal rate being 0.4 mm per day. There are three different stages of hair development (Fig. 7.3).

Anagen: This is the growth phase; 80–90% of scalp hair is in this phase at any one time. The length of this phase depends on the hair site: it lasts between 3 and 7 years for scalp hair, but only for 4 months for eyebrow hair.

Catagen: The resting phase, which normally lasts for 3–4 weeks. During this stage, the synthesis of the

hair follicle stops. 10–20% of scalp hair is in catagen at any one time, with 50–100 follicles entering the phase every day.

Telogen: The shedding phase; less than 1% of scalp hairs are in telogen at any one time. Hairs undergoing telogen are distinguished by a short club root.

Hair growth is not usually in phase, but if synchronized during the resting stage, will be uniformly shed 3 months later (telogen effluvium). This synchronization results from childbirth, high fever, surgery, drugs or other stress. Anagen effluvium (abrupt cessation of hair growth) occurs after ingestion of drugs such as cytotoxins, heparin and warfarin, carbimazole, colchicine and vitamin A. It may also follow ingestion of drugs such as thallium.

Nails

Consisting of a dense plate of hardened keratin between 0.3–0.5mm thick, the nail is a leftover of the mammalian claw. Its function is to protect the tip of the finger and facilitate grasping.

131

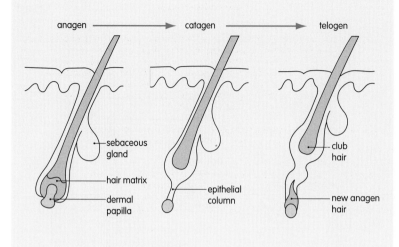

Fig. 7.3 Stages of hair development. (Adapted with permission from *Dermatology: an Illustrated Colour Text,* 2nd edn, by D.J. Gawkrodger, Churchill Livingstone, 1997.)

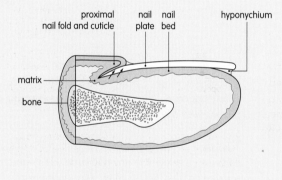

Fig. 7.4 Structure of the nail. (Adapted with permission from *Dermatology: an Illustrated Colour Text,* 2nd edn, by D.J. Gawkrodger, Churchill Livingstone, 1997.)

Structure of the nail

The nail is composed of a nail bed, nail matrix and a nail plate (Fig. 7.4) The nail matrix is composed of dividing keratinocytes which mature and keratinize into the nail plate. Underneath the nail plate lies the nail bed; this structure produces a small amount of keratin. The pink appearance of the nail plate is caused by the dermal capillaries which underlie the nail, and the white lunula at the base of the nail plate is the distal, visible part of the nail matrix. The thickened epidermis which underlies the free margin of the nail at the proximal end is called the hyponychium.

Nail growth

The fingernails grow at 0.1 mm per day; the toenails grow more slowly. Any pathological process which disturbs nail growth leaves visible clinical signs in the nail. Systemic illness may lead to transverse grooves in the nail called Beau's lines, which indicate an interruption to the growth of the nail matrix. Cytotoxic drugs cause black transverse bands in the nail, heavy metal poisoning causes white transverse bands, and trauma to the nail matrix can cause white spots within the nail or splinter haemorrhages.

Clubbing of the nail is caused by many disorders (Fig. 7.5); the nail matrix increases in vascularity and

Fig. 7.5 Some causes of finger clubbing. (Adapted with permission from *Principles of Clinical Medicine*, 2nd edn, P.J. Kumar and M.L. Clarke, Bailliere Tindall, 1990.)

Causes of finger clubbing	
respiratory	lung cancer, cystic fibrosis, interstitial lung disease, idiopathic pulmonary fibrosis, sarcoidosis, lipoid pneumonia, empyema, pleural mesothelioma, pulmonary artery sarcoma, cryptogenic fibrosing alveolitis, pulmonary metastases, bronchiectasis and lung abscess
cardiac	cyanotic congenital heart disease, other causes of right-to-left shunting, and bacterial endocarditis
gastrointestinal	ulcerative colitis, Crohn's disease, primary biliary cirrhosis, cirrhosis of the liver, achalasia and peptic ulceration of the oesophagus
malignancy	thyroid cancer, thymus cancer, Hodgkin's disease and disseminated chronic myeloid leukaemia
miscellaneous	acromegaly, thyroid acropachy and pregnancy

feels fluctuant. In addition, the normal angle between the base of the nail and the nail fold is lost, the nail curvature increases in all directions and the end of the finger may expand.

Sebaceous glands

Derived from epidermal cells, sebaceous glands are closely associated with hair follicles and produce an oily sebum (Fig. 7.6). This sebum flows into the hair follicles, and from there travels to the surface of the skin, where it oils both the hair and the keratinized surface of the skin to help waterproof and protect them from dehydrating and cracking. The secretions are in general highly toxic to bacteria.

The sebaceous glands are sensitive to androgens and become active at puberty. They are most numerous over the scalp, face, chest and back, and are not present on hairless skin.

Sweat glands

These glands are located within the dermis, and are present over the majority of the body—there are an estimated 2.5 million on the skin surface. The glands are composed of coiled tubes which secrete a watery substance, and are classified into two different types: eccrine and apocrine.

Eccrine glands

These sweat glands are found all over the skin, especially in the palms, soles, axillae and forehead, but are not present in mucous membranes. Eccrine glands are under psychological and thermal control and are innervated by sympathetic (cholinergic)

Location of sebaceous and sweat glands	
Type of gland	**Location**
sebaceous	associated with hair follicles; found on scalp, face, chest and back. Are not found on skin which is hairless
eccrine sweat	widely distributed, but most numerous on palms, soles, axillae and forehead
apocrine sweat	open into hair follicles; profuse around axillae, perineum and areolae

Fig. 7.6 Location of sebaceous and sweat glands. (Adapted with permission from *Principles of Clinical Medicine*, 3rd edn, P.J. Kumar and M.L. Clarke.)

nerve fibres. The watery fluid which the glands secrete contains chloride, lactic acid, fatty acids, urea, glycoproteins and mucopolysaccharides.

Apocrine glands

These are large sweat glands, the ducts of which empty out into the hair follicles. They are present in the axillae, anogenital region and areolae. They become active at puberty and produce an odourless, protein-rich secretion which gives out a characteristic odour when acted upon by skin bacteria. The apocrine glands are a phylogenetic remnant of the mammalian sexual scent gland. Wax in the ears is produced by a modified version of the same gland. Apocrine glands are also present on the eyelids. These glands are under the control of the sympathetic (adrenergic) nerve fibres.

 The slightly acidic pH of the skin (between 6 and 7) is maintained by sebum, sweat and the intercellular lipids of the stratum corneum. This lower pH level discourages microbial growth on the skin's surface.

Nerves in the skin

Functions of the skin include perception of touch and temperature, and so the organ is richly innervated. The densest concentrations of nerve endings are found in areas where sensation is of paramount importance: hands, face and genitalia. There are different types of sensation detectors found in the skin (Fig. 7.7). Free sensory nerve endings are found within the dermis and epidermis, and detect pain, itch and temperature. They contain neuropeptide transmitters such as substance P. Corpuscular receptors which are specialized for certain types of sensation are also found in the dermis: these are

Pacinian corpuscles, which detect pressure and vibration, and Meissner's corpuscles, which are sensitive to touch, and are found in the dermal papillae of the feet and hands. Innervation to hair-bearing and non-hair-bearing skin is also different.

Merkel cells are derived embryologically from the neural crest and play a role in sensation by acting as mechanoreceptors. They also contain neurotransmitters.

The sensory nerve fibres that innervate the skin are both myelinated and unmyelinated, and their cell bodies are contained within the dorsal root ganglion.

Vessels in the skin

The skin has a rich blood supply. A superficial artery plexus is formed at the papillary and reticular dermal boundary by branches of the subcutis artery. Branches from this plexus form capillary loops in the papillae of the dermis, each with a singular arterial and venous vessel: arteriovenous anastomoses. The veins drain into mid-dermal and subcutaneous venous plexus.

Dilatation or contraction of the arteriovenous anastomoses plays a direct role in thermoregulation of the skin. The changes in blood flow through the capillary loops help to control direct heat loss through the surface of the skin via convection and radiation (Fig. 7.8). The arteriovenous anastomoses are under the control of the sympathetic nervous system.

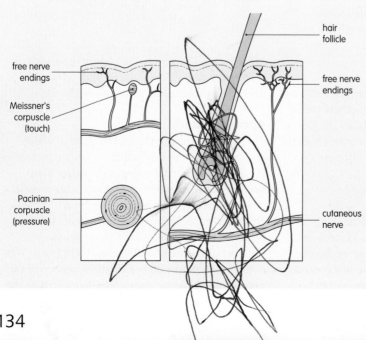

Fig. 7.7 The different types of nerve detectors within the skin. (Adapted with permission from *Dermatology: an Illustrated Colour Text,* 2nd edn, by D.J. Gawkrodger, Churchill Livingstone, 1997.)

Lymphatic drainage of the skin occurs through lymphatic meshes that originate in the papillae and go on to become larger lymphatic vessels which subsequently drain into regional lymph nodes.

Functions of the skin

Skin performs several functions. These include:
- Providing a mechanical barrier to antigens and bacteria, thus forming a protective cover for the body.
- Contributing to thermoregulation.
- Synthesizing vitamin D within the epidermis upon exposure to sunlight.
- Providing protection against excessive water absorption or loss.
- Providing protection, via skin pigmentation, against ultraviolet light.
- Distinguishing between pain, touch and temperature sensations.

Keratinocyte function

The main function of keratinocytes is to produce the high molecular weight polypeptide chains called keratin. The stages of keratinocyte maturation have been described. Each different stage of keratinocyte maturation produces different molecular weight keratins (e.g. 50, 55, 57 and 67 kDa), hence different keratins are found in each separate layer of the epidermis. The hardiness of keratin is caused by the strong covalent bonds which link the cysteine molecules, and the keratin found in the epidermis contains less cysteine and more glycine molecules than the stronger keratin which makes up hair.

Melanocyte function

Melanocytes are found within the basal layer of the epidermis and produce melanin, a brown pigment which protects against harmful ultraviolet rays from the sun—the melanin forms a protective cap over the nuclei of keratinocytes in the epidermis. The hereditary determination of number and size of melanosomes, the membrane-bound storage organelles, is responsible for the varying shades of the skin across different races, not the number of melanocytes. In addition, the amount of melanin in the skin can be temporarily increased in response to exposure to the sun's rays, as pre-formed melanin is photo-oxidized, stimulating melanocytes to produce more melanin, resulting in a 'tan'.

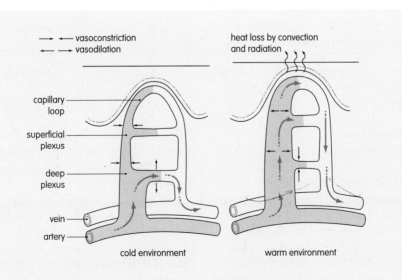

Fig. 7.8 Regulation of temperature by arteriovenous anastomoses. (Adapted with permission from *Dermatology: an Illustrated Colour Text,* 2nd edn, by D.J. Gawkrodger, Churchill Livingstone, 1997.)

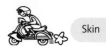

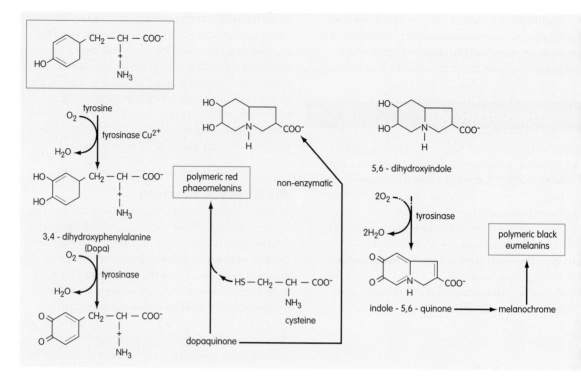

Fig. 7.9 Biosynthesis of melanin from tyrosine. (Adapted with permission from *Dermatology: an Illustrated Colour Text*, 2nd edn, by D.J. Gawkrodger, Churchill Livingstone, 1997.)

As well as absorbing the energy of ultraviolet radiation, melanin also acts as a free radical scavenger and as an energy sink. Melanin itself is produced from tyrosine (Fig. 7.9), and comes in two separate forms, eumelanin and phaeomelanin. Eumelanin is the more common form and pigments the skin a brown–black colour. Phaeomelanin produces a yellow–red coloration, the pigment produced in red-haired people. Most melanins are a mixture of the two different forms.

Fibroblast function

Fibroblasts produce and secrete the components of the extracellular matrix, the intricate meshwork of fibrous proteins embedded in a gel-like substance. The extracellular matrix holds the cells together, so the majority are not in direct physical contact with each other. Nutrients, waste products and other water-soluble materials diffuse through the gelous matrix between the blood vessels and cell tissues.

The main components of the extracellular matrix produced by fibroblasts are collagen, elastin and structural proteoglycans such as glycosaminoglycans (GAGs). Their functions are discussed in Chapter 1.

Types of collagen	Location
type I	reticular dermis
type III	papillary dermis
types IV and VII	basement membrane structures
type VIII	endothelial cells

Fig. 7.10 Types of collagen found in the skin.

Collagen is the major structural protein of the dermis, and makes up 70–80% of its dry weight. Of the 15 different types of collagen, five are found in the skin (Fig. 7.10).

The cable-like structure of collagen fibres provide tensile strength; the collagen is resistant to longitudinal stress. In disorders where there is pathology of the collagen, such as scurvy (a disease caused by vitamin C deficiency), the tissues which rely on collagen for strength become very fragile. In skin the blood vessels are easily damaged, and bleeding is very noticeable in the mucous membranes, especially in the gums.

Elastin is a rubber band-like protein fibre which facilitates the stretching and recoiling of structures. It plays an important role in the inflation and deflation of the lungs: in the skin, it maintains normal elasticity and flexibility.

The structural proteoglycans which make up the ground substance of the skin are mainly GAGs; these proteins provide the viscosity and hydration of the skin.

Thermoregulation

Thermoregulation is dependent on metabolic and physical factors. The evaporation of sweat from the skin's surface aids cooling of the skin, and the variations in the arteriovenous anastomoses also play an important role in temperature regulation (p. 135). Both of these mechanisms help to maintain the body's core temperature of 37°C in differing climates and during physical exertion.

Immune functions of the skin

The skin's structures, cells, functional systems and immunogenetics all play a role in the cutaneous immunity system (Fig 7.11).

Epidermal barrier

This physical structure provides an impenetrable barrier to most micro-organisms that come into contact with it. In addition to this external structure, the vessels of the dermis are important routes through which immune cells can travel to where they are needed.

Langerhans cells

Situated in the epidermis, these dendritic, bone marrow-derived cells are the first line of defence against micro-organisms which penetrate the epidermal barrier. They can be distinguished

Immune components of the skin		
Type of defence	**Different components**	**Action**
structural	skin	impenetrable physical barrier to most outside organisms
	blood and lymphatic channels	provide transport network for cellular defence
cellular	Langerhans cells	play important role in antigen presentation
	T lymphocytes	facilitate immune reactions, including cell destruction. Self-regulating through the action of suppressor T cells
	mast cells	facilitate inflammatory reaction of the skin
	keratinocytes	produce inflammatory cytokines; have the ability to express surface immune reactive molecules
systematic	skin-associated lymphoid tissue	as skin contains the above immune cells and structural defences, it can be classified as a fully functioning immunological unit
	cytokines and eicosanoids	cytokines are cell mediation molecules produced by components of the cellular defence system; eicosanoids are non-specific inflammatory mediators produced by mast cells, macrophages and keratinocytes
	complement cascade	activation of the complement cascade initiates a variety of destructive mechanisms, including opsonization, lysis, chemotaxis and mast cell degranulation
	adhesion molecules	increase the number of cellular defence facilitators in a particular area by binding T cells
immunogenetic	major histocompatibility complex (MHC)	facilitates immunological recognition of antigens. Located on HLA gene cluster; the appearance of specific HLA genes is associated with certain pathologies, e.g. ankylosing spondylitis is associated with HLA B27

Fig. 7.11 Immune components of the skin.

137

histologically by Birbeck granules, a cytoplasmic organelle found only in this type of cell. The Langerhans cells play a defensive role in antigen presentation.

 Other dendritic cells can be distinguished in the epidermis, which also appear to present antigen. If they lack the Birbeck granules, however, they aren't Langerhans cells.

T lymphocytes

These cells are produced in the bone marrow and mature in the thymus gland; they circulate throughout the body's tissues and come into direct contact with invading foreign antigens. Once activated by this binding process, the T cells proliferate and carry out a cell-mediated immune attack on the antigens.

There are four different types of T cells (Fig. 7.12), distinguished by different functions and varying surface receptors and identified by monoclonal antibodies. The other family of lymphocytes, B lymphocytes, is not normally seen within the skin but can be present in some types of skin pathology.

Mast cells

Mast cells are found within the dermis and are involved in the immediate (Type I) hypersensitivity reaction of the skin. They can be recruited to inflammation sites within the dermis.

Keratinocytes

As well as being responsible for keratin, keratinocytes also produce proinflammatory cytokines, such as interleukin-1 (IL-1). Keratinocytes can also express surface immune reactive molecules such as major histocompatibility complex (MHC) class II antigens (e.g. HLA DR), and intercellular adhesion molecules such as ICAM-1.

MHC class II antigens are also expressed on B lymphocytes, Langherhans cells, some T lymphocytes, macrophages and endothelial cells. They play an important role in immunological recognition, and are also responsible for the mechanism behind transplant rejection. The tissue type antigens of each person are also found within the MHC, which is situated within the HLA gene complex on chromosome 6. Certain HLA genes are associated with an increased risk of developing specific diseases, including some which are classified as 'autoimmune' (Fig. 7.13).

The adhesion molecules, in particular ICAM-1, are found on the cell surface of lymphocytes and some endothelial cells and keratinocytes. They bind with T cells by interacting with leucocyte-functional antigens, and so increase the site's cell traffic.

Lymphoid tissues of the skin

Lymphoid tissue is a term used to describe tissues that collectively store, produce and process lymphocytes. The skin, with its rich blood supply and generous lymphatic drainage, together with the circulating T lymphocytes and *in-situ* immune cells, can be classified as lymphoid tissue.

Cytokines and eicosanoids

The cytokines include γ-interferon, IL-1, IL-2 and IL-3. Produced mainly by T lymphocytes, these soluble molecules mediate actions between cells. They are also produced by Langerhans cells,

T lymphocytes found in the skin	
Helper	Facilitates immune reactions
Delayed hypersensitivity	Specifically sensitized
Cytotoxic	Kills infecting cells
Suppressor	Regulates other lymphocytes

Fig. 7.12 T lymphocytes found in the skin.

NLA antigens associated with skin diseases	
Skin disease	HLA antigen
psoriasis	B13, Bw37, Cw23
Reiter's disease	B27
dermatitis herpetiformis	B8

Fig. 7.13 HLA antigens associated with skin diseases.

keratinocytes, fibroblasts, endothelial cells and macrophages.

Eicosanoids are produced from arachidonic acids by mast cells, macrophages and keratinocytes. They are non-specific inflammatory mediators; prostaglandins, thromboxanes and leukotrienes are all eicosanoids.

Hypersensitivity reactions of the skin

A hypersensitivity reaction is one in which the adaptive immune response is exaggerated or inappropriate; an allergy is the acquisition of an inappropriate specific immune reaction to a normally harmless substance in the environment. There are four main types of hypersensitivity response, all of which are exhibited in the skin (Fig. 7.14).

If a patient who has high circulating levels of a certain antibody is injected with the appropriate antigen, an Arthus reaction will occur—a type III hypersensitivity reaction. This involves a red oedematous area which develops over the site of the injection within 4–12 h.

Skin secretions

The components of sweat, sebum and epidermal lipids differ in content (Fig. 7.15). Sweat is a watery isotonic liquid which is delivered to the skin's surface. It has a low pH of between 4 and 6.8 which

Hypersensitivity reactions of the skin	
Type I (Intermediate)	Fc receptors bind IgE to the surface of mast cells; when an antigen is encountered, the IgE molecules cross-link. This action stimulates the release of inflammatory mediators such as histamine, prostaglandins and leukotrienes. The response occurs within minutes, although there is a delayed component present, and results in urticaria in the skin. Massive histamine release can cause anaphylaxis. The most common allergens that provoke an allergic reaction are pollen grains, bee stings, pencillin, certain foods, moulds and house dust mites.
Type II (Antibody-dependent cytotoxicity)	When antigens bind to target skin cells on the basement membrane, a reaction occurs whereby cytotoxic killer-T cells or complement activation destroy the foreign body. The powerful effects of complement cascade activation include opsonization, lysis, mast cells degranulation, smooth muscle contraction and chemotaxis. Haemolytic anaemia and transfusion reactions are examples of type II hypersensitivity, as is the pathology involved in pemphigus: IgG antibodies which are directed against keratinocyte surface-antigens result in lysis of the keratinocytes causing intra-epidermal splitting. This results in characteristic skin blisters of pemphigus.
Type III (Immune complex disease)	When antigens and antibodies bind in the blood, an immune complex is formed which is deposited in the walls of small blood vessels such as those found in the skin. Although these complexes are usually removed by the reticuloendothelial system, a leucocytoclastic vasculitis can sometimes occur; vascular damage caused by complement activation and lysosomal enzymes released from polymorphs. This vasculitis is seen in systemic lupus erythematosus, dermatomyositis and microbial infections such as infective endocarditis.
Type IV (Cell-mediated or delayed)	Pre-sensitized T cells come into secondary contact with the antigen after it has become bound to an antigen presenting cell. The T cells release cytokines which in turn activate other T cells and macrophages—the process takes some time and the damage to tissue is most pronounced after 48–72 hours. Disorders which contain a variant of Type IV hypersensitivity in their pathology include allergic contact dermatitis, leprosy and tuberculosis.

Fig. 7.14 Hypersensitivity reactions of the skin. (Adapted with permission from *Dermatology: an Illustrated Colour Text*, 2nd edn, by D.J. Gawkrodger, Churchill Livingstone, 1997.)

Fig. 7.15 Components of sebum and epidermal lipid.

Components of sebum and epidermal lipid		
Component	Sebum (%)	Epidermal lipid (%)
glyceride/free fatty acids	58	65
wax esters	26	0
squalene	12	0
cholesterol esters	3	15
cholesterol	1	20

Action of hormones on the skin		
Hormone	Site of production	Action on skin
corticosteroids	adrenal cortex	vasoconstriction, decreased mitosis of basal cells, anti-inflammatory role
androgens	adrenal cortex, gonads	stimulates growth of terminal hair, stimulates sebum production
oestrogens	adrenal cortex, ovaries	stimulates melanin production
melanocyte stimulating hormone (MSH)	pituitary gland	stimulates melanin production
adrenocorticotrophic hormone (ACTH)	pituitary gland	stimulates melanin production
Epidermal growth factor (EGF)	skin	stimulates cell differentiation, plays a role in calcium metabolism
vitamin D	skin	no effect on skin, plays a role in bone metabolism

Fig. 7.16 Hormones and the skin. (Adapted with permission from *Dermatology: an Illustrated Colour Text*, 2nd edn, by D.J. Gawkrodger, Churchill Livingstone, 1997.)

makes the skin slightly acidic, and this discourages microbial growth. The minimum insensible loss through perspiration per day is 0.5 l, and the maximum daily output is 10 l, which is limited by the body's capability of sweating 2 l/h. Men sweat more than women.

As well as lowering the skin's pH and cooling the skin, sweat hydrates the outer layers of the epidermis and aids the hands and soles of the feet in gripping.

Hormonal production and the skin

The skin manufactures vitamin D in the dermis but is also affected by many other hormones (Fig. 7.16).

- List the four different sections of the epidermis and describe the stage of keratinocyte maturation for each one.
- Define where you would find lanugo, vellus and terminal hair.
- List ten causes of clubbing.
- Differentiate between eccrine and apocrine sweat glands.
- Describe the different functions of Merkel's cells, Meissner's corpuscles and Pacinian corpuscles.
- Differentiate the two forms of melanin.
- List the various products of fibroblasts and their functions.
- Describe the four different types of hypersensitivity reaction.
- List the functions of sweat.
- Explain the systemic importance of vitamin D production.

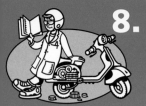

8. Disorders of the Skin

Terminology of skin disorders

Dermatologists use very specific terms to describe skin lesions (local involvement) and eruptions (widespread involvement). These terms are split into macroscopic and microscopic.

Macroscopic appearances

Macule (Fig. 8.1A)
An area of colour or textural change; macules are seen in vitiligo (hypopigmentation), freckles (hyperpigmentation) and capillary haemangioma (erythematous). They are flat lesions.

Papule (Fig. 8.1B)
A solid elevation of skin less than 5 mm in diameter. They can appear in various guises: dome-shaped (xanthomas), flat-topped (lichen planus) or spicular (accompanying hair follicles).

Nodule (Fig. 8.1C)
An elevation greater than 5 mm in diameter that may be either solid or oedematous. Nodules are seen in rheumatoid arthritis and a dermatofibroma is an example of the lesion.

Plaque (Fig. 8.1D)
A plaque is an extended pustule, palpable as a plateau-like elevation of skin no more than 5 mm in elevation but in general measuring more than 2 cm in diameter. Plaques are commonly seen in psoriasis and mycoides fungoides infection.

Vesicle (Fig. 8.1E)
Less than 5 mm in diameter, a vesicle is a skin blister filled with clear fluid. Vesicles may be subepidermal or intraepidermal, and may be singular or grouped.

Pustule (Fig. 8.1F)
Similar to a vesicle, a pustule is filled with a visible collection of pus rather than free fluid, and may, but not always, indicate an infection. A furuncle is an example of an infected pustule, whilst the pustules that appear in psoriasis are sterile.

Bulla (Fig. 8.1G)
A bulla is a vesicle that is greater than 5 mm in diameter. They occur in bulbous pemphigoid and pemphigus vulgaris.

Blister (Fig. 8.1H)
A lesion of any size which is filled with clear fluid and which forms because of cleavage of the epidermis. It may be a result of constant abrasion of the skin or as part of a pathological process. The cleavage may be intraepidermal or subdermal.

Wheal (Fig. 8.1I)
Wheals are transitory, and consist of a compressible, red or white, papule or plaque of oedema. They are usually indicative of urticaria.

Scale (Fig. 8.1J)
Scales are flat flakes of abnormal skin that indicate disordered keratinocyte maturation and keratinization. They vary in appearance, from large and polygonal like fish scales in ichthyosis, to silvery and white in psoriasis.

Lichenification
This is chronic thickening of the skin with increased skin markings, caused by constant rubbing or scratching.

Excoriation
A superficial linear abrasion caused by scratching.

Onycholysis
Onycholysis is the separation of the nail from the nail bed, leading to the nail plate becoming thickened, crumbly and yellow. Subungual hyperkeratosis subsequently occurs. It is a feature of many disorders, including psoriasis, fungal infections and trauma.

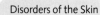

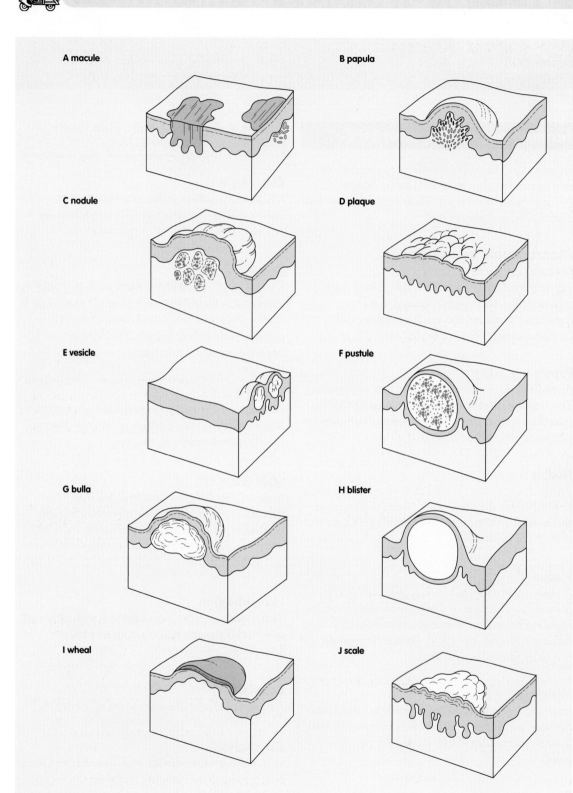

Fig. 8.1 (A) macule; (B) papule; (C) nodule; (D) plaque; (E) vesicle; (F) pustule; (G) bulla; (H) blister; (I) wheal; (J) scale. (Adapted with permission from *Dermatology: an Illustrated Colour Text,* 2nd edn, by D.J. Gawkrodger, Churchill Livingstone, 1997.)

Microscopic appearances

Hyperkeratosis

This is hypertrophy of the corneous layer of the skin, which leads to thickening of the epidermis.

Parakeratosis

Parakeratosis is a pathological process where the nuclei of the cells in the stratum corneum persist. It is seen in disease states such as psoriasis.

Acanthosis

This is hypertrophy of the stratum spinosum of the epidermis.

Dyskeratosis

This term describes a process in which keratinocytes mature early, becoming keratinized before they reach the surface of the skin. Cells within the epidermis become rounded, and may break away from other cells.

Acantholysis

This is a pathological process whereby the prickle cells of the stratum spinosum separate, leading to atrophy of the epidermis. Acantholysis is seen in diseases such as pemphigus vulgaris and keratosis follicularis.

Papillomatosis

This is a term used to describe diseases characterized by a number of papillomas.

Lentiginous

This term describes skin that is covered by lentigines: brown macules which resemble freckles, except with the regular border and rete—ridges which freckles lack.

Spongiosis

This is an inflammatory intercellular oedema of the epidermis.

Exocytosis

This term describes a process whereby material is released into extracellular space by fusion of an intracellular membrane-bound vesicle.

Erosion

A destructive lesion of the skin which affects only the epidermis, and which heals without scarring.

Ulceration

The formation of an ulcer (a lesion on the surface of the skin formed by sloughing of inflammatory, necrotic tissue).

Inflammation and skin eruptions

Psoriasis

Psoriasis is an inflammatory dermatosis with a chronic course. It is presents with erythematous, well-demarcated, silvery-scaled plaques.

Classification of types

There are six different variants of psoriasis: plaque, flexural, palmoplantar pustulosis, guttate, scalp and acrodermatitis of Hallopeau (Fig. 8.2).

Plaque

This is the most commonly seen type of psoriasis. Well-defined red plaques topped with silvery-white scales are usually seen over the extensor surfaces of the limbs, i.e. elbows and knees, with smaller lesions over the limbs and trunk (Plate 1). The plaque discs can be large or small, and may itch.

Flexural

The lesions in flexural psoriasis are clearly demarcated, pink and glazed, and lack the scales of plaque arthritis. The sites normally affected include the groin, perianal regions and genital skin. Less commonly, the inframammary skin folds and the umbilicus may be affected.

Palmoplantar pustulosis

This type of pustular psoriasis affects the palms and soles. The sterile pustules, which are related in severity to disease activity, can appear white, yellow or brown when dried. When accompanied by universal scaling on the trunk and limbs (erythrodermic psoriasis), the pustular psoriasis is known as generalized pustular psoriasis, which is a serious and potentially fatal condition. It is seen either spontaneously or after administration of potent oral or topical corticosteroids, and involves treatment and problems similar to that of widespread burn management. Palmoplantar pustulosis usually affects cigarette-smoking, middle-aged women, some of whom also have classic plaque psoriasis elsewhere.

145

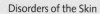

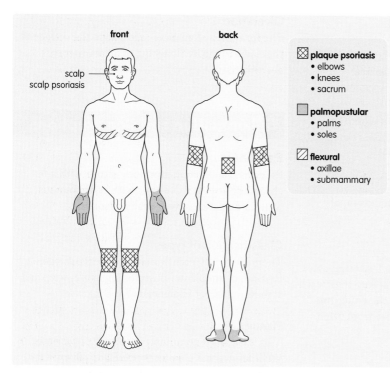

Fig. 8.2 Distribution of the different types of psoriasis.

plaque psoriasis
- elbows
- knees
- sacrum

palmopustular
- palms
- soles

flexural
- axillae
- submammary

front
back

scalp
scalp psoriasis

Guttate

Guttate psoriasis is characterized by 'drop-like' eruptions which appear symmetrically on the trunk and limbs. It may follow a streptococcal throat infection and is more common in young adults.

Scalp

Scalp psoriasis may often be the only clinical sign of psoriasis. Hyperkeratized plaques can be seen at the hair margin; the scales appear thicker and are better demarcated than dandruff.

Acrodermatitis of Hallopeau

Although the nails are affected by psoriasis in half of all sufferers, acrodermatitis of Hallopeau is a rare, indolent variant that only affects the fingers and nails.

Epidemiology

Two per cent of the western world suffers from psoriasis; it is less common in Asia and Africa. The male: female ratio is 1:1, and the disease commonly presents in the second and third decade, though onset may occur at any age. It is rare in children aged 8 years and under.

Aetiology

Psoriasis has a strong genetic link, with identical twin studies showing a concordance of 80%, and 35% of patients showing a family history. The inheritance is polygenic: HLA antigens CW6, B13 and B17 have strong correlations with the disorder, and environmental factors are thought to trigger the disease. Drugs such as beta-blockers, lithium and antimalarials may precipitate the disorder, or make existing psoriasis worse. Trauma to the upper layers of the skin, such as a scratch or a surgical scar, may lead to the formation of psoriatic skin at the site of damage: this is termed the Koebner phenomenon (Plate 2). Sunlight aggravates psoriasis in 10% of individuals, although for most it is beneficial.

Pathology

Active, psoriatic skin has a cell turnover rate which is 20–30 times faster than that of normal skin. The epidermal turnover time dramatically decreases from the normal 30 days to 3–4 days. Because of the increase in cell production, acanthosis results, which manifests as the scaly plaque of psoriasis. Parakeratosis also occurs (Fig. 8.3).

Complications

Erythroderma

Classified as inflammatory dermatosis that involves more than 90% of the skin surface, erythroderma needs prompt hospital admission as the systemic complications can be fatal. Erythrodermic psoriasis can be precipitated by the withdrawal of steroid treatment or an intercurrent drug eruption.

Psoriatic arthritis

Around 5% of patients with psoriasis develop a joint disease. A distal arthritis that causes swelling of toes and digits (called dactylitis) is the most common form, but a rheumatoid-like arthritis may also develop, with a similar polyarthritic pattern. Severe psoriasis may cause mutilans arthropathy, a destructive arthritis that erodes the small bones of the hands and feet, leading to progressive deformity. In addition, patients with psoriasis who are HLA B27-positive may develop ankylosing spondylitis.

Bacterial infection

Although this is rare, staphylococci can infect psoriatic plaques.

Management

The management of psoriasis is split into topical and systemic treatments. Topical treatments are usually the first line of treatment, with systemic therapy used for psoriasis that is not responsive to topical treatment, of life-threatening severity or which severely restricts the patient's quality of life.

Topical

Tar-based preparations These treatments are distilled from coal tar and are frequently used for in-patient care. Often combined with ultraviolet B (UVB) exposure or dithranol (see below), the tar preparations appear to work by altering the DNA synthesis of the skin. The disadvantages of this treatment are that the tar preparations stain, can cause a burning sensation and have a strong odour.

Dithranol Again, a messy and smelly treatment, dithranol interferes with skin mitosis. Lassar's paste is the most common preparation of dithranol used in hospitals, and is applied over psoriatic plaques. As normal skin is irritated by the preparation, surrounding skin can be protected by the application of white paraffin (e.g. Vaseline). The dithranol only needs to be applied to the skin for 30 min per day— under this regime the psoriasis will usually clear up within 3 weeks.

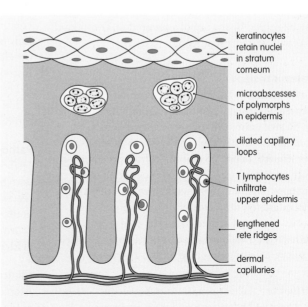

keratinocytes retain nuclei in stratum corneum

microabscesses of polymorphs in epidermis

dilated capillary loops

T lymphocytes infiltrate upper epidermis

lengthened rete ridges

dermal capillaries

Fig. 8.3 Histological changes in psoriasis.

Vitamin D analogues   Topical synthetic vitamin D analogues inhibit cell proliferation and promote keratinocyte differentiation, thus reversing some of the structural abnormalities of the skin present in psoriasis. The analogues have a similar efficacy to dithranol.

Topical corticosteroids   Use of topical steroids should only be considered for stubborn plaques, or for the treatment of steroids on the face, genitals or flexures, as they are non-irritant. Their use must be strictly monitored as the side effects caused by steroid usage include:

- Atrophy of the skin.
- Induction of acne or perioral dermatitis.
- Precipitation of unstable psoriasis upon treatment withdrawal.
- Allergic contact dermatitis.
- Infection (fungal, bacterial or viral) precipitated by steroidal treatment.
- Reduced efficacy after prolonged use (tachyphylaxis).
- Systemic effects of steroidal treatment—growth retardation, Cushingoid appearance and endocrine effects caused by systemic absorption of steroid.

Topical steroids are available as creams, ointment, lotion and gels (for scalp).

Salicylic acid ointment   This is used to treat psoriasis of the scalp, palms and hands. The scalp can also be helped by the use of a coconut oil compound or a tar-containing shampoo.

Systemic therapy

Methotrexate   This drug acts by inhibiting cell mitosis; it is usually administered orally, although it can be given intramuscularly or intravenously. Contraindications include a history of alcoholism, liver disease, peptic ulceration, colitis, pregnancy and acute infection; normal liver, kidney and marrow function must be established before the treatment begins, and monitored carefully throughout the course. The most serious side effects of methotrexate include hepatic fibrosis and cirrhosis. Results are usually observed within 2–4 weeks.

Retinoids   Acitretin, a vitamin A analogue, can be used to treat both plaque and pustular psoriasis. It

may also be used as a topical treatment or may be combined with UVB or PUVA therapy. Acitretin is teratogenic; if given to women of childbearing age, effective contraception must be started 1 month before beginning treatment, continued throughout, and for 3 years after stopping the course due to the long half-life of the drug.

Cyclosporin   This immunosuppressant clears psoriasis when taken in high doses. It is nephrotoxic, however, and renal function should be carefully monitored throughout the course. The long-term effects of taking cyclosporin are not yet known.

Fumaric acid derivatives   Although the short-term effectiveness of these drugs is good, 75% of patients on this treatment complain of acute side effects, including gastrointestinal symptoms and flushing. Many patients therefore stop taking the drug: there is also no evidence to support use in long-term maintenance treatment.

Eczema and contact dermatitis
Definitions
Eczema and contact dermatitis are used interchangeably to describe the same condition; a non-infective inflammatory condition.

Atopic eczema
Aetiology
Atopic eczema often occurs in patients with a medical or family history of asthma, hay fever or conjunctivitis and affects 10–15% of children in Europe. An atopic (the inherited tendency to develop asthma, atopic eczema or hay fever) family history is positive in 65% of patients; 60% of those likely to present with atopy will do so in the first year of life. In three-quarters of patients, the disorder will remit by the age of 15 years.

Pathogenesis
High levels of circulating IgE antibodies, coupled with defective T cell function, are thought to cause reactions to commonly encountered allergens such as house dust mites. The resulting inflammation is pruritic, and affects both the dermis and the epidermis (Fig. 8.4).

Clinical features
Atopic eczema usually presents in the first 6 months of life as a symmetrical erythematous eruption

Fig. 8.4 Histological changes in eczema. (Adapted with permission from *Dermatology: an Illustrated Colour Text,* 2nd edn, by D.J. Gawkrodger, Churchill Livingstone, 1997.)

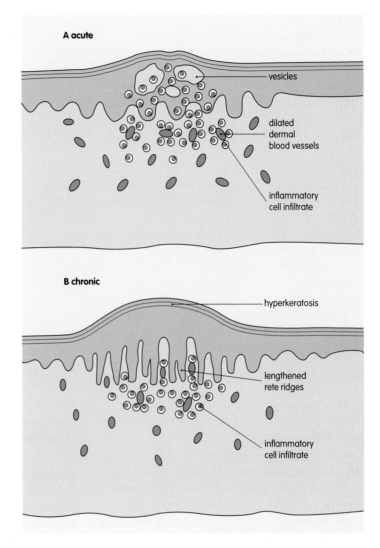

A acute
- vesicles
- dilated dermal blood vessels
- inflammatory cell infiltrate

B chronic
- hyperkeratosis
- lengthened rete ridges
- inflammatory cell infiltrate

affecting the face, trunk and limbs (Plate 3). As the child reaches 2 years, the eruption increasingly affects the flexures (Fig. 8.5). Lichenification, excoriations and dry skin occur, all of which are aggravated by the child scratching or rubbing the affected skin. The pruritis may affect sleep.

Management

Conservative management Educating the patient and family is important in the management of atopic eczema: the good prognosis should be stressed. Various lifestyle changes can be undertaken to lessen skin irritation: loose-fitting cotton clothing, avoidance of heat and irritants (e.g. wool, and in adults job-related substances), trimming down of nails to avoid excessive scratching. If pets are thought to aggravate the disease provisions should be made, and efforts to minimize the presence of house dust mites can be helpful. Similarly, if a history suggesting a food allergy is given, the offending food should be avoided.

Both local and national support groups exist for patients with atopic eczema; details of both should be made available to the patient.

Topical therapy *Emollients:* Aqueous cream, emulsifying ointment and bath oil emollients moisturize the skin, which in turn lessens the pruritis.

Topical steroids: Because of the side effects of topical steroids, hydrocortisone ointment should be started

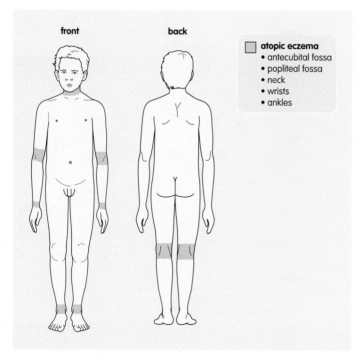

front   back

atopic eczema
- antecubital fossa
- popliteal fossa
- neck
- wrists
- ankles

Fig. 8.5 Distribution of eczema.

at the lowest potency and gradually increased in strength until an effective dose is found. It should be applied twice a day.

Antibiotics and antiseptics: These are used to treat the infective complications of eczema: bacterial (usually *Staphylococcus aureus*) and viral (viral warts, molluscum contagiosum or herpes simplex) infection may exacerbate the disorder. Eczema infected with herpes simplex is termed eczema herpeticum.

Medicated bandages: Bandages impregnated with coal tar or ichthammol paste that are left on overnight may be useful in excoriated or lichenified eczema. With exudative eczema, non-medicated wet dressings may help.

Systemic therapy *Antihistamines:* Sedative antihistamines (promethazine or trimeprazine) given at night may decrease the need to scratch.

Oral antibiotics and antiviral agents: Flucloxacillin is often given to treat the secondary infection of eczema eruptions. In-patient treatment with aciclovir is used to manage eczema herpeticum.

Other systemic treatments: Severe and resistant eczema can be treated by PUVA or a 6-week course of cyclosporin.

Contact dermatitis

Eczema precipitated by an exogenous substance is termed contact dermatitis. Clinically similar to atopic eczema, it is caused by skin irritants rather that allergens, and is a major cause of illness in industry (Plate 4). Atopic patients are more prone to development of contact dermatitis.

The site of presentation may give a clue to the causative factors of contact dermatitis (Fig. 8.6). The most important skin irritants include chemicals, solvents, detergents, abrasives and water itself; the most common allergy is nickel, which affects one in 10 women and one in a 100 men. Patch testing is useful in determining the irritant involved, and management is largely based on subsequently avoiding it once identified. Topical steroids are the secondary line of treatment.

Other forms of dermatitis

The other forms of endogenous dermatitis are listed in Fig. 8.7.

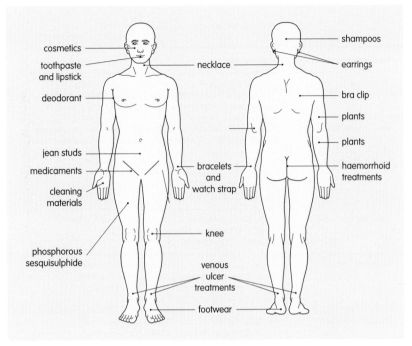

Fig. 8.6 Distribution of contact dermatitis. (Note that medical ointments and creams may cause rashes wherever applied.) (Redrawn with permission from *Dermatology: an Illustrated Colour Text*, 2nd edn, by D.J. Gawkrodger, Churchill Livingstone, 1997.)

cosmetics
toothpaste and lipstick
deodorant
jean studs
medicaments
cleaning materials
phosphorous sesquisulphide
necklace
bracelets and watch strap
knee
venous ulcer treatments
footwear
shampoos
earrings
bra clip
plants
plants
haemorrhoid treatments

Urticaria and angioedema

These two conditions are associated with acute oedema. Urticaria, commonly known as hives, is characterized by transient, pruritic wheals that are caused by extravascular plasma leakage in the dermis; angioedema is a more widespread collection of extravascular fluid that involves the dermis and subcutis.

Pathology

The lesions arise from the release of histamine and various other substances caused by mast cell degranulation. This release is mediated through one of several pathways: IgE-mediated (type I) sensitivity (p. 139), complement activation, direct release (usually drug-related), or blocking of the prostaglandin pathway (caused by drugs such as aspirin and NSAIDS).

Clinical features

Seventy-five per cent of urticaria cases are classified as chronic, idiopathic or acute. Wheals rapidly appear and disappear on the skin, usually within 24 h, and leave no residual mark. The lesions vary in size, shape and number, and may be accompanied by angioedema of the tongue and lips. Often no underlying cause is found and the disorder usually spontaneously resolves within a few months. With acute cases, the onset can usually be traced to an allergen that provokes a sudden IgE-mediated (type I) hypersensitivity reaction.

Management

Investigations should be instigated to detect provoking factors if the cause remains unclear from the history and examination. Dermographism (wheals induced by firm stroking of the skin that is present in 5% of the population) can be demonstrated, and cold urticaria can be induced by applying ice to the skin for 1 min. Hereditary angioedema can be detected by a low serum level of C_1 esterase inhibitor.

The mainstay of treatment is the use of antihistamines (terfenadine, astemizole, cetirizine or acrivastine), although management should also involve the avoidance of provoking factors. Systemic steroids may be used to treat severe acute angioedema, but not the chronic version. Acute anaphylactic shock or

Fig. 8.7 Other endogenous forms of dermatitis.

Endogenous forms of dermatitis	
Type of dermatitis	**Comments**
seborrhoeic dermatitis	disease of adults; *Pityrosporum ovale* plays an important role; dry, persistent redness and scaling seen on face; pruritis ani and chronic otitis externa are common symptoms
venous dermatitis of legs	feature of chronic venous insufficiency in legs; caused by venous hypertension in deep veins owing to valve incompetence
hand dermatitis	includes pompholyx, a vesicular pattern of dermatitis; may also be caused by discoid dermatitis, primary irritant hand dermatitis, allergic contact dermatitis and hyperkeratotic eczema
asteatotic dermatitis	seen mainly in the elderly, particularly in the winter, and usually on the legs; consists of fine scaling, minor erythema and superficial fissuring
neurodermatitis	localized lichenification seen in adult women on occipital scalp, nape, neck and arms; lesions are well-defined ovoid or elongated plaques; hyperpigmentation is common; itching intermittent and intense
discoid dermatitis	multiple, well-defined discoid lesions with prominent oedema; may be atopic, or may be precipitated by emotional stress
generalized exfoliative dermatitis	also known as erythroderma; skin is erythematous, oedematous and scaly; may be complicated by reversible loss of body hair; disease tends to be self-limiting

airways obstruction (caused by angioedema) should be treated immediately with a 1-mg injection of adrenaline—this treatment saves lives.

Lichenoid eruptions
Lichen planus
This is a fairly common disorder that affects the flexor surfaces, mucous membranes and genitalia. It presents as pruritic, papular violaceous lesions which may coalesce to form small plaques (Plate 5). A white lace-like pattern may form on the top of plaques; this is called Wickham's striae. Lichen planus may also present as annular, atrophic (rare), bullous or follicular lesions. Half of all patients recover spontaneously within 9 months, but in some the lesions may persist for up to 18 months. Although the disease is self-limiting, symptomatic treatment involves the use of topical steroids or PUVA in resistant cases.

Lichen sclerosus
Characterized by white, lichenoid and atrophic lesions that appear on the genitalia, lichen sclerosus is an immune-associated disorder which has a male: female ratio of 1:10. It is an uncommon disorder which usually presents in middle age. Management of genital lichen sclerosus involves topical steroids, with an antiseptic or antibiotic if necessary. Non-genital lichen sclerosus does not require treatment.

Lichen nitidus
This is a rare lichenoid eruption that features tiny monomorphic papules; these contain a lymphocytic infiltrate that causes the expansion of single dermal papillae, visible under microscopy. It is asymptomatic and requires no treatment.

Papulosquamous eruptions
Pityriasis rosea
A pityriasis rosea eruption is usually preceded by a 'herald patch'—a single erythematous oval macule which appears 4–14 days before the generalized eruption of multiple, smaller plaques over the trunk,

upper arms and thighs. The rash is symmetrical and may follow the distribution of the ribs, forming a 'Christmas tree' pattern.

Individual lesions are either 'medallion' plaques, an oval, rose-coloured patch which is slightly raised around the edges and which may have a fine collar of scales, or maculopapules (Plate 6). Pityriasis rosea usually affects those aged between 15 and 40 years; it is uncommon to be affected by a second eruption after the first clears up. This usually takes 1–2 months. The aetiology of the disease is unclear, but is thought to be viral in origin. Lesions may be pruritic; the itch can be relieved by a mild topical steroid. As the eruption is self-limiting, no other treatment is required.

Tinea versicolor

Otherwise known as pityriasis versicolor, this disorder is caused by fungal infection. It presents as irregular brown or pinkish macules that coalesce to form larger, superficially scaly lesions. Eruption sites include the neck, shoulders, upper arms and upper trunk.

Tinea versicolor mostly affects young adults and is more common in tropical climates. Examination under Wood's light shows skin fluorescence and, under microscopy, skin scrapings demonstrate the spores and short, rod-like hyphae; the so-called 'grapes and bananas' appearance. The management involves application of a topical imidazole antifungal, treatment with 2.5% selenium sulphide, or oral itraconazole for resistant cases. If hypopigmentation changes have occurred in darker skin, the patient should be warned that this may take some time to heal.

Reiter's disease

This term is used to describe a collection of physical signs, which include polyarthropathy, urethritis, iritis and a psoriasiform eruption. It affects HLA B27-positive men, and usually follows a non-gonococcal urethritis or bowel infection. The skin lesions occurring in Reiter's disease include keratoderma blennorrhagicum and balanitis of the penis. Joint arthropathy and nail involvement may be severe. Management involves treating the initial infection, anti-inflammatory analgesia for the joint and topical steroids for skin lesions.

Parapsoriasis

Known also as chronic superficial dermatitis, this is an eruption of pink, oval or round plaques that are topped by scales. The lesions may be pre-malignant. They appear in mid to late adulthood, and are usually sited on the abdomen, buttocks or thighs. Some lesions progress to malignant, cutaneous T cell lymphomas (mycosis fungoides) although the majority of lesions remain benign. Biopsy is necessary to detect pre-malignant plaques; treatment is with topical steroids for benign parapsoriasis, and PUVA or UVB for pre-malignant plaques.

Photodermatoses
Idiopathic causes
Polymorphic light eruption

The most common of the photodermatoses, this dermatitis of variable severity features pruritic, urticarial papules, plaques and vesicles that appear on the skin 24 h after exposure to the light. Sunscreen is used as a protective measure and a course of PUVA exposure at the close of spring can often acclimatize the skin, so a patient will not suffer light-induced problems during the summer months.

Chronic actinic dermatitis

Known also as actinic reticuloid dermatitis, this is a rare disorder that affects men in mid to late adulthood. It is characterized by the development of thick, lichenified plaques on sun-exposed skin, and there may be a previous history of contact or photodermatitis. It is managed by avoidance of the precipitating sunlight, use of protective sunscreen and treatment with topical steroids. If the dermatitis is resistant to these measures, oral steroids or azathioprine may be necessary.

Solar urticaria and actinic prurigo

In solar urticaria, skin wheals appear within minutes of exposure to sunlight and clear within 1–2 h. With actinic prurigo, sun-induced papules and lichenified nodules first appear in childhood, and may resolve by adolescence. Both conditions are rare.

Other causes

Other causes of photodermatoses include:
- Porphyria—metabolite accumulation due to enzyme insufficiency.
- Pellagra—nicotinic acid deficiency.
- Genetic—e.g. xeroderma pigmentosum.
- Drug-induced—e.g. nifedipine, thiazides, angiotensin-converting enzyme inhibitors and NSAIDs.

Effects of sunlight on other dermatological conditions

Sunlight aggravates the following conditions:

- Lupus erythematosus.
- Facial herpes simplex.
- Rosacea.
- Psoriatic disease (a minority).
- Vitiligo.

It benefits the following conditions:

- Acne.
- Psoriasis.
- Parapsoriasis.
- Pityriasis rosea.
- Atopic eczema.

Infection and infestation

Bacterial infections
The normal skin microflora

Normal bacteria resident on the skin include staphylococci, micrococci, corynebacteria and propionibacteria. In addition to bacteria, other micro-organisms present in healthy skin include yeasts and mites. The numbers of micro-organisms vary depending on site (e.g. forearm *versus* moist environs of axillae) and individual.

Diseases caused by overgrowth of normal flora
Erythrasma

An overgrowth of normal commensals can lead to this dry, red, scaly eruption which usually affects the skin folds; the affected skin will fluoresce under Wood's light. Erythrasma will clear up when treated with imidazole cream, topical fusidic acid or oral erythromycin.

Trichomycosis axillaris

This term refers to the yellowish substance formed on axillary hair as a result of corynebacteria overgrowth. Antimicrobial cream will usually clear the problem.

Pitted keratolysis

A proliferation of micrococci on the foot, encouraged by tight-fitting footwear and sweaty feet, may lead to foul-smelling, discoloured and pitted nails—micrococci can destroy the nail's keratin. Better hygiene will limit the problem, and topical neomycin or a 0.01% aqueous potassium permanganate foot soak may also help.

Staphylococcal infections
Impetigo

Impetigo can be caused by both staphylococcus or streptococcus infection. It presents as superficial skin blisters, which are easily ruptured to leave a crusted yellow exudate (Plate 7). The lesions are highly contagious and spread rapidly; they may complicate other skin disorders such as atopic eczema and herpes simplex. The management involves removing the residual crusts by soaking them in saline. If the infection becomes generalized, systemic antibiotics are necessary. With the most serious form of impetigo, that caused by *Streptococcus pyogenes*, oral penicillin is given to prevent glomerulonephritic complications.

Ecthyma

Ecthyma results from the growth of staphylococci in the skin of debilitated, immunosuppressed or diabetic patients after minor trauma. The bacterial infection leads to development of a number of shallow (and occasionally deep) round ulcers, usually on the legs. The ulcers leave scarring upon healing after treatment with systemic and topical antibiotics.

Folliculitis

Caused by infection with *S. aureus* or Gram-negative bacteria, folliculitis is caused by the pustular infection of multiple hair follicles. The pustules have erythematous edges and often contain an emerging hair shaft. Management is with topical and systemic antibiotics; to prevent recurrence, the patient should be educated about improved hygiene.

Scalded skin syndrome

This is a serious condition, usually caused by an autoimmune response to specific strains of staphylococcus infection. It usually affects infants, and causes severe erythema and the shedding of large sheets of epidermis from the body. The disorder responds well to prompt treatment with flucloxacillin or erythromycin, although a drug-induced adult variant of the condition (toxic epidermal necrolysis) is often fatal.

Streptococcal infections
Erysipelas
Presenting with localized erythema, swelling and tenderness, erysipelas is an acute infection of the dermis, caused by *S. pyogenes*. The inflammation is well-defined and may have palpable borders. The eruption follows a general malaise, with flu-like symptoms.

In healthy individuals, the eruptions clear in 2–3 weeks after treatment with oral penicillin to prevent streptococcal septicaemia. Penicillin can also be used prophylactically with recurrent attacks; these lead to lymphatic damage and irreversible oedema.

Necrotizing fasciitis
This serious infection may occur after minor trauma; it must be treated immediately to prevent serious skin necrosis in the affected area. The infection is characterized by a high fever and an ill-defined erythema that usually occurs on the leg. Systemic antibiotics and surgical debridement of the resultant necrotic tissue aid recovery.

Mycobacterial infections
Lupus vulgaris
The most common *Mycobacterium tuberculosis* skin infection, lupus vulgaris, arises as a postprimary infection and usually begins in childhood. Over time, initial painless, red brown nodules coalesce to form larger plaques, most commonly seen on the head and neck. Complications include the destruction of deeper skin tissues and the development of squamous cell carcinoma in longstanding lesions. A biopsy will aid the diagnosis, and the Mantoux test is positive. Treatment is with a three-drug programme, usually rifampicin, isoniazid and pyrazinamide. After an 8-week course, the pyrazinamide is stopped, and the other drugs are continued for 6–9 months depending on the response.

Scrofuloderma
This is an infection that occurs on the skin superficial to a lymph node affected with tuberculosis, or an affected bone or joint. A dull red nodule develops, which ulcerates and can lead to fistulae, granulation and scarring.

Warty tuberculosis
This results from the inoculation of tuberculosis into the skin of previously infected patients. It forms warty plaques on the hands, knees and buttocks; the condition is now extremely rare in the western world, but is still common in developing countries.

Spirochaetal infections
Secondary syphilis
The secondary stage of syphilis begins 1–3 months after the primary chancre, and is characterized by pink or copper-coloured papules that appear on the trunk, palms, limbs and soles. If left untreated, the papules will resolve in 1–3 months.

Yaws/bejel/pinta
These non-venereal treponemal infections are endemic in tropical developing countries. In all three, the serology is positive for syphilis, and the infection may be treated with penicillin.

Lyme disease
This condition is caused by *Borrelia burgdorferi* and is spread by tick bite. Lyme disease is characterized by a slowly expanding erythematous ring at the site of the initial tick bite. Complications include arthritis, neurological pathology and cardiac problems, although penicillin or tetracycline are normally successful treatments.

Other bacterial infections
Anthrax
Primarily an animal disease, anthrax causes haemorrhagic bullae at the site of inoculation. The lesion is accompanied by oedema and fever. The diagnosis is by culture of the blister fluid and the disease is treated by intramuscular injections of penicillin or intravenous tetracycline (followed by oral administration).

Gram-negative infections
Gram-negative bacilli, such as *Pseudomonas aeruginosa*, may infect skin wounds such as leg

ulcers. They may also cause nail discoloration, folliculitis and cellulitis (Plate 8).

Viral infections
Viral warts
Also known as verrucae, viral warts are benign cutaneous tumours caused by infection with human papilloma virus (HPV). The virus spreads through direct contact, sexual contact and also through water (e.g. local swimming baths). There are over 50 HPV subtypes, with different types being responsible for specific lesions: hand warts, plantar warts, genital warts, etc.

Common warts appear as dome-shaped papules with a papilliferous surface (Plate 9). Between 30 and 50% of common warts resolve spontaneously within 6 months; hand and foot warts can be treated with an abrasive stone or scalpel to pare down keratotic skin to allow easier treatment with drugs, cryotherapy and cautery.

Molluscum contagiosum
Caused by a DNA poxvirus, molluscum contagiosum mainly affects children and teenagers. The lesions appear as multiple pearly-pink umbilicated papules, a few millimetres in diameter, which spread through direct contact or through a medium such as towels. They commonly occur on the face, neck and trunk and are treated by expressing the 'cheesy' contents through forceps pressure, curettage or cryotherapy. As this treatment can be painful, with young children it is easier to teach the parent how to squeeze the affected lesions after a warm bath to soften the skin.

Herpes simplex
A common infection, caused by herpesvirus hominis, herpes simplex has two types of primary infection. Type 1 primary infection is facial or non-genital, and is sometimes accompanied by fever, malaise, lymphadenopathy and occasionally gingivostomatitis. If symptomatic, the illness lasts 2 weeks.

Type 2 primary infection occurs after sexual contact in young adults; lesions develop on the vulva, vagina, penis or in the perianal region. If the infection occurs in pregnant women, it is an indication for caesarian delivery: neonatal infection with herpes simplex is commonly fatal.

After the initial attack, the virus becomes latent, residing in the dorsal root ganglion. Reactivation leads to lesions at a similar site each time, often manifesting on the lips, face or genitals. The vesicular eruption may be preceded by a tingling or burning, crusts form within 1–2 days and the lesions clear after a week.

Treatment involves the use of aciclovir cream, with more severe infections requiring the use of systemic aciclovir. Treatment of genital herpes can also include the use of famciclovir; barrier contraception should be used by those infected, and sexual intercourse should be avoided altogether during symptomatic episodes of the disease.

Herpes zoster
Otherwise known as shingles, this infection occurs in a dermatomal distribution and follows a previous infection with the varicella zoster (chickenpox) virus. Reactivation of the virus leads to a self-limiting, vesicular eruption accompanied by local lymphadenopathy, pain numbness and paraesthaesia. The thoracic dermatomes are most often involved (Plate 10), although involvement of the ophthalmic division of the trigeminal nerve is common in the elderly, and may result in corneal ulcers.

Treatment is with analgesia and calamine lotion to dry the lesions. If secondary bacterial infection occurs, topical antiseptic or antibiotic is necessary. Severe cases require oral aciclovir.

Fungal infections
Human fungal infections are called mycoses: they are classified into superficial, cutaneous infections (tinea, candidosis and pityriasis versicolor) and deep, systemic infections (actinomycosis, sporotrichosis and blastomycosis, etc).

Dermatophyte infections
These fungi reproduce by producing spores: they cause tinea infection or 'ringworm'. The usual sites of dermatophyte infection are the nail, hair and stratum corneum. There are three different types of dermatophyte which cause tinea in humans: *Microsporum*, *Trichophyton* and *Epidermophyton*.

Microsporum
Infecting skin and hair, *Microsporum* fluoresce under Wood's light and usually cause infection during childhood. Along with *Trichophyton* fungi, they cause tinea capitis (ringworm of the scalp). Two *Microsporum* are responsible: *M. audouini*, which spreads from child to child, and so is responsible for epidemics in schools, and *M. canis*, which is passed on from family pets, mainly kittens and puppies.

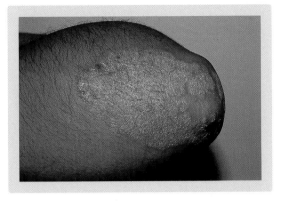

Plate 1 Plaque psoriasis.

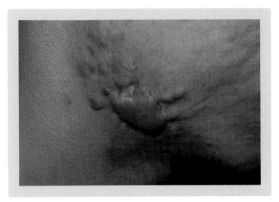

Plate 2 The Koebner phenomenon.

Plate 3 Atopic/flexural eczema.

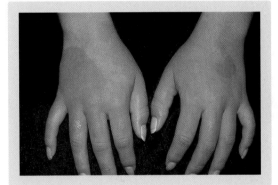

Plate 4 Contact dermatitis.

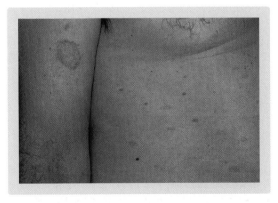

Plate 6 Pityriasis rosacea.

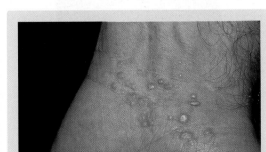

Plate 5 Lichen planus.

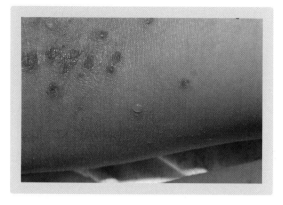

Plate 7 Impetigo.

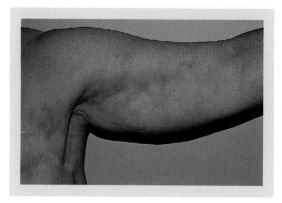

Plate 8 Cellulitis.

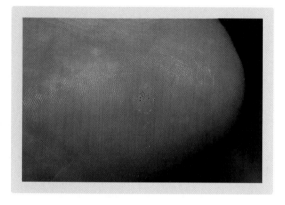

Plate 9 Simple viral wart.

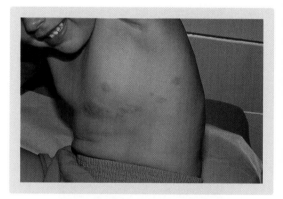

Plate 10 Herper zoster.

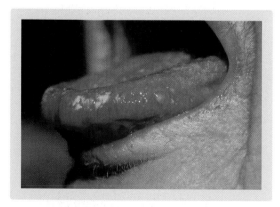

Plate 11 *Candida albicans*.

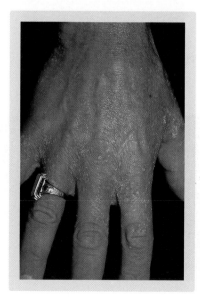

Plate 12 Scabies infestation.

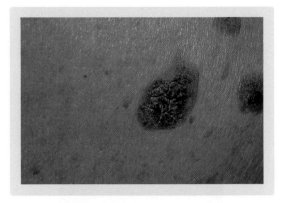

Plate 13 Seborrhoeic warts.

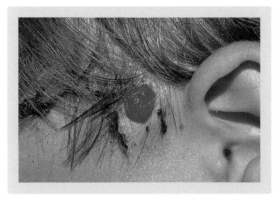

Plate 14 Pyodermic granuloma.

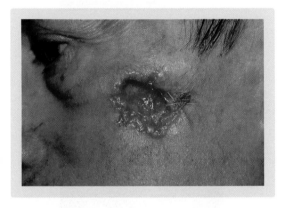

Plate 15 Basal cell carcinoma.

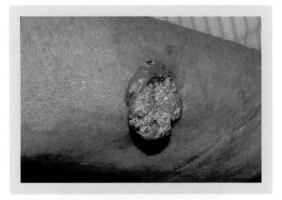

Plate 16 Squamous cell carcinoma.

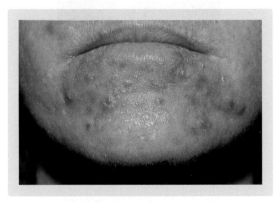

Plate 17 Papulopustular acne.

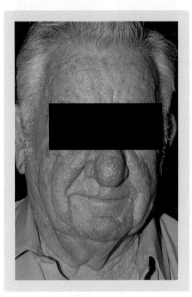

Plate 18 Rosacea.

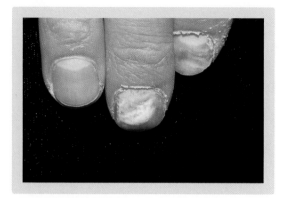

Plate 19 Fungal infection of the nails.

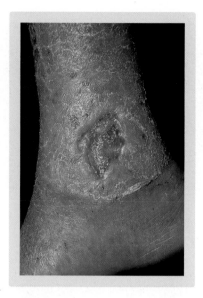

Plate 20 Venous ulcer.

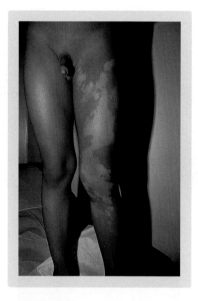

Plate 21 Vitiligo.

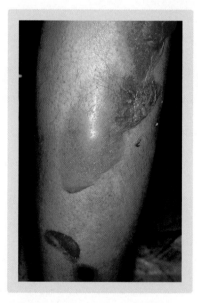

Plate 22 Bulbous pemphigoid.

Trichophyton

Trichophyton causes many types of tinea; this type of dermatophyte spore cannot be detected by Wood's light and requires examination of skin scrapings under microscopy for diagnosis. The commonest example is *T. rubrum* which causes tinea cruris (groin), tinea pedis (foot), tinea barbae (beard), tinea facei (glabrous skin of the face) as well as infection of hands, feet and nails.

Epidermophyton

Epidermophyton causes tinea cruris (ringworm of the groin) and tinea pedis (ringworm of the foot).

Candida albicans infections

Candida albicans is an opportunistic organism normally resident in the mouth and gastrointestinal tract. There are a number of predisposing factors that increase the risk of *Candida albicans* infection:

- Pregnancy.
- Oral contraceptive pill.
- Wide spectrum antibiotics.
- Corticosteroid treatment.
- Immunosuppressive drugs.
- Diabetes mellitus.
- Hypothyroidism.
- Blood dyscrasias.
- HIV infection.
- Poor hygiene.
- Humid environment.

Infection can occur as a genital, intertriginous, mucocutaneous, oral, paronychial or systemic eruption. It usually presents as white plaques, which can be itchy and sore (Plate 11). With systemic infection, red nodules can be seen in the skin. Management involves improved hygiene and the cessation of systemic antibiotics if appropriate.

Topical therapy includes magenta paint and, more commonly, imidazoles. Amphotericin, nystatin and miconazole are used for oral candida. Systemic therapy includes oral nystatin, itraconazole and fluconazole. Vaginal candida can be treated by a single dose of clotrimazole or econazole as a pessary.

Infestations
Insect bites

Insect bites can cause a chemical, irritant or immune-mediated response in the skin, caused by the introduction of foreign material into the body. Depending on the type of bite, the lesion can present as anything from itchy wheals to large bullae. Lesions are identified as insect bites by their pattern—either grouped or linear lesions which track up a limb. Secondary infection of the bite may occur.

Management involves elimination of the cause (bedbugs, cat fleas, etc.). Symptoms may be treated with hydrocortisone cream or calamine lotion.

Pediculosis (lice)

Lice infestations are of two types: pubic louse or body louse (Fig. 8.8). The latter is most common as head lice, which often cause epidemics in school children: they are spread by direct contact and the

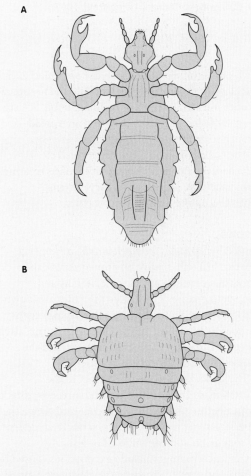

Fig. 8.8 (A) Body louse (*Pediculus humanus*). (B) Female pubic louse. (Adapted with permission from *Dermatology: an Illustrated Colour Text*, 2nd edn, by D.J. Gawkrodger, Churchill Livingstone, 1997.)

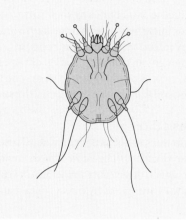

Fig. 8.9 Female scabies mite. (Adapted with permission from *Dermatology: an Illustrated Colour Text*, 2nd edn, by D.J. Gawkrodger, Churchill Livingstone, 1997.)

lice lay eggs (nits) on hair. Body lice are found in the homeless, or those with poor hygiene, and are spread through infested clothing or bedding. Pubic lice are generally found in young adults and are spread through sexual contact.

The lice cause itching, which can lead to secondary infection. Management involves treatment with malathion, lindane or carbaryl lotions, depending on the type of infestation.

Scabies

Caused by *Sarcoptes scabiei hominis*, a mite (Fig. 8.9) that can only survive on human skin, scabies infestation develops as a chronic, itching and contagious disease. The female mite burrows down into the skin at a rate of 2 mm a day, laying eggs as she goes. After 3 days the eggs hatch, maturing after 2 weeks. The mites mate; the males die and the females continue the cycle.

The skin takes 4–6 weeks to react to the infestation, so the infection may be spread by direct contact before the problem is recognized. Once the hypersensitivity reaction occurs, scratching reduces the mite population down to 12 or less.

Clinical symptoms include excoriations caused by itching, and scaly burrows, measuring up to 1 cm in length, which are seen on the skin of infected individuals (Plate 12). They are usually found on the wrists, ankles, nipples and genitalia, and the mite may be visible at the end of the burrow as a small white dot. Extraction of the mite for microscopy confirms the diagnosis.

In institutions (nursing homes, hospitals, etc.) or in immunosuppressed patients, proliferation of the scabies mite leads to the formation of large, encrusted eruptions; this is known as 'Norwegian scabies'. Secondary infection is also common with scabies infestation. Management includes contact tracing and the use of lindane, malathion and permethrin lotion to treat infected patients and contacts. Hydrocortisone, benzyl benzoate and 10% sulphur ointment can also be used.

Tropical skin infections and infestations

Although not endemic in the western world, tropical skin diseases can be seen in visitors and immigrants, and an awareness of the diseases listed below is useful in western medicine.

Leprosy

Caused by *Mycobacterium leprae*, leprosy is spread via nasal droplets and takes several years to incubate. Depending on the degree of type IV hypersensitivity in an infected individual, the patient will develop either tuberculoid leprosy (strong cell-mediated immunity) or lepromatous leprosy (weak cell-mediated immunity). Tuberculoid leprosy affects nerves (anaesthesia, muscle atrophy) and skin (red plaque facial lesions). Lepromatous leprosy mainly affects the skin, causing multiple, symmetrical macules, papules, nodules and plaques on the face (leonine facies), arms, legs and buttocks.

Leprosy results in bone damage because of repeated trauma (tuberculoid) and saddle nose defect (lepromatous). If left untreated, ichthyosis, testicular atrophy, leg ulcers, acute skin lesions and nerve destruction may result. Treatment lasts between 6 months and 2 years, and involves use of rifampicin, dapsone and clofazimine.

Leishmaniasis

This disease is caused by a protozoon transmitted to humans through the bite of sand flies. There are three types of leishmaniasis: cutaneous (endemic to the dry deserts around the Mediterranean), American (endemic to South and Central American tropics) and visceral (endemic to India).

Filariasis

Caused by the nematode worm *Wuchereria bancrofti*, filariasis is characterized by gross oedema of the legs and scrotum, termed 'elephantiasis'. It is treated with diethylcarbamazine.

Larva migrans

This is seen in holiday makers returning from tropical beaches, where they may have been infested with a hookworm larva. These larvae emerge from eggs present in the faeces of infested cats and dogs; they penetrate the skin and migrate in a serpentiginous fashion, causing intensely itchy red burrows. The disease is self-limiting as the larvae die within a few weeks, but may be successfully treated with topical 10% thiabendazole cream, or oral albendazole, when symptomatic.

Onchocerciasis

Caused by *Onchocerca volvulus*, this filarial infestation is common in Africa and South America where the filariae are transmitted through gnat bites. The adult worm may grow up to 7 cm long, with microfilariae found in the dermis and, more seriously, in the eye, causing blindness.

Granulomatous nodules are present on the skin, following an itchy, papular eruption. Onchocerciasis can be treated with a single dose of ivermectin, followed by repeated doses at 6-month intervals until the worm has been eradicated.

Tumours of the skin

Benign tumours of the skin

Epidermal tumours

Seborrhoeic wart

Otherwise known as a basal cell papilloma, seborrhoeic warts are common, pigmented tumours of unknown aetiology which affect the elderly or the middle-aged. The tumour consists of basal keratinocytes. They are multiple or solitary, round or oval in shape, and begin as a small, lightly pigmented papule before becoming darkly pigmented, warty nodules which measure up to 6 cm in diameter (Plate 13).

The lesions appear to be stuck onto the skin, and have well-defined margins and keratin plugs. They are found on the trunk and face, and are usually treated by liquid nitrogen cryotherapy, curettage or shave biopsy.

Skin tags

Benign, pedunculated fibroepithelial polyps, skin tags are common lesions found in middle-aged to elderly patients. They are most commonly found in the neck, axillae, groin and eyelids, and if removal is required (usually on cosmetic grounds), the polyp stalk is cut and the lesion removed. Skin tags can also be removed by cryotherapy.

Epidermal cysts

These cysts are filled with keratin and arise from the epidermis or outer root of the hair follicle (pilar cyst). They are usually found on the scalp, face and hands, and are firm, mobile lesions, up to 3 cm in diameter. Excision will clear the lesion; bacterial infection may be a complication.

Milium

These are small (1–2 mm in size), keratin-filled, white cysts usually found around the eyelids or on the cheeks. They can appear at any age, and may follow the healing of subepidermal blisters. They can be successfully excised using a sterile needle.

Dermal tumours

Dermatofibroma

Normally asymptomatic, dermatofibromas are common nodules present in the dermis, which may or may not be pigmented. They usually occur on the legs, and are more common in women than men. If the diagnosis is in doubt, an excisional biopsy should be performed.

Pyogenic granuloma

This is an acquired haemangioma (despite the name, it is neither pyogenic nor granulomatous), which presents as a bright-red, blood-encrusted nodule on the finger, lip, foot or face (Plate 14). The lesion, which develops rapidly over a few weeks, is pedunculated and bleeds easily. Pyogenic granuloma develops in children and young adults and is treated by excision. The excised material is examined histologically to exclude malignant melanoma.

Keloid

A keloid is a lesion arising from the excessive development of connective tissue that occurs after injury to the skin or inflammation. Unlike usual skin scarring, a keloid progresses beyond the limit of the original injury, and presents as a hard nodule or plaque which is most commonly found on the upper back, chest and ear lobes.

Keloids are more common in the Afro-Caribbean population, and are treated by steroid injections into the lesion.

Clinical features of melanocytic naevi	
Type of melanocytic naevi	Clinical features
congenital	present at birth; usually greater than 1cm in diameter; can become prominent and hairy; vary from light brown to black; 5% carry risk of malignancy
junctional	flat macules up to 1cm in size; round or oval; light to dark brown in colour; usually found on palms, soles and genitalia
intradermal	dome-shaped papule or nodule; seen on face and neck; may or may not be pigmented
compound	macules usually smaller than 1cm; vary in pigmentation; occur anywhere; larger lesions may develop warty surface
spitz	firm, red–brown nodule; usually occur in children on face; growth initially rapid; dermal vessels are dilated
blue	usually solitary; blue in colour; common on hands and feet
halo (Sutton's)	seen on trunk of adolescents and children; indicative of destruction of naevi cells by body's defence system; white halo of pigmentation surrounds existing naevus; there is an association with vitiligo
Becker's	rare; unilateral lesion in adolescent males; hyperpigmented, becoming hairy; found on back and chest

Fig. 8.10 Clinical features of melanocytic naevi.

Campbell-de-Morgan spot

Also known as cherry angiomas, these are capillary proliferations which present as bright-red papules in the middle-aged and elderly population. They are found on the trunk and can be excised by hyfrecation or cautery.

Lipoma

Lipomas present as soft subcutaneous masses found on the trunk, neck and upper extremities. The fatty nodules may be multiple, and are sometimes painful, in which case they can be removed by excision.

Naevi
Melanocytic naevi

Aetiology   Commonly known as 'moles', melanocytic naevi are present in most Caucasian adults. The number of naevi appears to be influenced by a genetic component.

Pathology   The naevus cells are thought to derive from melanocytes and histologically there are three different types of naevi (Fig. 8.10):

- Junctional—naevus cells cluster at the dermatoepithelial junction.
- Intradermal—naevus cells cluster in the dermis.
- Compound—naevus cells cluster at both sites.

Clinical features   Only congenital naevi are present at birth; other types develop during childhood and adolescence. Pregnancy or excessive sun exposure may cause the development of further naevi in later life. The number of melanocytic naevi present in Caucasians is usually between 10 and 30.

Complications   Dysplastic naevi which change size, shape or colour, and those which itch, become inflamed or encrusted must be examined carefully as these alterations suggest malignant melanoma.

Management   Naevi are excised for biopsy, because of cosmetic reasons, repeated inflammation or those which, because of their site, experience recurrent trauma. Naevi may also be removed prophylactically, e.g. a large hairy congenital naevus which has an increased risk of malignant change.

Vascular naevi

These naevi are often present at birth. Most lesions are caused by superficial capillary networks; larger angiomas are caused by deeper, multivascular plexuses.

Port-wine stain   Also known as naevus flammeus, this is a large, irregular, red–purple macule that can affect the face asymmetrically. In later life it may become darker and nodular.

Salmon patch   The most common vascular naevus, this lesion presents in half of all newborns. The pink patches situated on the upper eyelid often clear rapidly, but those at the back of the neck—'stork-mark' patches—may persist.

Strawberry naevus   Also known as a capillary–cavernous haemangioma, strawberry naevi usually develop soon after birth, growing to a maximum size at 1 year. The naevus begins to involute at 2 years, and has usually resolved by the age of 7 years. Strawberry naevi can occur anywhere on the surface of the skin, and leave an atrophic area behind after healing.

Cavernous haemangioma   A similar lesion to a strawberry naevi, this lesion presents as a nodule and may not involute completely. The risk of trapped platelets may lead to thrombocytopenia, and so a course of prednisolone, or even surgery, may be necessary.

Epidermal naevi   These linear lesions are warty and pigmented, presenting at birth or in early childhood. They can range from a few centimetres long to involving the whole of a limb; they may recur after excision. A scalp variant, naevus sebaceous, may become neoplastic and should be removed.

Connective tissue naevi   Presenting as smooth, skin-coloured papules or plaques, these lesions are rare. They may be singular or multiple.

Malignant melanoma
Epidemiology

A malignant tumour of melanocytes is known as a melanoma: this is the most lethal of skin tumours. The aetiology is unknown, but intensive exposure to ultraviolet light over short periods, such as that experienced whilst sunbathing, is thought to have a positive correlation with the development of melanomas. There are 10 cases in every 100 000 population per year, and the incidence is rising rapidly. The male: female ratio is 1:2, and melanomas can develop in anyone over the age of 20 years. Melanomas tend to develop on areas exposed to the sun: the back is the most common site in men and the leg in women, where half of all cases occur.

Pathology

Thirty per cent of lesions develop on the site of a pre-existing melanocytic naevus; the risk of neoplastic change is greatest in congenital naevi. Individuals with multiple melanocytic naevi (over 100), previous malignant melanoma, and those with a fair complexion (especially people with red hair and blue eyes) who burn easily in the sun are also at increased risk.

Local invasion is staged by the Breslow scale, where the depth of the lesion is measured in millimetres.

Clinical features

There are four main variants of malignant melanoma, listed in Fig. 8.11.

The prognosis relates to the depth of tumour (Fig. 8.12).

Management

Malignant melanomas are treated by surgical excision. A margin of healthy skin is excised alongside the tumour: 1 cm for tumours less than 1 mm thick, 3 cm for a tumour more than 1 mm thick. Close follow-up is needed to detect recurrence, which may occur locally or through metastases. Public heath education in the general population will help to detect early malignant changes and prevent excessive sun-exposure in the future.

Varicants of malignant melanoma		
Variant	Percentage of new UK cases	Clinical features
superficial spreading	50	occurs commonly in women; mainly on lower leg; macular; variable pigmentation; can regress
lentigo	15	develops in longstanding lentigo maligna (macular lesion arising in elderly or on sun-dam aged skin); most common on face
acral lentiginous	10	affects palms, soles and nail beds; often diagnosed late so has poor survival rates; most common malignant melanoma in mongoloids
nodular	25	occurs commonly in men; usually arises on trunk; pigmented nodule which may rapidly grow and ulcerate

Fig. 8.11 Main variants of malignant melanoma.

Prognosis and tumour depth	
Depth of tumour (mm)	5-year survival rate (%)
<1.49	93
1.5–3.49	67
>3.5	38

Fig. 8.12 Prognosis related to tumour depth.

Malignant epidermal tumours
Basal cell carcinoma
Aetiology
Otherwise known as rodent ulcers, basal cell carcinoma is the most common type of skin cancer. They arise from basal keratinocytes in the epidermis, and are most common in middle to late life.

Basal cell carcinoma is most commonly caused by excessive sun-exposure, but can also result from ingestion of arsenic, irradiation and chronic scarring. There is also some evidence of genetic predisposition. Fair-skinned individuals are most at risk, and the incidence is greater in men than women.

Pathology
The tumour is composed of basophilic cells which bud down from the epidermis to invade the dermis. They may also invade in a lobular fashion (Fig. 8.13).

Clinical features
The lesions tend to arise in sun-exposed areas of the face, such as the nose, eyelids and temple. They grow slowly and are locally invasive: lesions may have existed for 2 or more years before the patient presents (Plate 15).

Management
If possible, complete excision is the best treatment; this can be difficult if lesions are around the eye or nasolabial fold. Incisional biopsy and radiotherapy may be used in those over 60 years. Cryosurgery may also be used on superficial trunk lesions.

Squamous cell carcinoma
Aetiology
These arise from well-differentiated keratinocytes and usually develop in an area of damaged skin. The risk factors for squamous cell carcinoma include:
- Chronic sun-exposure causing actinic damage.
- Irradiation.
- Chronic ulceration/scarring.
- Industrial and tobacco carcinogens.

Other diseases such as viral infections (viral warts) and genetic disorders (xeroderma pigmentosum) may predispose to squamous cell carcinoma. The lesions usually occur in those over 55 years, and are

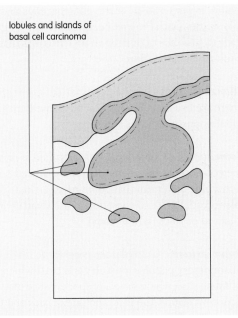

Fig. 8.13 Histopathology of basal cell carcinoma. (Adapted with permission from *Dermatology: an Illustrated Colour Text,* 2nd edn, by D.J. Gawkrodger, Churchill Livingstone, 1997.)

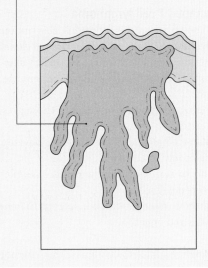

Fig. 8.14 Histopathology of squamous cell carcinoma. (Adapted with permission from *Dermatology: an Illustrated Colour Text,* 2nd edn, by D.J. Gawkrodger, Churchill Livingstone, 1997.)

more common in men than women. The tumour may metastasize.

Pathology
The dermoepidermal junction is destroyed by the malignant keratinocytes, which then invade the dermis (Fig. 8.14).

Clinical features
The lesions, which are usually found on sun-exposed sites such as the face, neck, forearm and hand, begin as small papules which progress to ulcerated, crusted lesions. Squamous cell carcinomas may also present as a dome-shaped nodule (Plate 16). Primary sites of metastatic basal cell carcinoma are usually found around the edges of ulcers, scars or in areas of irradiation.

Management
Surgical excision is the first line of management, although tumours of the face and scalp may be treated by incisional biopsy and radiotherapy. Lymph nodes should be examined for metastases.

Other tumours of the skin
Intraepidermal carcinoma (Bowen's disease)
This form of cancer is common in elderly women, and presents as either solitary or multiple lesions. The trunk and lower legs are mainly affected, with lightly pigmented scaly lesions, reaching several centimetres in size developing at these sites. Histologically, there are atypical but non-keratinized keratinocytes present, and a thickening of the epidermis. Arsenic exposure is a major risk factor, and conversion to squamous cell carcinoma may rarely occur. Treatment is by excision, curettage or cryotherapy.

Keratoacanthoma
This is a non-malignant, rapidly growing tumour that arises in sun-exposed areas. It forms a dome-shaped papule complete with a central keratin plug, which may leave a crater if removed. The lesion resembles a squamous cell carcinoma histologically; it is differentiated by a more symmetrical pattern. The lesion will resolve spontaneously within a few

months, but leaves scarring; removal of the keratoacanthoma is preferable.

Cutaneous T cell lymphoma

Also known as mycosis fungoides, this tumour is due to a lymphoma that develops in normal skin tissue. It grows slowly, and may lead to secondary skin deposits. The four stages of development are as follows:

- Premycotic plaques—similar to those present in psoriasis.
- Infiltrated plaques—fixed plaques develop, most commonly on the trunk.
- Tumour stage—within the plaques nodules and ulcers develop.
- Systemic disease—tumour spreads to lymph nodes and organs.

Treatment is aimed at containing the lymphoma—topical steroids can be used to control the premycotic plaques. UVB therapy, PUVA, topical nitrogen mustard, photopheresis, radiotherapy and chemotherapy are also used, to varying effect.

Kaposi's sarcoma

A multicentric tumour seen in around 33% of patients with AIDS. Arising from vascular endothelium, and presenting as a purple nodule or plaque on the face, mouth, limbs or trunk, it may also infect internal organs. This sarcoma may result from infection with herpesvirus 8. A variation of Kaposi's sarcoma, seen in elderly Jewish men from Eastern Europe, is more benign and is not associated with HIV.

Disorders of specific skin structures

Sweat and sebaceous glands
Acne vulgaris
Pathology

Acne is one of the most common diseases of skin. Its various lesions (comedomes, papules, pustules, cysts and scars) result from chronic inflammation of the pilosebaceous apparatus, and it affects mainly the face, shoulders and trunk. It commonly presents around puberty, and so appears in women earlier than men, although both sexes are affected equally. Acne is essentially caused by excessive production of

sebum, hyperkeratosis of the pilosebaceous duct and colonization with *Propionibacterium acnes*. This leads to a release of inflammatory cytokines that results in inflammation.

Clinical features

There are five main lesions in acne: comedomes, papules, pustules, cysts and scars.

Comedomes   Comedomes are classified as either open or closed. Open comedomes are dilated pores with a plug of keratin that contains melanin (blackheads). Closed comedomes are small cream-coloured papules (whiteheads).

Other lesions   Comedomes progress to inflammatory papules, pustules and cysts which are found on sites which have a preponderance of sebaceous glands: the face, shoulders, back and upper chest (Plate 17). Cysts are the most destructive of the lesions in acne: upon healing, they leave scars that may be 'ice-pick', keloidal or atrophic.

Complications

Although acne itself is a relatively harmless disease, the psychological effects it has on young patients cannot be overestimated. Patients severely devalue their own self-image because of the disorder, and consequently suffer shame and lack of self-confidence. Upon successful physical treatment of acne, the psychological symptoms often improve.

Management

There are a variety of treatments for acne, listed in Fig. 8.15.

Rosacea

Rosacea is an erythematous, pustular dermatitis that affects the face. The aetiology is unknown; histology shows dilated dermal blood vessels, sebaceous gland enlargement and inflammatory cell changes.

Clinical features

The first sign of rosacea is facial flushing. This is followed by the development of erythema, telangiectasia, papules and pustules (Plate 18). It occurs most commonly in middle age, although all age groups can be affected.

Treatment of acne vulgaris	
Treatment	**Comments**
benzoyl peroxide cream	eradicates *P. acnes*; bleaches clothes, may cause irritation and contact allergies
tretinoin	treats comedomes before they evolve, but may cause irritation
antibiotics	first-line: tetracycline; second-line: erythromycin and trimethoprim; antibiotics are suppressive, not curative; they are thought to affect lipase-producing bacteria present in pilosebaceous follicles
anti-androgens	used in combination with an oestrogen in women only; anti-androgen suppresses sebum production
retinoid	isotretinoin reduces sebum production, inhibits *P. acnes* and is anti-inflammatory; women must not be pregnant and must take oral contraceptive pill throughout 6-month course as retinoids are teratogenic; side effects can be severe
triamcinolone acetonide	steroid injected into acne cyst to aid healing
non-drug therapies	excision, cryotherapy, removal of comedomes using an extractor

Fig. 8.15 Treatment of acne vulgaris.

Complications
Complications include lymphoedema of the face, enlargement of the connective tissue and sebaceous glands of the nose (rhinophyma-hyperplasia), and blepharitis and conjunctivitis.

Management
Metronidazole gel is used twice a day; if the rosacea proves resistant, oral tetracycline is started. Isotretinoin can also be used. Surgical correction is required for rhinophyma-hyperplasia.

Others
Perioral dermatitis
A side effect of topical steroids, perioral dermatitis presents as papules and pustules around the mouth and chin. It is treated effectively with oral tetracycline.

Hydradenitis suppurativa
This is the term used to describe chronic inflammation of the apocrine sweat glands. Nodules, abscesses, cysts and sinuses develop in the axillae, groin and perineum, and may result in permanent scarring. Treatment depends on the severity of the

condition and includes topical antiseptics, systemic antibiotics and excision.

Hyperhidrosis
Hyperhidrosis is excessive sweating caused by eccrine gland overactivity. It usually arises from heightened emotion, but hypoglycaemia and shock may also stimulate the sweat glands. It can be managed by the application of 20% aluminium chloride in alcohol.

Hair disorders
Alopecia
Classification
Diffuse non-scarring   This is diffuse hair loss across the whole scalp. It may be androgen-dependent (common male pattern baldness: Fig. 8.16), where the follicles are slowly converted from terminal to vellus hairs, and is present in 80% of men by the age of 70 years. Androgenetic alopecia also occurs in postmenopausal women to a lesser extent.

Diffuse non-scarring alopecia is also caused by endocrine disorders: underactivity of the thyroid, pituitary and adrenal glands can all cause alopecia, as can dietary protein, iron or zinc deficiency. Telogen effluvium can result in diffuse non-scarring

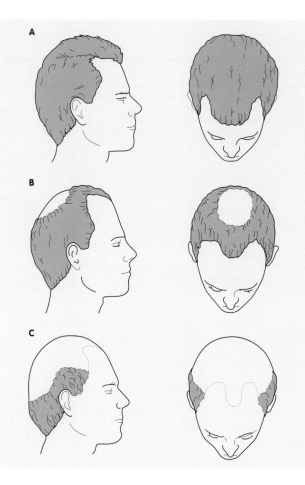

Fig. 8.16 Male pattern baldness. (A) Bitemporal recession; (B) vertex involvement; (C) most severe pattern of male baldness. (Adapted with permission from *Dermatology: an Illustrated Colour Text*, 2nd edn, by D.J. Gawkrodger, Churchill Livingstone, 1997.)

alopecia, as can the ingestion of certain drugs such as heparin and warfarin.

Localized non-scarring   Patchy hair loss may be caused by infection (tinea capitis), trauma or alopecia areata. This condition can cause patchy baldness or complete hair loss and is associated with autoimmune disorders. It is characterized by pathognomonic 'exclamation mark' hairs— dystrophic, depigmented hairs which are short and taper towards the margins of hair loss. The hair loss appears to be caused by the anagen stage being prematurely arrested, and begins at 20–30 years. If the alopecia areata is localized, regrowth may occur, but the course of the disorder is unpredictable. It can be treated to some extent by triamcinolone acetonide and PUVA.

Scarring (cicatricial) alopecia   Scarring results from the destruction of hair follicles, which can occur with burns, irradiation, infection (shingles,

kerion or tertiary syphilis), lichen planus, lupus erythematosus and pseudopelade—a term used to describe the end-stage of a destructive inflammatory process of unknown aetiology in the scalp.

Excess hair
Hirsutism
The excessive growth of male pattern hair in a female is known as hirsutism. It can be idiopathic, presenting with terminal hair development in the beard area and around the nipples, or more frequently drug-induced. Other causes of hirsutism are listed in Fig. 8.17.

Hypertrichosis
This term describes excessive growth of terminal hairs in a non-androgenic distribution. It can be classified into localized (caused by melanocytic naevi, chronic scarring and inflammation) or generalized (caused by anorexia nervosa, malnutrition,

Fig. 8.17 Other causes of hirsutism.

Other causes of hirsutism	
Cause of hirsutism	**Example of disease**
endocrine	acromegaly
	Cushing's syndrome
	virilizing tumours
	congenital adrenal hyperplasia
ovarian	polycystic ovaries
iatrogenic	excess androgens
	excess progesterones
idiopathic	end-organ hypersensitivity to androgens

underlying malignancy and drugs). Investigation is important in finding the underlying cause.

Others
Hair shaft defects
Usually genetic in origin, these defects are rare but can result in brittle, beaded and broken hair shafts.

Dandruff
The normal scalp is layered with fine scales of keratin; dandruff is simply a physiological exaggeration of the normal exfoliative process. Certain conditions (i.e. seborrhoeic dermatitis of the scalp and psoriasis) can produce severe scaling of the scalp that may be mistaken for dandruff.

Tinea capitis
Tinea capitis is ringworm of the scalp that may cause alopecia.

Nail disorders
Congenital disease
Nail-patella syndrome
Inherited in a Mendelian dominant fashion, nail-patella syndrome is a disorder in which the nails and the patella are rudimentary or absent. The thumb is always affected; other digits may or may not be spared.

Paronychia congenita
The nails are thickened and discoloured in this autosomal dominant disorder; there may also be palmar–plantar keratoderma, with or without hyperhidrosis. There is a risk of malignant mucosal dysplasia.

Trauma
Subungual haematoma
These traumatic lesions occur when the nail has undergone increased pressure (e.g. fingernail trapped in the door; toenail stood on). The possibility of a malignant cause must always be considered with a subungual haematoma, however.

Splinter haemorrhages
Although commonly due to trauma, splinter haemorrhages may also be indicative of infective endocarditis.

Ingrown toenails
Two factors contribute to ingrown toenails: ill-fitting shoes predispose to deformities of the feet and, if the wrong method of cutting toenails is employed, spicules of bone are left, which damage the nail fold. The nail of the big toe is most often involved, and intense discomfort is experienced.

Onychogryphosis
Chronic trauma predisposes to onychogryphosis, a condition in which the hallux toenails become grossly thickened and horn-like.

Brittle nails
Usually caused by heavy exposure to detergents and water, this is a common complaint. It may also be caused by iron deficiency, hypothyroidism and digital ischaemia.

Nail involvement in the dermatoses
Psoriasis
Psoriatic nail involvement causes pitting, nail thickening, onycholysis, discoloration and subungual hyperkeratosis.

Alopecia areata
Fine pitting and rough nail surfaces are features of alopecia areata.

Eczema
Nail features of eczema include coarse pitting, transverse ridging, dystrophy and shiny nails caused by rubbing.

Lichen planus
Lichen planus leads to a thinned nail plate, longitudinal grooves, adhesions between the nail fold and the nail bed and loss of nail.

Infections
Tinea unguium
Caused by fungus, this infection spreads to the free edge of the nail and spreads distally to involve the whole nail. As a result, the nail becomes thickened, yellow and crumbly, and subungual hyperkeratosis can be seen (Plate 19). Toenails are involved more than fingernails, but very rarely are all the nails on one hand and foot involved. Treatment is with oral terbinafine or itraconazole.

Chronic paronychia *(Candida albicans)*
This is often seen in wet-workers. The nail becomes boggy, the cuticle is detached and pressure on the nail will cause pus to be extruded. Secondary involvement of the nail matrix can result in an abnormally ridged nail, and the nail plate may become infected.

  Management involves avoiding wet work by wearing rubber gloves, simple antiseptics and clotrimazole or amphotericin B lotion. Cauterization of the subcuticular space may be necessary in resistant cases: this is performed by inserting a cotton wick soaked in phenol into the space for 1 min.

Acute bacterial paronychia
Originating at the junction of the posterior and lateral folds, this infection leads to pus formation.

Management includes drainage and sometimes oral erythromycin and flucloxacillin are used.

Tumours of the nails
Viral warts
Periungual warts often occur; treatment is the same as for warts elsewhere.

Periungual fibromas
These are a complication of tuberous sclerosis, and appear during puberty.

Myxoid cysts
These mucous cysts are found adjacent to the proximal fingernail fold; they contain clear fluid and are fluctuant. They can be treated with cryotherapy, steroid injection or excision.

Malignant melanoma
If a pigmented streak appears in the nail, biopsy must be performed to exclude a malignant melanoma. Biopsies must also be performed on all atypical or ulcerating lesions around the nail fold.

Nail changes in systemic disease
Nails often show non-specific changes in systemic disease, the most important of which is clubbing. Discoloration, koilonychia, onycholysis, pitting and ridging are also important signs of systemic disease (Fig. 8.18).

Vascular and lymphatic disorders
Disorders of cutaneous blood vessels
Definitions
Erythema: redness of the skin caused by vasodilatation. It may be localized or generalized.

Flushing: sudden onset of erythema owing to vasodilatation. It is caused by a number of factors, including emotion (blushing), menopause, foods, drugs, rosacea, carcinoid syndrome and phaeochromocytoma.

Telangiectasia: visible dilatation of dermal venules or arterioles (spider naevi). They can result from skin atrophy, excessive oestrogen, connective tissue disease, rosacea, venous disease or they may be

Nail changes in systemic disease	
Nail change	**Causes**
Beau's lines (tranverse grooves)	severe systemic illness
brittle nails	iron deficiency, hypothryoidism, loss of blood supply to nails, exposure to water and *chemicals*
colour change	drugs, cyanosis, infection, trauma, renal failure, nicotine staining, psoriasis
clubbing	bronchial carcinoma, fibrosing alveolitis, asbestosis, infective endocarditis, congenital cyanotic defects, inflammatory bowel disease, thyrotoxicosis, biliary cirrhosis
koilonychia (spoon-shaped nail)	iron deficiency anaemia, lichen planus, chemical exposure
nail fold telangiectasia (dilated capillaries)	connective tissue disorders
onycholysis (separation of nail from bed)	psoriasis, fungal infection, trauma, thyrotoxicosis, drugs (tetracyclines)
pitting	psoriasis, eczema, alopecia, lichen planus
ridging (transverse and longitudinal)	eczema, psoriasis, lichen planus

Fig. 8.18 Nail changes in systemic disease.

congenital. The lesions can be treated by needle cautery, hyfrecation and laser treatment.

Purpura: this describes a discoloration of the skin caused by the extravasation of blood cells, which may be caused by a number of factors: vessel wall defects, defective dermal support, clotting defects or idiopathic pigmented purpura.

Raynaud's phenomenon
This is a three-stage process caused by paroxysmal vasoconstriction which affects mainly women. The fingers first turn white, due to ischaemia, then blue, due to cyanosis caused by pooled, deoxygenated blood in capillaries, then finally red, due to reactive hyperaemia as the capillaries reperfuse. Causes of Raynaud's phenomenon include:
- Arterial occlusion.
- Connective tissue disease.
- Hyperviscosity of blood.
- Neurological defects.
- Vasoconstriction caused by use of vibrating tools.
- Toxins and drugs.

As the phenomenon is often precipitated by cold, affected patients are advised to keep their hands warm. Nifedipine and diltiazem may also help.

Livedo reticularis
This is cyanosis occurring in a marble pattern on the skin. It is caused by reduced arteriole flow and poor skin circulation; reversible livedo is usually induced by cold and is seen in children, whilst fixed livedo is usually caused by vasculitis, and requires further investigation.

Chilblains
These are painful, purple–pink inflamed swellings found on the fingers, toes and ears, which are cold to the touch. The lesions may last for weeks and may be complicated by ulceration. Chilblains are much less common since the introduction of central heating.

Lymphatic disorders and the skin
Lymphoedema
Secondary lymphoedema is caused by inadequate lymphatic drainage, which may be due to:
- Recurrent infection.
- Blockage.
- Surgical or irradiation destruction.

Primary lymphoedema may follow infection and usually presents in adolescence. Lymphoedematous areas are at increased risk of infection, and prophylaxis with penicillin may be necessary.

Lymphangitis

Presenting as a tender red line extending from a focus of infection, lymphangitis describes lymphatic vessel infection. It is treated with intravenous antibiotics.

Leg ulcers

Aetiology

Leg ulcers can be caused by venous disease, arterial disease, vasculitic disease or neuropathy (Fig. 8.19). They affect 1% of the adult population and are twice as common in women as in men.

Pathology

Venous ulcers   Valve incompetence in perforating veins leads to increased capillary hydrostatic pressure and permeability. Fibrin deposits form adjacent to the capillaries, which interfere with nutrient exchange and lead to ulceration. Usually presenting in middle age to later life, risk factors for development of venous ulcers include obesity and venous thrombosis. The first signs are a feeling of heaviness in the legs caused by oedema; discoloration of the skin and eczema may subsequently occur. Fibrosis of the dermis and subcutis

(lipodermatosclerosis) leads to ulceration, which often follows minor trauma. The ulcer usually affects the medial, and sometimes the lateral, malleolus (Plate 20). Ulcers are exudative to begin with, but may then enter a granulomatous, healing phase, which takes months. Some larger venous ulcers may never heal. The post-ulcer leg has a slender, sclerosed ankle caused by fibrosis.

Arterial ulcers   Arterial disease leads to ischaemia, with reduced temperature in the leg and hair loss, toenail dystrophy and cyanosis. Leg ulcers form on the foot or mid-shin, and are sharply defined; surrounding pulses are reduced or absent.

Vasculitic ulcers   Vasculitic ulcers begin as a purpuric patch, which becomes necrotic leading to punched-out lesions.

Neuropathic ulcers   These occur on the foot and are a result of neurological disease.

Complications

Neglected ulcers may enlarge and become difficult to manage. Specific complications of venous ulcers include infection, lymphoedema, contact dermatitis (sensitivity to topical treatment) and, rarely, malignant change to squamous cell carcinoma.

Management

Treatment of underlying factors—obesity, cardiac failure, anaemia and arthritis—is helpful; other treatments include:

- Compression bandages to increase venous return and reduce oedema. This treatment is contraindicated in arterial ulcers, so Doppler studies must be carried out to exclude coexisting arterial disease before treatment is initiated.
- Elevation, exercise and diet to encourage normal blood flow.
- Topical therapy—antiseptics, desloughing agents, colloid or gel dressings, low-adherent bandages and medicated dressings, etc.
- Oral therapy—mainly analgesia, diuretics and antibiotics to treat secondary infection.
- Reconstructive vein surgery is only helpful in younger patients.

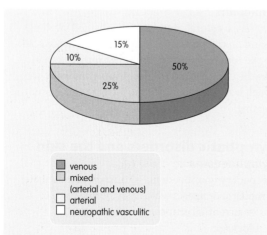

Fig. 8.19 Percentages of leg ulcers caused by venous disease, arterial disease, vasculitic disease or neuropathy.

Types of vasculitis	
	Clinical features
Henoch–Schönlein purpura	cutaneous signs accompanied by arthritis, abdominal pain and haematuria; it often follows a streptococcal infection and mainly affects children
nodular vasculitis	painful subcutaneous nodules are found on the lower legs
polyarteritis nodosa	an uncommon necrotizing vasculitis which affects middle-aged men; subcutaneous nodules develop, together with hypertension, renal failure and neuropathy
Wegener's granulomatosis	a rare and potentially fatal vasculitis; malaise, lung involvement and glomerulonephritis are accompanied by cutaneous vasculitis in 50% of patients
giant cell arteritis	affects the elderly, who present with scalp tenderness owing to temporal artery involvement which can cause scalp necrosis; prednisolone should be given, or sight may be lost

Fig. 8.20 Types of vasculitis.

Vasculitides and reactive erythema
Vasculitis

This term refers to inflammation of small to medium-sized blood vessels. It is commonly caused by circulating immune complexes, which lodge in the vessel walls and activate complement, causing damage to the vessel walls. The disease is usually detected through characteristic skin changes; palpable purpura over the legs and buttocks which is often painful. Vasculitis may affect only the skin, or may also spread to the joints, kidneys, lungs, gut and nervous system (Fig. 8.20). Cutaneous vasculitis is treated successfully with dapsone and oral steroids.

Erythema multiforme

This is an immune-mediated disease characterized by target lesions consisting of red rings with a pale central area that may blister. Mucosa may be involved. The disease is caused by circulating immune complexes that are deposited in blood vessel walls; histological features include a necrotic epidermis, oedema in the dermis, an inflammatory infiltrate and vasodilatation. Underlying causes include viral, bacterial and fungal infections, drugs, pregnancy and malignancy.

Management is by treatment of the underlying cause, and systemic steroids to modify the acute symptoms.

Erythema nodosum

This is an inflammation of subcutaneous fat, and causes painful red–blue nodules on the calves and shins. The female: male ratio is 3:1. Circulating immune complexes play an important role in the pathology, and the causes of erythema nodosum include infection, drugs, inflammatory bowel disease and sarcoidosis.

Joint pain and fever often accompany the nodules, and the disease usually clears spontaneously after 2 months, so treatment is rarely needed.

Sweet's disease

Sweet's disease is an acute, febrile, neutrophilic dermatosis which is characterized by red, annular plaques on the face and limbs. The lesions are accompanied by fever and a raised neutrophil count. Treatment with prednisolone is usually effective.

Graft-versus-host disease

When donor lymphocytes react against host tissue, it is known as graft-*versus*-host disease. It usually happens with bone marrow transplants, and causes fever, malaise and an acute eruption which may progress to toxic epidermal necrolysis. A skin biopsy helps with the diagnosis, and systemic steroids are usually necessary in management.

Disorders of pigmentation

Hypopigmentation
Vitiligo
Aetiology
This is a common acquired idiopathic disorder that leads to patchy, scaled macules (Plate 21). There is an association with pernicious anaemia, thyroid disease and Addison's disease, with about 30% of patients having a positive family history. The onset is usually between 10 and 30 years of age; the male: female ratio is 1:1, and it affects around 0.5% of the population.

Clinical features
Vitiligo may be precipitated by trauma or sunburn. The well-defined white macules are usually symmetrical, and frequently affect the hands, wrists, knees, neck and areas surrounding orifices.

Complications
As melanocytes are absent from lesions, care must be taken when skin is exposed to the sun.

Management
Camouflage cosmetics often prove unsatisfactory. Sunscreen helps to reduce the contrast between tanned skin and patches of vitiligo and, in darker skin, topical steroids may induce repigmentation. When vitiligo is nearly universal and very noticeable, induced depigmentation of remaining normal skin can be caused by 20% hydroquinone ointment.

Albinism
Albinism is an autosomal recessive disorder, which has a prevalence of 1 in 20 000. In this condition, melanocytes fail to synthesize melanin, leading to a lack of pigment in the skin. As well as the skin being pale, the hair is also white and the eye lacks pigmentation. Patients suffer from photophobia, nystagmus and poor sight. As the body has no protection against ultraviolet rays, the sun should be strictly avoided as the risk of squamous cell carcinoma is greatly increased.

Phenylketonuria
This is an autosomal recessive metabolic defect. The enzyme that converts phenylalanine into tyrosine is missing, which leads to the accumulation of metabolites in the brain. If left untreated, mental retardation and choreoathetosis occur. The hair and skin are fair because melanin synthesis is impaired. In addition, atopic eczema is common. Treatment is through a diet low in phenylalanine.

Hyperpigmentation
Freckles and lentigines
Freckles are small, light brown macules in sun-exposed areas, which darken upon intense ultraviolet exposure: they have normal numbers of melanocytes but, upon stimulation, synthesis of melanin is increased. They are common and are frequently seen on many faces over the summer months. Lentigines are dark brown macules that do not darken in the sun: they have an increased number of melanocytes. Lentigines may respond to cryotherapy.

Chloasma
Induced by pregnancy, or by taking the oral contraception pill, chloasma is a symmetrical facial pigmentation that often involves the forehead. It improves spontaneously, although sunscreens and camouflage cosmetics may help.

Drug-induced pigmentation
Pigmentation is a common effect of some drugs: phenothiazines, minocycline, amiodarone, clofazimine, chlorpromazine and antimalarials are all examples.

Other causes
Peutz–Jager syndrome causes lentigines to form around the lips, mucosa and fingers; these lesions are associated with the small bowel polyps of the disease. Addison's disease leads to melanogenesis through the production of excess adrenocorticotrophic hormone; pigmentation occurs on buccal mucosa, palmar creases, scars and flexures.

Blistering disorders

Pemphigus
Pathology
This potentially fatal disease affects both sexes equally, and usually presents between young and middle age. Ninety per cent of patients have

Fig. 8.21 Clinical patterns of pemphigoid.

Clinical patterns of pemphigoid	
Type of pemphigoid	Clinical features
bullous	large, tense blisters which usually affect elderly patients; trunk, limbs and flexures are affected; 10% of patients have oral lesions; may be preceded by urticaria; may be localized to a single site (Plate 22)
cicatricial	ocular and oral mucosa affected; post-pemphigoid scarring may affect sight
pemphigoid (herpes) gestationis	bullous lesions which are associated with pregnancy; clears after delivery but may recur in subsequent pregnancies

circulating IgG autoantibodies, which bind to the skin's intracellular matrix, inducing the release of proteolytic enzymes from adjacent keratinocytes. This subsequently causes intraepidermal split, resulting in thin-walled, fragile blisters. Pemphigus also has an association with other autoimmune disorders.

Clinical features

The disease presents in one-half of patients as an eruption of shallow blisters around the mouth; further lesions follow several months later on the face and trunk of all affected individuals. Blisters invariably rupture, so the disease tends to present with skin erosions more predominant than blisters. This is in contrast to pemphigoid where the blister walls are thicker and more robust.

Management

Systemic steroids, usually oral prednisolone, are given in a high dose to control the blistering, often in tandem with an immunosuppressive drug such as azathioprine. The steroids are continued at a lower dose for years; at this stage, the mortality and morbidity from steroid side effects and immunosuppression is equal to that of the disease itself.

Pemphigoid
Pathology

Affecting the elderly, pemphigoid is characterized by a chronic blistering eruption. The pathology is similar to that of pemphigus, with the exception that IgG antibodies are deposited at the basement membrane. There are circulating IgG antibodies present in 70% of patients. The damage is deeper than in pemphigus, and therefore the blisters have a thicker wall and are less likely to rupture.

Clinical features

Pemphigoid has three different patterns (Fig. 8.21).

Management

Oral prednisolone is prescribed at a lower dose than for pemphigus; the disease is self-limiting in half of all cases, and in the other half steroids can be stopped after 2 years. Azathioprine may also be prescribed.

Dermatitis herpetiformis
Pathology

This disease features a symmetrical eruption of pruritic blisters, and usually presents in the third or fourth decade. IgA can be seen at the dermal papillae when viewed through immunofluorescence; jejunal villus atrophy is also present in the majority of cases. The clinical signs respond well to a gluten-free diet, suggesting that gluten sensitivity is present in both the gut and the skin. The male: female ratio is 2:1.

Clinical features

The first sign of dermatitis herpetiformis is usually a group of small, itchy vesicles that erupt on the scalp, elbows, knees and buttocks. Although small bowel

Classification of ichthyoses			
Type of ichthyosis	Mode of inheritance	Incidence	Clinical features
ichthyosis vulgaris	autosomal dominant	1:250 births	disorder of epidermal cornification; onset between 1 and 4 years; granular layer is reduced or absent; dry skin with white scales on back and extensor surface of limbs; palmar and plantar markings are increased
X-linked ichthyosis	X-linked	1:7000 births	onset is early; scales are dark and widespread, with face, neck and scalp all involved; caused by deficiency of steroid sulphatase
bullous ichthyosiform erythroderma/ epidermolytic hyperkeratosis	autosomal dominant	1:100000	presents at birth; skin is red, moist and eroded in parts; erythema eventually replaced by scales; flexures particularly affected; hyperkeratosis develops in childhood
non-bullous ichthyosiform erythroderma	autosomal dominant	1:100000	presents at birth; collodion baby (newborn with tight, shiny skin causing feeding difficulties and ectropian); progresses to reddening and thickening of skin with fine, white scales; acanthosis is present

Fig. 8.22 Classification of ichthyoses.

pathology is often present, gastrointestinal symptoms are uncommon.

Inherited disorders of the skin

The ichthyoses
The ichthyoses are a group of disorders characterized by dry and scaly skin. The inheritence is autosomal dominant, with the exception of X-linked ichthyosis. The different types of ichthyoses are listed in Fig. 8.22.

Management
Regular use of emollients and moisturizing creams are the mainstays of treatment. Neonatal ichthyoses must be managed in a paediatric intensive care unit, as fluid losses may be huge and thermoregulation is disturbed.

Keratoderma
This disorder is characterized by gross hyperkeratosis of the palm and soles. It can also be acquired or inherited. Tylosis describes the typical diffuse pattern of hyperkeratosis found; in some patients it is associated with oesophageal carcinoma. Keratoma is treated with keratolytics such as salicylic acid ointment or urea cream.

Epidermolysis bullosa
Minor injury or trauma induces blistering in patients with epidermolysis bullosa. The disease ranges in severity from simple epidermolysis bullosa, the most common type, which features blisters limited to areas affected by friction, to junctional epidermolysis bullosa, a rare and potentially fatal disorder where large blisters are seen around the bodily orifices at birth. Dystrophic epidermolysis bullosa, which can be inherited in either an autosomal recessive or autosomal dominant manner, causes severe blistering and deformity of the nails. In the recessive form, oesophageal stricture and fusion of fingers and toes may occur. The disease is managed in specialized centres, and management relies on the avoidance of trauma and secondary infection.

Neurofibromatosis
Two forms of neurofibromatosis (NF) are recognized: NF1 (von Recklinghausen's peripheral neurofibromatosis) and NF2 (bilateral acoustic

central neurofibromatosis). The disease is inherited in an autosomal dominant fashion, and affects 1 in 3000 births. Skin involvement includes:

- *Café-au-lait* spots—light brown macules which appear in childhood; six or more macules more than 2.5 cm in diameter are diagnostic.
- Axillary freckling.
- Cutaneous neurofibromata—smooth sessile nodules which may become pedunculated; gross cutaneous nodular overgrowth leads to elephantiasis neuromatosa.
- Lisch nodules—pigmented hamartomas in the iris.
- Oral lesions.

In 10% of patients, IQ is 70 or less. In 6% the development of malignant sarcomas is a serious complication. Genetic counselling is an important part of management for patients; excision of nodules may also be appropriate.

Tuberous sclerosis

This rare disorder is passed on in an autosomal dominant manner, and is characterized by hamartomas in organs and bone. The cutaneous features include:

- Ash-leaf patches—present in infancy, these are ovoid or elongated hypopigmented macules which fluoresce under Wood's light.
- Adenoma sebaceum—an acne-like eruption of fibromatous papules around the nose in late childhood and adolescence.
- Periungual fibromata—fibrous pink projections which are visible under the nail folds.
- Shagreen patch—angiofibromatous plaque sited on the lower back.

Management involves genetic counselling, support groups and cauterization of adenoma sebaceum.

Xeroderma pigmentosum

Caused by defective repair of ultraviolet-damaged DNA, this condition is characterized by photosensitivity that begins in infancy. The persistent ultraviolet-damaged skin results in the development of skin tumours, which may cause death by 30 years. Affected patients must avoid sunlight. The condition is rare, and is autosomal recessive in inheritance.

Pseudoxanthoma elasticum

Pseudoxanthoma elasticum describes a group of four disorders caused by abnormalities in elastin and collagen. It is characterized by loose, wrinkled skin which contains papules and is most often found in the flexures of the neck. The disorders are inherited in both an autosomal dominant and recessive pattern.

Connective tissue disorders in the skin

Lupus erythematosus
Aetiology

Ninety per cent of patients with systemic lupus erythematosus (SLE) have circulating antinuclear antibodies detectable in their serum; antibodies to nucleolar and cytoplasmic antigens are also present. SLE is associated with HLA B8 and DR3; patients may also have T suppressor cell dysfunction.

In discoid lupus erythematosus, only 25% of patients have circulating antinuclear antibodies.

Pathology

The lesions of discoid lupus erythematosus are annular lesions with an erythematous margin, which show epidermal atrophy, hyperkeratosis and basal layer degeneration.

SLE shows similar lesions accompanied by dermal oedema, inflammation and occasionally vasculitis. Immunoglobulins and complement are deposited at the junction of the epidermis and dermis in the lesions (and in sun-exposed skin in SLE); they can be viewed by direct immunofluorescence.

Clinical features

Skin involvement, which is present in 75% of patients with SLE, includes:

- Erythematous butterfly rash present on the face.
- Photosensitivity.
- Discoid lesions.
- Diffuse alopecia.

Other systemic features (Fig. 8.23) must also be present to diagnose SLE.

Clinical features of discoid lupus erythematosus include the discoid lesions which appear on the face, scalp or hands. The lesions have a well-defined

Systemic features of systemic lupus erythematosus	
System	**Clinical features**
musculoskeletal	arthritis
	tenosynovitis
cardiovascular	pericarditis
	endocarditis
respiratory	pneumonitis
	effusion
	infarction
central nervous system	psychosis
renal	glomerulonephritis
blood	anaemia
	thrombocytopenia

Fig. 8.23 Systemic features of systemic lupus erythematosus.

margin, and are red, atrophic and scaly. Follicular keratin plugs may be seen.

Complications
In addition to the systemic features listed in Fig. 8.23, post-healing scarring may lead to alopecia and hypopigmentation in pigmented skin.

Management
Discoid lupus erythematosus can be treated with potent topical steroids; systemic therapy involves administration of chloroquine or immunosuppressive agents. Regular ophthalmic checks are also necessary to detect retinal involvement. Sunscreen is used to protect photosensitive skin.

Systemic sclerosis
This is a multisystem disorder which affects the skin in the following ways:
- Raynaud's phenomenon.
- Resorption of finger pulps.
- Tight, waxy and stiff skin on the fingers, forearms and calves.
- Perioral furrowing.
- Telangiectasia.

Systemic features, such as renal involvement, may cause death. Treatment is based mainly on education and support, although nifedipine may aid Raynaud's phenomenon.

Localized scleroderma (morphoea)
This disease, of unknown aetiology, causes tight bands of sclerosis on the skin, accompanied by indurated plaques. The lesions, which affect the trunk and limbs, eventually become pale and shiny, leading to hairless and atrophic areas of skin. The disease resolves spontaneously within a few months.

Dermatomyositis
The skin changes in dermatomyositis involve:
- Lilac–blue discoloration around the eyelids, cheek and forehead, with or without oedema.
- Blue–red papules or linear lesions on the dorsum of the hands, elbows and knees.
- Pigmentation.
- Nail fold telangiectasia.
- Photosensitivity.
- Contractures.

There is also an association with malignancy. Further information on dermatomyositis can be found on p. 46, Chapter 2.

Skin manifestations of systemic disease

Skin signs of endocrine and metabolic disease
Diabetes mellitus
Cutaneous signs of diabetes mellitus include:
- Candida or bacterial infection—caused by poorly controlled blood sugar levels.
- Ulcers—caused by neuropathy or arteriopathy of the feet.
- Eruptive xanthomas—associated with secondary hyperlipidaemia.
- Diabetic dermatopathy—pigmented scars on the shins which are associated with diabetic microangiography.
- Necrobiosis lipoidica—yellow–red atrophic plaques seen on shins.
- Granuloma annulare—popular annular lesions found on hands, feet and face which fade within a year.

Thyroid disease

Cutaneous signs of thyroid disease are listed in Fig. 8.24.

Hyperlipidaemia

Cutaneous signs of hyperlipidaemia usually involve xanthomatous deposits. The xanthomas are controlled by treating the underlying hyperlipidaemia.

Cutaneous signs of thyroid disease	
Thyrotoxicosis	**Myxoedema**
skin becomes soft and pink	alopecia
hyperhidrosis	coarse and thickened hair
alopecia	skin becomes dry, yellow and puffy
pigmentation	asteotic eczema
onycholysis	xanthomas
clubbing	
pretibial myxoedema	
palmar erythema	

Fig. 8.24 Cutaneous signs of thyroid disease.

Skin signs of nutritional deficiency and gastrointestinal disease
Malnutrition

Different forms of malnutrition lead to varying skin manifestations (Fig. 8.25).

Inflammatory bowel disease

The skin changes in Crohn's disease and ulcerative colitis vary (Fig. 8.26).

Skin signs of malignancy
Acanthosis nigricans

An uncommon condition associated with malignancy, acanthosis nigricans is characterized by thickening and pigmentation of the skin around the flexures and neck. The skin becomes velvety and papillomatous, and warty lesions develop around the mouth, on the palms and soles. Rarely, the condition may present in childhood; this is an inherited form of the disorder and is not associated with malignancy. When presenting in older patients, a carcinoma, which is most commonly of the gastrointestinal tract, must be excluded.

Paget's disease of the nipple

A unilateral plaque-like lesion that forms on the nipple areola commonly indicates the spread of an intraductal carcinoma of the breast; an eruption resembling eczema around the perineum or axilla may be caused by intraepidermal malignant spread. With both presentations, a skin biopsy should be performed to confirm the diagnosis.

Cutaneous signs of malnutrition		
Deficiency	**Disease**	**Cutaneous signs**
protein	kwashiorkor	altered pigmentation desquamation ulcers (with brown/red hair in Afro-Caribbeans)
vitamin C	scurvy	purpura swollen, bleeding gums Indurated (woody) oedema
nicotinic acid	pellagra	scaly dermatitis pigmentation
iron		alopecia koilonychia pruritus angular cheilitis

Fig. 8.25 Cutaneous signs of malnutrition.

Skin changes in inflammatory bowel disease	
Inflammatory bowel disease	**Cutaneous signs**
Crohn's disease	perianal abscesses sinuses fistulae erythema nodosum Sweet's disease pyoderma gangrenosum aphthous stomatitis glossitis
ulcerative colitis	erythema nodosum Sweet's disease pyoderma gangrenosum

Fig. 8.26 Skin changes in inflammatory bowel disease.

Erythema gyratum repens

This is an extremely rare disorder that is caused by malignancy, usually of the lung. Scaly concentric rings, which resemble wood-grain and which rapidly change pattern, appear on the body.

Necrolytic migratory erythema

This disorder is characterized by serpiginous erythematous plaques which usually begin in the perineum. The eruption is caused by a glucagon-secreting tumour of the pancreas, and is associated with weight loss, anaemia, diabetes and angular stomatitis.

Secondary tumour deposits in skin

Skin metastases often present late in a diagnosis of malignancy, and so carry a poor prognostic value. They usually appear as firm, pink nodules and are found most commonly on the scalp, umbilicus and trunk. Tumour tissue may metastasize to the skin from the following primary tumours:
- Breast.
- Gastrointestinal tract.
- Ovary.
- Lung.
- Malignant melanomas, lyphomas and leukaemias may also involve the skin.

Conditions occasionally associated with malignancy

In addition, other conditions which may be associated with malignancy, but also with more benign diagnoses, include:
- Generalized pruritis.
- Acquired ichthyosis.
- Hyperpigmentation.
- Pyoderma gangrenosum.
- Dermatomyositis.
- Erythroderma.
- Hypertrichosis.

A careful history and examination should be obtained from all patients who present with the above but who have no obvious underlying cause.

Skin changes in pregnancy

The following skin changes commonly occur in pregnancy:
- Increased pigmentation (especially in the nipples).
- Proliferation of melanocytic naevi.
- Development of spider naevi and abdominal striae (stretchmarks).
- Pruritus.
- Telogen effluvium may also occur in the postpartum period.

Drug-induced skin disorders

Most drugs will list an eruption as a side effect, and drug reactions are both common and frequent. Beware of a patient who claims to be 'allergic' to a drug; true allergies are uncommon, and a mild eruption may be the cause of such a statement.

Mechanisms of drug-induced skin disorders

There are several mechanisms that produce a drug-induced skin disorder (Fig. 8.27).
The four most important drug reactions are listed in Fig. 8.28.

Fig. 8.27 Mechanisms that produce drug-induced disorders.

Mechanisms that produce drug-induced disorders	
Mechanism	**Example**
excessive therapeutic effect	an overdose of anticoagulants may lead to subcutaneous bleeding and purpura
pharmacological side effects	dry lips and mucosa resulting from use of isotretinoin; bone marrow suppression with use of cytotoxic drugs
hypersensitivity	true allergy; may occur via any of the four skin type reactions
skin deposition of drug or metabolites	gold
facilitative effect	use of a drug upsets biological balance; use of wide-spectrum antibiotics may result in *Candida*, etc.
idiosyncratic reaction	reaction peculiar to individual

Important drug reactions			
	Toxic erythema	**Fixed drug eruption**	**Toxic epidermal necrolysis**	**Psoriasiform and bullous eruptions**
---	---	---	---	---
aetiology	caused by drugs (ampicillin, sulphonamides and carbamazepine), scarlet fever or viral infection	quinine, phenolphthalein and sulphonamides often responsible	drug-induced epidermal necrosis	lithium and chloroquine exacerbate psoriasis; β-blockers, gold and methyl dopa may precipitate an eruption
clinical features	eruption which may be morbilliform or urticarial; may be accompanied by fever or followed by skin peeling; eruption affects trunk more than limbs	round, red–purple plaques which occur on same site each time drug is taken; lesions may blister and cause pigmentation	intraepidermal split in skin: skin red, swollen and separates as in scold	psoriatic eruption
complications	recurrence of symptoms drug taken to alleviate	recurrence of symptoms drug taken to alleviate	problems in fluid and electrolyte balance; mortality around 25%	recurrence of symptoms drug taken to alleviate
management	stop precipitating drug; clears up within 1–2 weeks	stop precipitating drug	in-hospital management in intensive care unit	stop precipitating drug; emollients if necessary

Fig. 8.28 Important drug reactions.

- Differentiate between vesicles, pustules, bullae and blisters
- Describe the pathology of dyskeratosis.
- List the five different types of psoriasis and describe the differences between them.
- Name the topical treatments for eczema.
- Describe the different pathways through which histamine is released in urticaria.
- List the physical features of Reiter's disease.
- Name the condition which sunlight aggravates.
- List the staphylococcal infections that affect the skin.
- Describe the course of an infection with herpes simplex.
- List the factors which predispose to *Candida albicans*.
- Describe the treatments available for scabies.
- Describe the different types of naevi and their distribution.
- Name the risk factors for malignant melanoma.
- List the differences between basal cell and squamous cell carcinoma.
- What is the classification of alopecia?
- List the causes of hirsuitism.
- What is Raynaud's phenomenon?
- Describe the differing pathologies of leg ulcers.
- List the cutaneous forms of malnutrition.
- Name the skin changes in pregnancy.

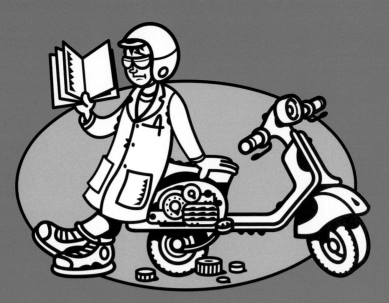

CLINICAL ASSESSMENT

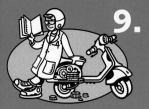

9. Common Presentations of Muscle, Bone and Skin Diseases

Common presenting complaints of the musculoskeletal system

Monoarticular arthritis

Monoarticular arthritis is a common presenting joint complaint (Fig. 9.1). It can be classified into acute and chronic forms.

Acute monoarticular arthritis

Ninety per cent of cases of acute monoarticular arthritis are caused by one of several causes. These include:
- Sepsis, e.g. from staphylococcal infection.
- Crystal-induced, e.g. gout.
- Trauma.

Chronic monoarticular arthritis

If monoarticular arthritis persists for more than 2 months, it is referred to as chronic (Figs 9.2 and 9.3). The causes of chronic monoarticular arthritis include those of both acute monoarticular arthritis and polyarticular arthritis.

Polyarticular arthritis

Polyarticular arthritis is inflammation of more than one joint. It can be classified into an acute or chronic form: when the condition lasts for more than 6–8 weeks, it is described as chronic.

Causes of acute polyarthritis include:
- Rheumatoid arthritis.
- The spondylarthritides.
- Viral arthritis (e.g. rubella and hepatitis B).
- Systemic lupus erythematosus.
- Acute rheumatic fever.

Causes of chronic polyarthritis include:
- Osteoarthritis.
- Rheumatoid arthritis.
- Some of the spondylarthritides (e.g. psoriatic arthritis, Reiter's syndrome).
- Sarcoid arthritis.
- Systemic lupus erythematosus.

The diagnosis of polyarticular arthritis is aided by a thorough history, as this type of arthritis is often associated with extra-articular features that would indicate the most likely cause (Fig. 9.4).

Back pain

There are four common types of presenting back pain (Fig. 9.5):
- Inflammatory—stiffness after inactivity, with pain relieved by use.
- Mechanical—pain that is aggravated by use. Can be associated with symptoms such as locking.
- Neuropathic/referred—pain that is difficult to localize: it may be dermatomal, aggravated by moving the source of the referred pain, rather than the actual site of pain, and may be relieved by rubbing.
- Destructive—progressive pain that may be worse at night. Destructive pain usually indicates serious pathology.

Inflammatory back pain is caused by:
- Ankylosing spondylitis.

Mechanical back pain is caused by:
- Acute back strain (damage to either ligaments or muscles).
- Postural damage.
- Prolapsed intervertebral disc.
- The spondylarthritides.
- Congenital hemivertebrae or sacrilization.
- Fibromyalgia.
- Spinal stenosis (accompanied by non-referred pain down into legs).
- Cauda equina syndrome (accompanied by sciatica to below knee).

Neuropathic/referred back pain is caused by:
- Nerve root compression caused by prolapsed intervertebral disc; tumour of a vertebra, nerve or fibro-osseous canal through which the nerve root leaves the spinal column; spondylosis, abscess or, less commonly, congenital diastematomyelia and tuberculosis.

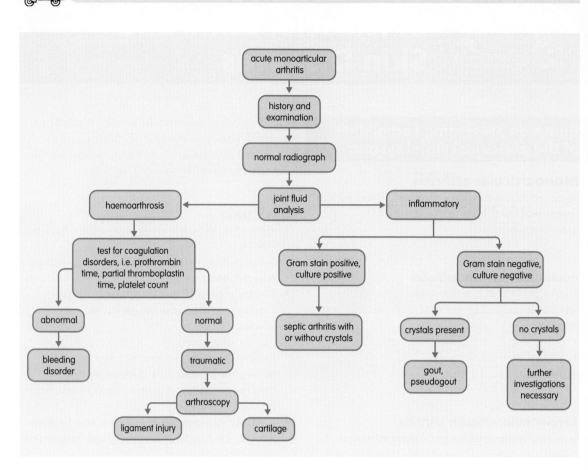

Fig. 9.1 Stages involved in determining a diagnosis of monoarticular arthritis.

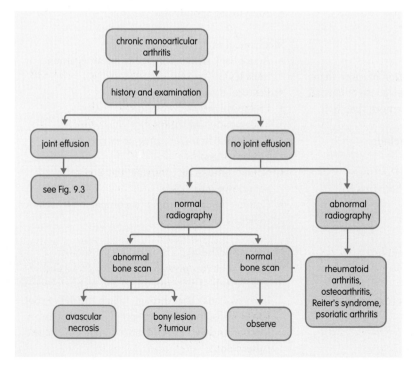

Fig. 9.2 Stages involved in determining a diagnosis of chronic monoarticular arthritis with no joint effusion.

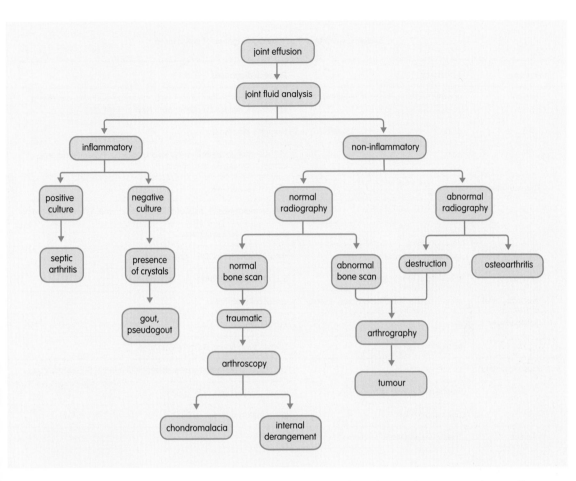

Fig. 9.3 Stages involved in determining a diagnosis of chronic monoarticular arthritis with an associated joint effusion.

- Referred pain caused by intracranial tunour, pelvic mass, osteoarthritis of the hip, retroperitoneal or urogenital pathology, aortic dissection.

Destructive back pain is caused by:
- Malignancy.
- Metabolic disturbance (i.e. osteoporosis).
- Sepsis.

Muscle weakness

Patients with muscle weakness can be divided into two categories: those with 'true' muscle weakness and those with normal muscle strength.

Muscle weakness may result from disorders occurring anywhere along the motor cortex, corticospinal tracts, anterior horn cells, peripheral nerves, neuromuscular junction and muscle.

(Only the last two of these sites will be considered here.)

Diagnosis of muscle weakness is aided by considering the distribution of the weakness (Fig. 9.6).

Further investigations, involving electromyography and muscle biopsy, are required for the definitive diagnosis of muscular weakness.

Common presenting complaints of the skin

Eruptions

Eruptions are generally classified according to their site on the body. They can occur on or in the:

Systemic symptoms that may aid diagnosis of polyarthritis		
System	**Symptoms**	**Possible diagnoses**
general	unexplained weight loss, fatiguability	systemic lupus erythematosus (SLE), rheumatoid arthritis, ankylosing spondylitis, Reiter's syndrome, sarcoidosis
eyes	dryness	Sjögren's syndrome
	pain	SLE, rheumatoid arthritis, ankylosing spondylitis, Reiter's syndrome, Behçet 's syndrome, sarcoidosis
mucocutaneous	dry mouth	Sjögren's syndrome
	rash	SLE, dermatomyositis, psoriasis, Reiter's syndrome, Sjögren's syndrome
	nail pitting	psoriasis, Reiter's syndrome
	subcutaneous nodules	rheumatoid arthritis, SLE, gout, sarcoidosis
respiratory	shortness of breath, pleuritic pain	SLE, rheumatoid arthritis
gastrointestinal	symptoms of inflammatory bowel disease	enteropathic arthritis
genitourinary	dysuria	Reiter's syndrome
	painful intercourse	Sjögren's syndrome, Behçet's syndrome
musculoskeletal	muscle weakness	polymyositis, dermatomyositis, rheumatoid arthritis, SLE, sarcoidosis
	muscle tenderness, stiffness	rheumatoid arthritis, SLE
	joint symptoms	inflammatory arthritis
nervous	headaches and visual problems	SLE

Fig. 9.4 Systemic symptoms that may aid in a diagnosis of polyarthritis.

- Face.
- Scalp.
- Feet.
- Hands.
- Anogenital folds.
- Axillae.
- Glans penis.

Facial eruptions are caused by:
- Acne vulgaris.
- Rosacea.
- Atopic dermatitis.
- Contact dermatitis.
- Systemic lupus erythematosus.
- Perioral dermatitis.

Scalp eruptions are caused by:
- Pityriasis capitis.
- Seborrhoeic dermatitis.
- Psoriasis.

- Tinea capitis.
- Discoid lupus erythematosus.

Eruptions of the hands and feet are caused by:
- Tinea.
- Psoriasis.
- Contact dermatitis.
- Endogenous dermatitis.

Anogenital fold eruptions are caused by:
- Candidosis (in females).
- Tinea (in males).
- Seborrhoeic dermatitis.
- Psoriasis.

Eruptions in the axillae are caused by:
- Seborrhoeic dermatitis.
- Psoriasis.
- Contact dermatitis.

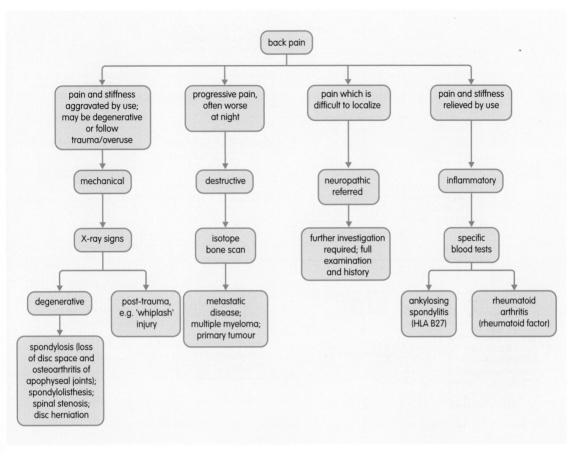

Fig. 9.5 Stages involved in determining diagnoses of mechanical, destructive, neurogenic/referred and inflammatory back pains.

Eruptions of the glans penis are caused by:
- Candidosis.
- Psoriasis.
- Lichen planus.
- Scabies.
- Intraepidermal carcinoma.

Blistering

Blistering can occur at several levels of cleavage in the skin. There are common and uncommon causes of blistering.

Common causes of blistering include:
- Friction.
- Insect bites and stings.
- Burns.
- Impetigo.
- Contact dermatitis.
- Drugs.

Uncommon causes of blistering include:
- Pemphigus vulgaris.
- Pemphigus foliaceus.
- Bullous pemphigoid.
- Cicatricial pemphigoid.
- Pemphigoid gestationis.
- Dermatitis herpetiformis.
- Linear IgA disease.

Hypopigmented lesions

These are classified into generalized hypopigmentation and patchy hypopigmentation (with or without inflammation, atrophy or induration).

The causes of generalized hypopigmentation include:
- Phenylketonuria.
- Hypopituitarism.
- Albinism.

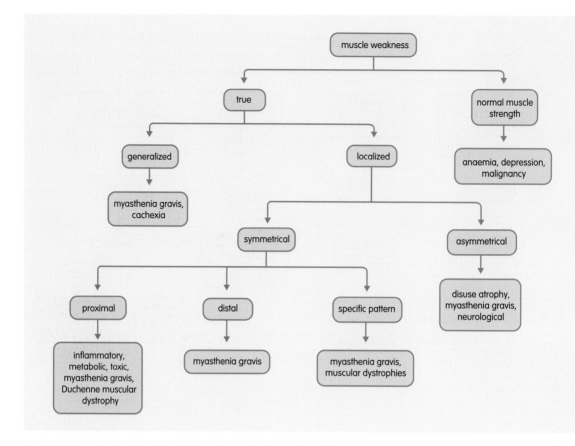

Fig. 9.6 Stages involved in determining a diagnosis of muscle weakness.

The causes of patchy hypopigmention include:
- Vitiligo.
- Achromic naevus.
- Piebaldism.
- Waardenburg's syndrome.
- Ash-leaf macules.
- Chemical-induced.

The causes of patchy hypopigmentation with inflammation include:
- Tinia versicolor.
- Leprosy.
- Pityriasis alba.

The common causes of patchy hypopigmentation with atrophy or induration include:
- Radiodermatitis.
- Morphoes.

- Lichen sclerosus.
- Burns.

Features which assist in the diagnosis of hypopigmentation can be found in Fig. 9.7.

Hyperpigmented lesions

Hyperpigmented lesions can be split into hyperpigmented naevi and all other causes.

A naevus consists of non-functional cells and may be defined as a congenitally determined tissue defect.

Hyperpigmented naevi include:
- Congenital melanocytic naevus.
- Acquired melanocytic naevus.
- Mongolian spot.
- Acquired blue naevus.
- Spitz naevus.

Fig. 9.7 Systemic symptoms that may aid in a diagnosis of hypopigmentation.

Systemic symptoms that may aid in a diagnosis of hypopigmentation	
Cause of hypopigmentation	Clinical signs
vitiligo	pernicious anaemia; Addison's disease; thyroid disease
albinism	white hair; lack of pigmentation in iris; poor sight; photophobia; nystagmus
phenylketonuria	if untreated, mental retardation; choreoathetosis

Fig. 9.8 Stages involved in determining a diagnosis of leg ulceration.

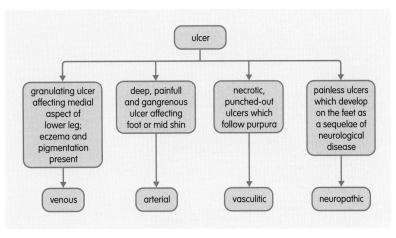

- Halo naevus.
- Pigmented hairy epidermal naevus.

The other causes of hyperpigmentation include:
- Tanning.
- Post-inflammatory pigmentation.
- Hypoadrenalism.
- Hyperoestrogenism.
- Chloasma.
- Metabolic causes (e.g. cirrhosis, haematochromatosis).
- Chemicals and drugs.
- Freckles.
- *Café-au-lait* macules.
- Peutz–Jegher syndrome.
- Simple lentigo.
- Actinic (solar) lentigo.

Skin ulcers

Ulcers are skin defects caused by the loss of the entire epidermis and dermis due to trauma, sloughing or necrosis. They may be venous, arterial or neuropathic (Fig. 9.8).

Hair loss or gain

Hair loss (or alopecia) can be classified as diffuse localized, localized scarring and localized non-scarring (Fig. 9.9). Excess hair is usually termed hirsutism (excessive female growth of terminal hair in a male pattern) and hypertrichosis (excessive growth of terminal hair in a non-androgenic pattern) (Fig. 9.10).

Causes of hirsutism are split into five categories:
- Pituitary.
- Adrenal.
- Ovarian.
- Iatrogenic.
- Idiopathic.

Hypertrichosis is classified into localized and generalized.

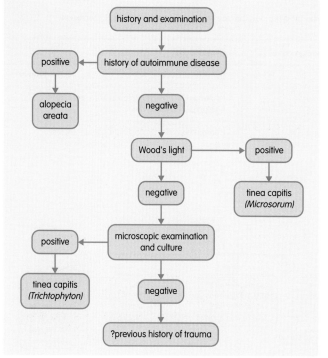

Fig. 9.9 (A) Stages involved in determining a diagnosis of localized non-scarring alopecia.

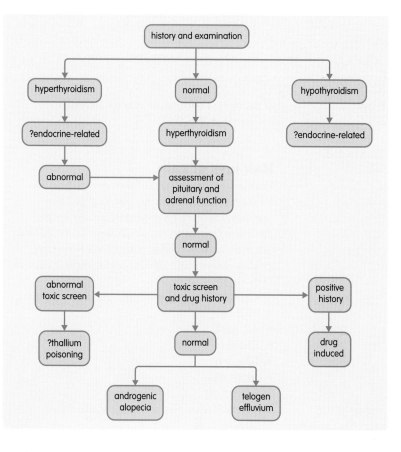

Fig. 9.9 (B) Stages involved in determining a diagnosis of diffuse non-scarring alopecia.

Fig. 9.10 Stages involved in determining a diagnosis of hirsutism/hypertrichosis.

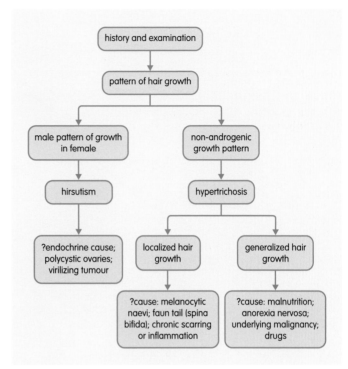

- Name the causes of acute polyarthritis.
- List the four types of back pain.
- Name the causes of anogenital fold skin eruptions.
- What are the common causes of blistering?
- Which naevi are classified as hyperpigmented?

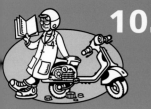

10. History and Examination

Taking a history

Things to remember when taking a history
First contact
When meeting a patient for the first time, you should:

- Always introduce yourself by name and status, e.g. medical student.
- Mention the consultant's name, as this reassures the patient you are genuine and provides a common link between you.
- Check that the patient is sitting/lying comfortably before you begin.
- Try to put the patient at ease by sitting a reasonable distance away, and take the interview at a relaxed pace; do not worry about any silences between your questions.
- Dress appropriately, as many patients feel uncomfortable giving personal details to young people—especially if they are scruffy and unshaven! Therefore you will obtain better histories if you are suitably dressed.

The patient's surroundings
Try to observe the patient walking into the consulting room, as any disabilities can be seen more easily during movement.

On the ward, look around the bedside for any clues to the patient's level of disability, or see what the patient brings to the consultation, e.g. an inhaler, oxygen, walking stick/frame, sputum pot, reading material, etc.

The patient's appearance and behaviour
Everyone subconsciously makes assumptions about people based on their appearance—you should try to be aware of someone's physical features and clothing.

Watch the patient's behaviour for clues while taking the history, e.g. is there agitation or distress, can you see any tremors, abnormal behaviour, or abnormal eye and body movements?

Structure of a history for muscles
Presenting complaint
When a patient presents with a muscular complaint, determine the symptoms experienced by the patient, e.g. muscle weakness. This should be recorded in the patient's own words, rather than medical jargon.

History of presenting complaint
Nature of complaint
A patient with proximal weakness, i.e. weakness involving the upper parts of the arms and legs, will describe difficulties in:

- Getting out of the bath.
- Ascending stairs.
- Getting up out of chairs.

A patient with weakness of the hands may find it difficult to brush the hair.

Distal weakness in the limbs is suggested by:
- Difficulties in opening jars.
- Footdrop, in some cases.
- Tripping over rugs.

Patients with myotonia may present with an inability to let go upon shaking hands.

Onset of complaint
The onset of a muscular complaint will depend on the patient's lifestyle, e.g. athletes will notice a change in muscle strength at an early stage.

Onset is usually gradual in the muscular dystrophies, inflammatory myopathies and myasthenia gravis. However, the inflammatory myopathies, periodic paralyses and myasthenia gravis may also present suddenly.

The age of onset is also important, e.g. an underlying malignancy should be excluded in elderly patients presenting with myasthenic symptoms.

Pattern of symptoms
In the case of the inflammatory myopathies and muscular dystrophies, weakness is progressive as opposed to intermittent, as in the periodic paralyses.

Precipitating or relieving factors

Exercise: An important precipitating factor, particularly in the metabolic myopathies, periodic paralyses and myasthenia gravis, is exercise. The symptoms of Lambert–Eaton myasthenic syndrome improve with exercise.

Temperature: The myotonia associated with Thomsen's disease and paramyotonia congenita is worse in the cold.

Other associated symptoms

Muscle pain may be a feature of the viral myalgias (very common), metabolic myopathies and alcohol excess myopathy. Dysphagia, dysarthria and respiratory symptoms may be present, depending on the muscle groups involved.

Bone pain is suggestive of osteomalacia-induced myopathy.

Past medical history

A history of HIV infection should be excluded, as the infection itself, or its treatment, e.g. zidovudine, may be responsible for myopathy.

Drug history

A range of drugs, e.g. steroids, cholesterol-lowering agents, chloroquine and lithium, can result in proximal myopathy.

Family history

If other family members are affected by a muscular disorder, a family tree should be constructed. The sex of the patient and affected relatives should be noted.

Social history

Alcohol: When ascertaining the patient's social history, you should ask about alcohol consumption. How many units does the patient consume and how often?

Sexual practices: You should try to establish if the patient is at risk of infection with HIV.

Exercise: Ask the patient about exercise, as this can help exclude disuse atrophy.

Systems review

You should try to establish whether the patient has symptoms of other connective tissue disorders, e.g. dark urine is suggestive of myoglobinuria and is associated with metabolic myopathies and acute alcoholic myopathy.

Does the patient have symptoms of endocrine disease, e.g. Cushing's syndrome or thyroid abnormalities?

Summary of patient's history

Always write a summary of a patient's history when clerking. When presenting the case, begin with a brief overview of the patient: 'Mr Jones is a 63-year-old man with rheumatoid arthritis who presents with exacerbation of his joint pain'. This helps the listener to focus on the relevant parts of the subsequent history.

Structure of a history for joints
Presenting complaint

Presenting complaints of joint disorders are usually:
- Pain.
- Swelling.
- Stiffness.
- Deformity.
- Loss of function.
- Numbness or paraesthesia.

For each of these, ask when and where the symptom started, if anything makes it better or worse, and how daily life is affected.

History of presenting complaint
Past medical history

Enquire about any previous injuries, as some may predispose to new disorders.

Family history

Genetic disorders should be considered in joint complaints.

Social history

Information about the patient's social life, e.g. occupation and hobbies, can help to assist in a diagnosis.

The 'red flags' of musculoskeletal history—those signs which must not be missed—include:
- Pain which wakes the patient up at night.
- Severe, progressive pain which is unremitting.
- Pain accompanied by weight loss.

These features point to a diagnosis of malignancy or sepsis; both must be excluded.

Structure of a history for skin
Presenting complaint
Presenting complaints of skin disorders are usually:
- Rash.
- Itching.
- Psychological distress (severe acne, extensive psoriasis, etc.).

History of presenting complaint
For each of these, ask when and where the symptom started, if anything makes it better or worse (e.g. sunlight), and how daily life is affected. With lesions, ask how and where the problem started, how it first looked and if it has changed in appearance. Bear in mind that having a skin disease can be very stressful for patients, who frequently de-value their own body image and thus suffer psychological distress. However minor the problem may seem to you, it may genuinely cause the patient intense distress and psychosocial impairment.

Past medical history
Enquire about any previous skin disease or atopic syndromes such as hay fever, asthma or eczema. Coexisting medical conditions may also involve the skin.

Drug history
Skin eruptions are one of the common side effects of many prescribed drugs, so take a full drug history. Also enquire about over-the-counter drugs and alternative medicines (such as herbal remedies), as they may have been used inappropriately and may cause irritant or allergic reactions.

Family history
As well as a genetic component to skin disorders (tuberous sclerosis, psoriasis, etc.), disorders caused by infestation and infection may also have affected family members recently. A full family history is therefore important.

Social history
Occupational factors often lead to skin complaints; chemical engineers with contact dermatitis, health workers with latex allergies, etc. An enquiry into foreign travel may elicit the cause of an infection, as well as point towards a reaction to strong sunlight. A sexual history and contact tracing may be necessary in some disorders: HIV, syphilis, gonorrhoea, vulval disorders, etc.

Communication skills

The dynamic of effective communication
Being able to communicate effectively with patients is one of the most essential skills a clinician can have; after all, the history makes up 90% of the diagnosis. Encouraging the patient to tell their story, gently dissuading them from irrelevancies and being able to piece together the whole story smoothly and view it in context of the patient's life seems an awesome task at first, but one which comes with time and practice.

Communication is a dynamic process, and one which is affected by the behaviour and character of both doctor and patient. As a medical student you are faced with handicaps you must understand and deal with before you can establish effective communication with patients, namely:
- The perception that professionals don't show emotions.
- The pressure to feel as if you must be in control of the situation.
- The thought that you must have the answers and be able to act.
- The pressure from peers and tutors to match up to expectations.

Identifying and coping with pressures is the first step in effective communication.

The other factors that affect the doctor–patient dynamic are listed in Fig. 10.1. If they are ignored, a communication gap can ensue, i.e. you may think you've imparted appropriate information to the patient, but you may be unaware that the patient has not understood it.

Body language
Traditional images of doctors facing patients across huge desks are now outdated. To put the patient at ease, the doctor must appear approachable. If the patient is lying on a bed, sit down to take their history. If they are sitting in a chair on the wards, perch yourself on the bed next to them. Similarly, if taking a history from a child, get down on their level. Don't be afraid to kneel on the floor!

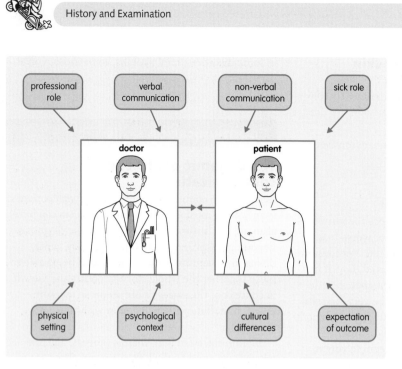

Fig. 10.1 Factors affecting the doctor–patient dynamic.

Non-verbal communication

A large proportion of communication between two people does not involve words. The most important components of non-verbal communication are:

- Eye contact.
- Facial expression.
- Non-verbal encouragement.

Eye contact

One of the most important tools in communicating is establishing and maintaining eye contact. It plays an important role in establishing trust, obviously an important part of the doctor–patient relationship. Although maintaining eye contact and taking notes is a difficult balancing act, try not to look away from the patient for too long to avoid appearing disinterested.

Facial expression

Most emotion is expressed through facial movements; you can generally tell if a patient is depressed or ecstatic just by looking at their face. By studying the patient's facial expression you can appropriately match your mood to theirs during the consultation.

Non-verbal encouragement

This may range from nodding your head while a patient relates their story, to uttering non-verbal sounds such as 'hmmmm' and 'uh-huh' during the history. Interaction with the patient while they are speaking encourages them to open up and disclose more information.

Verbal communication
Questioning the patient

There's a particular art to choosing which type of question to ask, and when to avoid asking at all. Questions are classified into open questions, closed questions and leading questions.

Open questions

These questions are the best kind with which to start a history, as they allow the patient to talk, e.g. 'Could you tell me about the pain you've been having?' Listening to the patient's explanation will then lead you into a specific line of questioning. There are times when you need to break in with closed questions, however, to clarify specific points and control the length of the interview.

Closed questions

These questions encourage the patient to give a short, often one-word answer, and are helpful in eliciting facts, e.g. 'Does the pain wake you up at night?'

Leading questions

These questions should be avoided as they tend to steer the patient towards an answer, e.g. 'I expect this is the worst pain you've ever had?' It's much better to substitute a closed question instead, e.g. 'On a scale of 1 to 10, with 1 being no pain and 10 being the worst pain you've ever had, where would you place this?'

Empathizing with the patient

Demonstrating appropriate empathy during the history-taking will often encourage the patient to disclose information they wouldn't otherwise have stated. Empathy can be expressed simply, e.g. 'I understand how hard this must be for you' or can have a hidden agenda, e.g. 'Are you worried that this might be anything in particular?' In this way it is easy to reassure and relax the patient if they have groundless fears.

Prompting the patient

Although it is better to avoid interrupting while taking a history, sometimes it is appropriate to prompt a patient into a new line of questioning, e.g. 'And could you tell me what happened when you got the pain?' Another way of subtly redirecting the patient's train of thought is to repeat what they've already told you, e.g. 'So, if I could just recap what you've said...?'

Clarifying statements

Don't be afraid to question the patient more closely about their symptoms; if they tell you they have lumbago, is that lower back pain or pain radiating down to their knee? If they're having problems with their waterworks, is that constipation, urinary incontinence or perianal numbness?

If you're having problems assessing your communication skills, ask a patient and their consultant for permission to tape yourself taking a history from them. Listen to it and analyse your performance; you may be surprised at how you come across! It is also useful to practise scenarios with friends using timed role play when revising for clinical exams.

General examination of joints and the musculoskeletal system

Clinical examination

It is useful to approach the clinical examination of a patient in a systematic way so that important signs are not missed. All findings should be recorded and summarized. You should make sure the patient feels at ease and explain instructions clearly. Remember to look at the patient's face when eliciting signs and explain your findings at the end of the examination.

When examining limbs, start with either the upper or lower limb, and examine both limbs at once. It is easier to find an abnormality when there is a normal structure available for comparison.

Joints should be examined from the front, back and sides.

General examination of joints

The routine for examination of joints involves:
- Inspection.
- Palpation.
- Movement.
- Stressing.

This routine is usually followed by X-rays. It is advisable to examine painful areas last.

Inspection

The area for examination should be adequately exposed and viewed in good light. Note should be made of:
- The alignment of the bones—look for any deformities and shortening. Subluxation is present when displaced parts of the joint surfaces remain partially in contact.
- The position of the joint and limbs at rest—is there any unusual posture?
- The joint contour to check for swellings and abnormalities—are there any effusions and general or localized swellings?
- Scars or sinuses—are these from operations (linear scar), injury (irregular scar) or suppurations (broad, adherent puckered scar)?
- The skin.
- Muscle wasting.

The terms valgus and varus refer to the deviation of the limb distal to a joint—away from or towards the midline, respectively (see Chapter 2).

197

Palpation

Palpation includes both measurements and sensibility.

Preferably with warm hands, initially feel gently and then more firmly. You should consider:

- Skin temperature changes by noting any warmth (inflammation, rapidly growing tumour) or coldness in local areas.
- Swellings—are they bony abnormalities or diffuse joint swellings?
- Areas of tenderness—these should be precisely located to relate them to anatomical structures.
- Pain—check the patient's face for apprehension.

Measurements

Measurements of limb length and width are carried out when there are discrepancies between both sides. Length is especially important in the lower limbs, and width provides information on muscle wasting, soft tissue swellings or bone thickenings. Refer to fixed points when measuring and check that the findings are reproducible.

Sensibility

An area's sensibility to light touch and to pinpricks should be assessed. You should precisely locate areas of blunting or loss of sensation.

Movement

Both active and passive ranges of movement must be recorded for the directional planes of each joint. These should be equal: passive movement exceeds active when there is muscle paralysis, or torn or slack tendons.

A goniometer, a hinged rod with a protractor in the centre, is the instrument used for measuring the range of joint movements. Measurements usually begin from the joint positioned in extension, and movement is expressed as degrees of flexion from this point.

The normal ranges of joint movements need to be fully understood, and both sides tested. Restricted movements in all directions are suggestive of arthritis, while restrictive movements in some directions and free movements in others suggest a mechanical disorder.

Pain and crepitations must also be noted. Joint crepitations are coarse and diffuse while those of the tendons are fine and located to the tendon sheath.

Stressing

Straining of the ligaments provides information about joint stability. When assessing ligaments, the muscles moving the joint must be relaxed as contracted ones can conceal unstable ligaments.

Pain is usually present in ligaments that have been recently injured, while those that are torn or stretched produce an increased range of movements.

The strength of muscle can be tested by asking the patient to move a joint against the resistance of the examiner. Muscle weakness is easily detectable and a very important sign of motor impairment.

Muscle power is graded according to the Medical Research Council as:

- 0, no power.
- 1, a flicker of contraction.
- 2, slight power to move a joint with gravity eliminated—this is when the joint is supported, usually by the edge of a bed or manually by the observer.
- 3, sufficient power to move a joint against gravity.
- 4, power to move a joint against gravity plus added resistance.
- 5, normal muscle power.

X-rays

Anteroposterior and lateral views of a joint are routinely taken during an X-ray examination, except for the hands and feet. Bones, joints and soft tissues are also examined.

Bones

It is important to observe the general outline of bones—are there areas of increased or decreased density?

Joints

When assessing joints you should check for:

- Narrowing of the joint space, indicating loss of cartilage thickness.
- Joint margin erosion, typical of rheumatoid arthritis.
- New bone-forming osteophytes, typical of osteoarthritis.
- Flattening or thickening of bone.
- Bone erosion or cavitation.

Soft tissues

In the soft tissues, areas of calcification, foreign bodies and increased density (suggestive of fluid) should all be noted.

Fig. 10.2 Movements at the cervical spine.

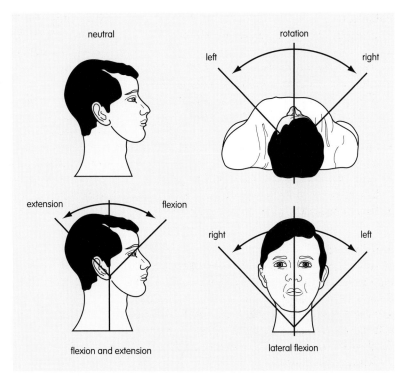

Regional examination of joints and the musculoskeletal system

The principles of general examination are applied to local areas. This section focuses on specific features that should be noted and manoeuvres that should be performed.

Examination of the back
Cervical spine
Inspection
During inspection of the cervical spine you should note any deformities such as torticollis, a 'cock-robin' posture (lateral flexion caused by cervical erosion from rheumatoid arthritis), and hyperextension (compensation for a small thorax in ankylosing spondylitis).

Palpation
During palpation of the cervical spine you should check for midline tenderness from a sprain or whiplash injury.

Movement
Movements of the cervical spine include flexion, extension, lateral rotation and lateral flexion. These movements are best seen from the side or front, and are expressed as a fraction of the usual range (Fig. 10.2). Restriction of movement occurs in arthritis and nerve compression.

Stressing
Stressing is not useful at the cervical spine.

Thoracic spine
Inspection
During inspection of the thoracic spine you should note any scoliosis (lateral fixed deviation) or kyphosis (anterior-facing concave curvature), which may be rounded or angular, due to collapsed vertebrae.

Palpation
During palpation, any tenderness of the thoracic spine can be because of collapse of T12 or L1 vertebrae, e.g. osteoporosis or trauma.

Movement
Movement of the thoracic spine is mainly rotational, but there is a small amount of flexion, extension and lateral flexion (Fig. 10.3).

Fig. 10.3 Movements at the thoracic and lumbar spine.

flexion

extension

lateralflexion

left   right

rotation

Stressing

Stressing is not useful at the thoracic spine.

Lumbosacral spine
Inspection

During inspection of the lumbosacral spine you should note any lordosis (posterior-facing concave curvature), scoliosis, vestigial ribs on the upper lumbar vertebrae, fusion of L5 with the sacrum (sacralization), and segmentation of S1 (lumbarization).

Palpation

During palpation, any tenderness of the lumbosacral spine may be because of ligament strain, pain from disc prolapse with spinal canal narrowing and nerve compression, or perianal anaesthesia from a cauda equina lesion.

Movement

Movement of the lumbosacral spine includes flexion, extension, lateral rotation and lateral flexion (see Fig. 10.3). Restriction follows different patterns, i.e.

general restriction in osteoarthritis, asymmetrical flexion in disc prolapse or scoliosis, and painful 'catch' on extension in muscle strain.

Stressing
Stressing is not useful at the lumbosacral spine.

Examination of the upper limb
Shoulder
Inspection
During inspection of the shoulder you should note its contour ('squaring off' in dislocation), swelling caused by effusion (synovitis in subacromial bursa and glenohumeral joint), deltoid muscle wasting, winging of the scapulae (congenital or muscular dystrophies), alignment of the clavicle and acromion, and the way in which the arms are held (chronic conditions and pain may affect this).

Palpation
During palpation of the shoulder, tenderness and pain may be localized to different areas in the rotator cuff disorders. It may be caused by glenohumeral or acromioclavicular arthritis, other arthropathies, or referred pain from other parts of the body.

Movement
Glenohumeral (abduction, adduction, flexion, extension, medial and lateral rotation) and scapular movements (elevation, retraction and rotation) (Fig. 10.4) are possible at the shoulder. You should eliminate scapular movement by pressing the scapula down at the top and asking the patient to move the shoulder. Check the power of deltoid (abduct the arm), serratus anterior (there is scapular 'winging' when both hands push firmly on a wall), and pectoralis major (push hands into waist). Check for abnormal movement between the acromion and the clavicle.

Stressing
Stressing is useful at the shoulder in checking for capsular lesions and osteoarthritis.

Elbow
Inspection
During inspection of the elbow you should look for 'gunstock' deformity (malunion of a previous

supracondylar fracture), joint effusion swellings, soft lumps posteriorly (olecranon bursitis), and pebbly osteophytes (osteoarthritis).

Palpation
During palpation of the elbow you should note any tenderness of the lateral epicondyle ('tennis elbow'), medial epicondyle ('golfer's elbow') and radial head (rheumatoid arthritis).

Movement
Flexion and extension movements are seen in the humeroulnar joint; supination and pronation can be seen in the radioulnar joints with the elbows flexed at 90° and held into the sides (Fig. 10.5). You should also test the median, radial and ulnar nerves.

Stressing
Stressing is not useful at the elbow.

Wrist
Inspection
During inspection of the wrist you should note any deformities or swellings of the tendon sheaths or joint capsule.

Palpation
During palpation of the wrist you should note any tenderness over the radial area (scaphoid fracture, de Quervain's tenosynovitis, osteoarthritis) or the ulnar area (tenosynovitis of extensors).

Movement
Flexion, extension, adduction and abduction movements may be seen at the radiocarpal joint, and supination and pronation at the inferior radioulnar joints (Fig. 10.6).

Stressing
Stressing is not useful at the wrist.

Hands
Inspection
During inspection of the hands you should look for mallet finger, trigger finger, dropped finger, swan-neck or boutonnière deformities, a Z deformity of

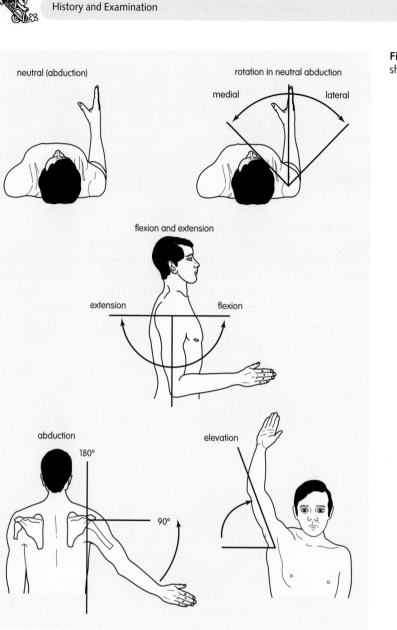

Fig. 10.4 Movements at the shoulder joint.

the thumb, ulnar deviation of the fingers (rheumatoid arthritis), Heberden's nodes at the distal interphalangeal joint, Bouchard's nodes at the proximal interphalangeal joints (osteoarthritis), ganglia and thickening of the palmar aponeurosis (Dupuytren's contracture).

Palpation
During palpation of the hands you should note any tenderness over the anatomical snuffbox, indicating a fracture of the scaphoid; tender joints occur in rheumatoid arthritis.

Movement
Flexion, extension, adduction and abduction movements can be seen at the metacarpophalangeal joints. There is also opposition of the thumb and little finger (Fig. 10.7). The interphalangeal joints only show flexion and extension.

Stressing
Stressing is useful at the hands—applying pressure on the fingers along their axis tests the mechanical stability of the metacarpals and phalanges.

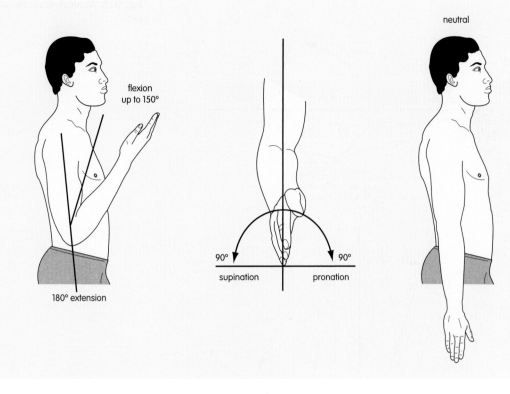

Fig. 10.5 Movements at the elbow joint.

Examination of the lower limb

Hip

Inspection

Inspection of the hip is not very useful unless it involves watching the gait.

Palpation

During palpation of the hip, you should note any pain at the front of the hip and the skin over the greater trochanter. You should measure the limbs to find their true length (from the anterior superior iliac spine to the medial malleolus, with the angle between the pelvis and limbs equal on both sides) or apparent length (from the xiphisternum to the medial malleolus, with the limbs lying parallel to the trunk).

Movement

Flexion, extension, abduction, adduction, medial rotation and lateral rotation are possible at the hip (Fig. 10.8). You should note any fixed deformities which may be flexed, abducted or adducted. Fixed flexion can be confirmed by performing Thomas's test. To perform Thomas's test, lie the patient flat on their back and place a hand under the lumbar lordosis. Flex the hip and knee of the leg unaffected by fixed flexion; if the other leg also flexes, fixed flexion of the hip on that side is confirmed and Thomas's test is positive. Performing a passive leg raise with the knee in extension will allow detection of nerve impingement caused by slipped disc; it also allows detection of quadriceps lag.

Stressing

Stressing is not very useful at the hip.

Knee

Inspection

During inspection of the knee you should look for genu valgum or genu varum, wasting of quadriceps femoris and swelling around the knee (thickened bone or synovium, fluid within the joint, bursitis).

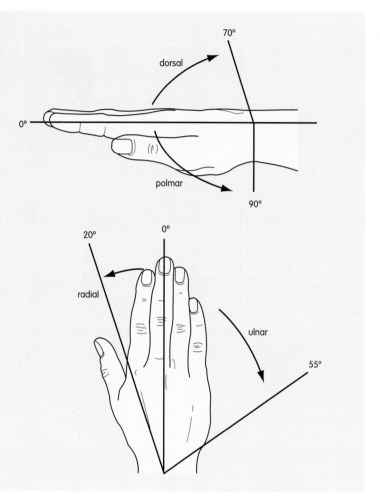

Fig. 10.6 Movements at the wrist joint.

Palpation
During palpation of the knee you should note any tenderness over the joint owing to torn menisci, synovitis or osteoarthritis. Loose bodies may be felt in the suprapatellar region.

Movement
Flexion and extension movements are possible at the knee (Fig. 10.9). Many of these movements can be hyperextended.

Stressing
During stressing of the knee you should check the collateral ligaments in full extension and the cruciate ligaments with the knee flexed at a right angle.

Ankle
Inspection
During inspection of the ankle you should check the hypertrophic calf muscles to be alerted to conditions such as Duchenne muscular dystrophy.

Palpation
During palpation of the ankle you should note any swelling near the joints that may indicate tenosynovitis.

Movement
Plantarflexion and dorsiflexion movements at the ankle are possible (Fig. 10.10). Inversion and eversion at the subtalar joint also occurs.

Fig. 10.7 Movements at: (A) the finger joint; and (B) the thumb joint.

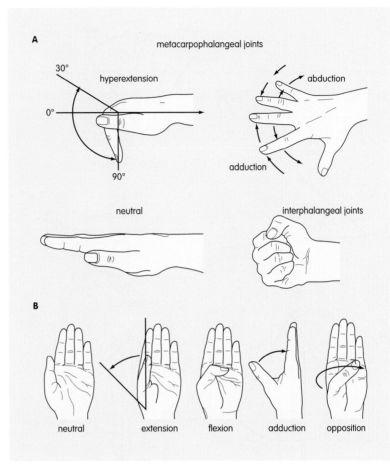

Stressing
Stressing of the ankle will enable checking of the integrity of the ligaments.

Feet
Inspection
During inspection of the feet you should look for congenital club foot, flat or hollow feet, claw toes, hammer toes, hallux valgus, hallux rigidus, bunions, calluses and toenail lesions.

Palpation
During palpation of the feet you should check for a hot, swollen, first metatarsophalangeal joint. This is apparent in gout. You should also check the metatarsal heads for prominence and pain.

Movement
Flexion and extension movements occur in the toes; inversion and eversion of the foot occurs at the midtarsal joint (Fig. 10.11).

Stressing
During stressing of the feet, longitudinal pressure will enable you to determine the integrity of the toes.

Examination of the thorax and abdomen
Thorax
Inspection
During inspection of the thorax you should look for deformities such as pectus carinatum (pigeon chest), pectus excavatum (funnel chest), scoliosis and 'gibbus' (sharp angular deformity caused by collapsed vertebrae from infection).

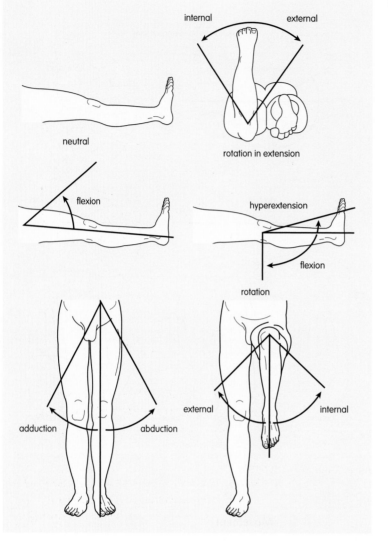

Fig. 10.8 Movements at the hip joint.

Palpation

During palpation of the thorax you should check for localized tenderness caused by broken ribs or metastasis.

Movement

Any restriction of expansion of the thorax to less than 5 cm is suggestive of ankylosing spondylitis.

Stressing

During stressing of the thorax, lateral compression can cause pain if there is a broken rib.

Abdomen

Inspection

During inspection of the abdomen you should look for urethral discharge or balanitis (Reiter's syndrome).

Palpation

During palpation of the abdomen you should check for splenomegaly (Felty's syndrome), enlarged inguinal lymph nodes (rheumatoid arthritis) and renal enlargement (ankylosing spondylitis).

You should ask about bowel habit. A rectal and stool examination may be useful for the diagnosis of

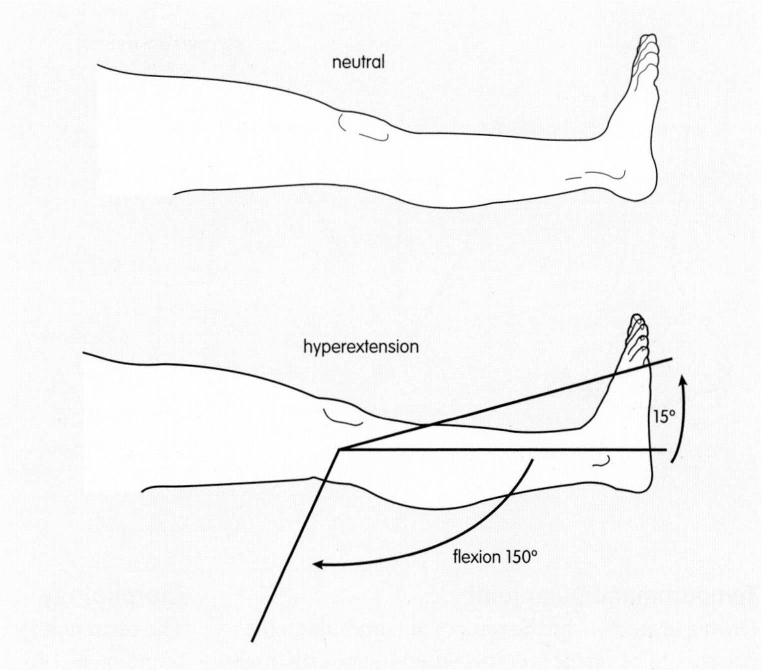

Fig. 10.9 Movements at the knee joint.

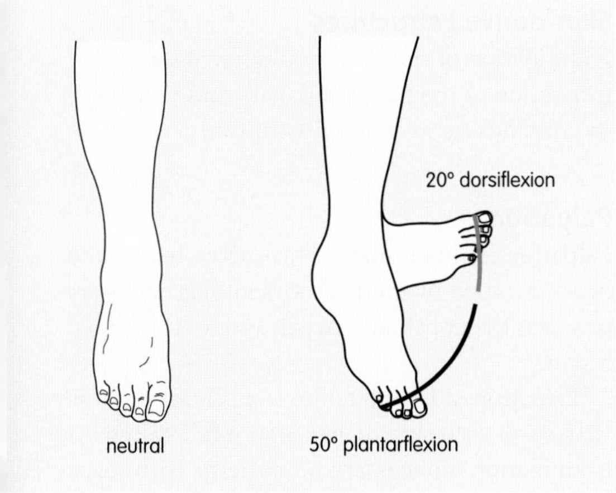

Fig. 10.10 Movements at the ankle joint.

the enteropathic arthropathies, ulcerative colitis and Crohn's disease.

Examination of the face

Eyes

During examination of the eyes you should check for any redness and dryness (Sjögren's syndrome), nodular scleritis and a thin blue sclera (rheumatoid arthritis), cataracts (steroid treatment for musculoskeletal disorders), iritis (ankylosing spondylitis), conjunctivitis (Reiter's syndrome), uveitis (Behçet's syndrome), and difficulty in closing the eyes (scleroderma).

Fundi

At the fundi, look for hyperviscosity (rheumatoid arthritis) or cytoid bodies composed of hard exudates [systemic lupus erythematosus (SLE)].

Mouth

At the mouth check for dryness and dental caries (Sjögren's syndrome), and ulcers (rheumatoid arthritis, SLE, Reiter's syndrome).

Facies

When examining the facies, check for parotid enlargement (Sjögren's syndrome), a cushingoid face (drugs used in rheumatoid arthritis and SLE), an expressionless, pinched 'bird-like' face (scleroderma), and alopecia (SLE and scleroderma).

Skin

You should check the skin for butterfly rash (SLE), urticaria and purpura (hypersensitive vasculitis in rheumatoid arthritis and SLE), malar telangiectasia, and skin tethering and pigmentation (scleroderma).

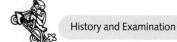
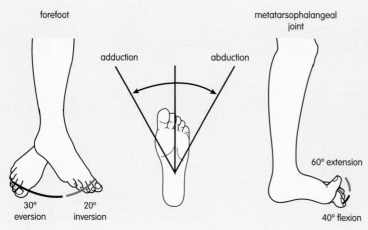

Fig. 10.11 Movements at the foot

forefoot

metatarsophalangeal joint

adduction   abduction

60° extension

30° eversion   20° inversion

40° flexion

Temporomandibular joint

During inspection of the temporomandibular joint you should listen for crepitus when the mouth opens or closes (rheumatoid arthritis).

Examination of the skin
Inspection

Ideally, examination of the skin should take place in natural daylight, with full exposure for atypical or widespread lesions. Inspection of the lesions involves noting the distribution and morphology of lesions.

Distribution

Different skin disorders commonly show different patterns of lesion distribution (see Chapter 8). It is important to determine whether the eruptions are symmetrical or asymmetrical, central or peripheral, localized or widespread, and on flexor or extensor surfaces. Some disorders may show specific patterns; shingles erupts in a dermatomal pattern, guttate psoriasis occurs on the trunk, contact dermatitis usually affects the hands or face, etc.

Morphology

The terminology used to describe skin lesions can be found on p. 143. It is important to note whether the lesions are grouped, linear, annular or whether they show the Koebner phenomenon.

Skin-derived structures

Examination of the skin should also involve inspection of the hair, scalp, nails and mucous membranes for associated symptoms.

Palpation

Palpation of skin lesions (a task often feared and hence avoided by medical students) is necessary to assess the constancy, depth and texture of a lesion.

Palpation of lymph nodes is essential in patients with suspected skin malignancy; a full systematic examination is necessary for patients with suspected lymphoma.

Pulses must be assessed in patients with leg ulcers.

- Name the main points for a good history-taking.
- Differentiate between open and closed questions.
- What factors are involved in the doctor–patient dynamic?
- List three methods of non-verbal communication.
- List the common points of inspection for all joints.
- Describe the normal appearance and range of movements possible at each joint.
- Explain how to examine the back, shoulder, elbow, hand, hip, knee and feet for signs of musculoskeletal disorders.
- What is Thomas's test?
- List the 'red flags' you should be aware of during a musculoskeletal history.
- Name the areas of palpation in skin examination.

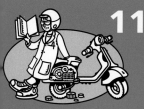

11. Further Investigations

Investigation of musculoskeletal function

Bone densitometry
Density of bone can be estimated by several techniques. These include:
- X-ray computerized tomography.
- Magnetic resonance imaging.
- Radioisotope scanning.

X-ray computerized tomography
X-ray computerized tomography (CT) involves X-ray scanning of part of the body from several angles with oscillators that detect the X-rays. Cross-sectional images are then compared and reconstructed by computer. These images can show variation in density between bone and surrounding tissue.

Magnetic resonance imaging
In magnetic resonance imaging (MRI) scanning, the part of the body under investigation is placed in a magnetic field. Hydrogen nuclei (protons) are lined up in the direction of this magnetic field, assuming a new orientation when the electromagnetic radiation is altered. On stopping the radiation, the protons return to their original position and emit radiofrequency signals as they do so. It is these signals that can be analysed and converted into a two-dimensional image.

MRI scanning can detect variations in density of tissues. It provides a means of scanning without the use of X-rays.

Radioisotope scanning
During routine investigations using radioisotope scanning, an intravenous injection of radiolabelled technetium is administered. Rays emitted from the technetium can be measured with a gamma camera or rectilinear scanner.

As the isotope diffuses from bone matrix to blood, its increased uptake provides a measure of hyperaemia of bone and increased osteogenic activity.

Electromyography
Electromyography is a technique used to record the electrical activity in muscle both at rest and during contraction.

Method
During electromyography, a needle electrode is inserted into muscle. Electrical activity in the muscle is displayed on a cathode ray oscilloscope and heard on a speaker.

Electromyography is used:
- To determine whether a disorder is caused by disease of the muscle or abnormalities of innervation.
- If there is an abnormality of innervation—this may be localized to the central nervous system, peripheral nerves or neuromuscular junction.
- To aid in the diagnosis of myopathy, myotonia and myasthenia.
- To obtain information about the distribution of a disorder so that a biopsy specimen can be taken from the appropriate site.
- To obtain information on the characteristics of motor units.

Assessment of muscle function
Normal muscle
Normal muscle at rest is electrically silent. The insertion of an electrode results in insertional activity because the muscle fibres are mechanically stimulated or damaged. If there is disease, the extent of this spontaneous activity may increase or decrease.

When insertional activity subsides, further activity may be seen only if the electrode is moved or the muscle contracts (Fig. 11.1).

Denervated muscle
Abnormal spontaneous activity of muscle at rest is termed fibrillation potentials. However, diseases of the neuromuscular junction and myopathies may also result in this pattern.

Myasthenia gravis
Single-fibre electromyography is used in the diagnosis of myasthenia gravis. This technique

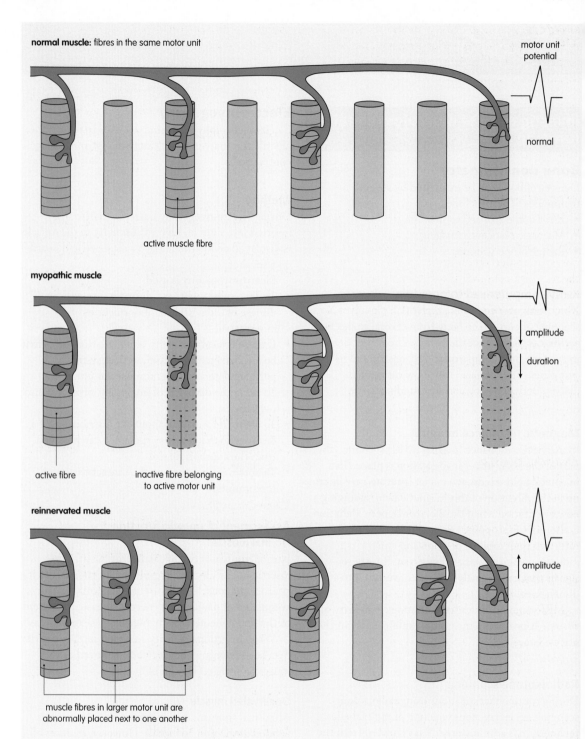

Fig. 11.1 Comparison of the motor unit action potentials recorded in normal muscle, myopathic muscle and reinnervated muscle.

records the time interval between the potentials of two fibres belonging to the same motor unit. In normal muscle this time interval is 10–50s but in myasthenia gravis it is increased.

Myopathic muscle
In myopathic muscle, the number of active muscle fibres in a motor unit is decreased (see Fig 11.1). This results in a reduced amplitude and action potential of shorter duration.

Reinnervated muscle
In reinnervated muscle, the muscle fibres are often reinnervated as a result of axonal sprouting of adjacent nerves (see Fig. 11.1). This results in a larger motor unit and therefore an increased amplitude of the recorded potential. In addition, there is an unusual arrangement of fibres in the same unit, which may now lie next to each other.

Limitations
Electromyography does not provide a specific diagnosis, as certain types of recording may occur in more than one disorder. It is, therefore, always important to confirm a diagnosis with clinical findings and laboratory results.

Muscle biopsy
Method
Muscle samples are usually taken by needle biopsy. Local anaesthesia is required for this procedure.

An open biopsy may be needed to diagnose focal abnormalities such as myositis.

Evaluation
A muscle biopsy is usually evaluated in one or more ways, including:
- Histology.
- Histochemistry.
- Electron microscopy.
- Assays of enzyme activities.

With these techniques it is possible to assess muscle fibre types, the presence of inflammation or degeneration, the presence of abnormal mitochondria and enzyme abnormalities.

Indications
Muscle biopsy differentiates between neuropathic and myopathic disorders. It is used to aid in the diagnosis of a range of inflammatory, dystrophic and metabolic myopathies.

Investigations of skin disorders

Surgical biopsies
Biopsies are classified as follows: excisional, incisional, punch, shave or curettage.

Excisional biopsy
Excisional biopsy is not only used to facilitate histological diagnosis of the lesion, but also to treat it effectively. The lesion is removed along with a defined margin of skin, which depends on the lesion. Benign and malignant skin lesions are both biopsied in this way.

Incisional biopsy
This is similar to excision biopsy, but less tissue is removed.

Punch biopsy
A biopsy in which a small (4mm) punch tool is used to remove a cylindrical section of skin for histological examination.

Shave biopsy
The lesion is shaved off parallel to the skin surface, with resultant bleeding treated by haemocauterization. This is only used for benign lesions, as some lesion remains; it is usually used for intradermal naevi and seborrhoeic warts.

Curettage
The lesion is removed using a curette spoon, with bleeding points cauterized. This method is used to biopsy seborrhoeic warts, pyogenic granulomas and viral warts.

Immunological tests
Prick tests
Prick tests are used to detect immediate (type I) hypersensitivity reactions, and involve injecting tiny amounts of antigen solutions into the skin of the forearm. After 15min, the skin is inspected and a wheal of 4mm or larger is regarded as a positive

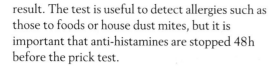

result. The test is useful to detect allergies such as those to foods or house dust mites, but it is important that anti-histamines are stopped 48h before the prick test.

Patch testing

This detects cell-mediated (type IV) hypersensitivity reactions by applying a standard battery of 23 test substances to aluminium discs which are then taped to the skin. The patches are left on for 2 days, after which erythematous patches are correlated to specific test substances. The skin is re-examined after 4 days, as some reactions take this long to occur. Patch testing is used in the investigation of contact dermatitis.

Immunofluorescence

Used to diagnose the autoimmune blistering disorders, this process targets specific immunoglobulins or complement fractions with an antibody labelled with fluorescein (a marker). The marker then shows up under fluorescent light.

An indirect method of immunofluorescence is also used, in which an animal substrate is used to reveal certain human serum antibodies tagged with anti-human immunoglobulin antibody under ultraviolet light.

Wood's lamp

This light emits ultraviolet radiation which causes certain fungal infections to fluoresce on skin and especially hair. It can also be used to detect hypopigmentation, such as that seen in vitiligo.

Microscopy

Skin scrapings treated with potassium hydroxide solution can be viewed under a light microscope to confirm fungal hyphae. Microscopy is also used in the diagnosis of scabies; the mite can be extracted from its burrow with a needle and viewed.

Routine investigations in musculoskeletal and skin disorders

Haematology
Erythrocyte sedimentation rate

The erythrocyte sedimentation rate (ESR) is the rate at which red blood cells settle out of suspension in blood plasma in anticoagulated blood. A standard ESR tube is used and the length of clear plasma at the top of the settled blood cells is measured at 1h. The normal rate is <10mm/h.

The ESR is raised in inflammatory conditions such as rheumatoid arthritis, systemic lupus erythematosus (SLE) and inflammatory myopathy.

C-reactive protein

C-reactive protein is normally present in small amounts in serum, and is synthesized in greater amounts by the liver in response to a variety of insults, including infection.

C-reactive protein is raised in inflammatory conditions. It is a more sensitive indicator than ESR, but the results are not available as quickly.

Haemoglobin

Anaemia—usually normochromic or normocytic—occurs in inflammatory conditions such as rheumatoid arthritis and SLE.

White blood cell count

The numbers of white blood cells are raised in infections such as septic arthritis.

Thyroid function

The thyroid function test is able to exclude myopathy caused by thyroid dysfunction; parathyroid hormone levels exclude myopathy associated with osteomalacia.

Blood biochemistry
Uric acid

Uric acid levels need be checked only if gout is suspected.

Muscle enzymes

Creatine kinase, a muscle enzyme, may be raised in inflammatory myopathy, muscular dystrophy, alcohol myopathy and metabolic myopathy.

Bone enzymes

Alkaline phosphatase, a bone enzyme, is raised in Paget's disease, osteomalacia and rickets, but not in osteoporosis.

Immunopathology
Autoantibodies
Autoantibodies that can be measured in musculoskeletal disorders include:

- Rheumatoid factor in rheumatoid arthritis, Sjögren's syndrome, SLE, polymyositis, dermatomyositis and sarcoidosis.
- Antinuclear antibodies (ANAs) in SLE (anti-Ro), Sjögren's syndrome, Still's disease, polymyositis (anti-Jo) and dermatomyositis.
- Anti-acetylcholine receptors in myasthenia gravis.

Synovial fluid analysis
Synovial fluid should be analysed for appearance, the presence of white blood cells, the presence of crystals, and should also be cultured for infections (Fig. 11.2).

Be aware that crystals found in gout are negatively birefringent whereas in pseudogout they are positively birefringent.

Imaging of the musculoskeletal system

The radiograph, or plain X-ray, is the imaging technique most commonly used to diagnose musculoskeletal disorders. It is simple, relatively cheap and quick. However, in some instances, the radiograph may not yield sufficient information; then, other imaging techniques, such as MRI, CT or radioisotope imaging, need to be employed.

Normal anatomy
The normal appearance of the musculoskeletal system during imaging is depicted in Figs 11.3–11.10. These include the:

- Skull (Fig. 11.3).
- Shoulder (Fig. 11.4).
- Elbow (Fig. 11.5).
- Hand (Fig. 11.6).
- Female pelvis (Fig. 11.7).
- Knee and leg (Fig. 11.8).
- Ankle (Fig. 11.9).
- Cervical spine (Fig. 11.10).

Bone disorders
Hereditary disorders
Hereditary bone disorders include:

- Congenital scoliosis (Fig. 11.11).
- Osteogenesis imperfecta congenita (Fig. 11.12).

Infections and trauma
Bone is prone to infection, called osteomyelitis (Fig. 11.13), and trauma.

Metabolic disease
Metabolic bone disorders include:

- Hyperparathyroidism (Fig. 11.14).
- Vitamin D deficiency (Fig. 11.15).
- Periarticular osteoporosis (Fig. 11.16).

Tumours
Hereditary bone tumours include:
- Osteosarcoma (Fig. 11.17).
- Giant-cell tumour (Fig. 11.18).

Synovial fluid changes in some rheumatic diseases				
Disease state	**Appearance**	**White blood cells (× 10⁶/L)**	**Crystals**	**Culture**
normal	clear viscous fluid	<200 mononuclear	none	sterile
osteoarthritis	increased volume; normal viscosity	3000 mononuclear	5% have pyrophosphate	sterile
rheumatoid arthritis	may be turbidly yellow or green; low viscosity	30 000 neutrophils	none	sterile
septic arthritis	turbid; low viscosity	50 000–100 000 neutrophils	none	positive
gout	clear; low viscosity	10 000 neutrophils	needle-shaped; negative birefringence	sterile
pyrophosphate arthropathy (pseudogout)	clear; low viscosity	10 000 neutrophils	brick-shaped; positive birefringence	sterile

Fig. 11.2 Synovial fluid changes in some rheumatic diseases. (Adapted with permission from *Clinical Medicine,* 3rd edn, by P. Kumar and M. Clark, Baillière Tindall, 1994.)

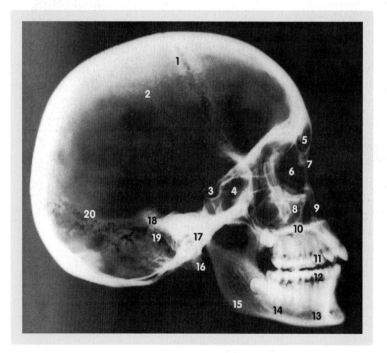

1	coronal suture
2	grooves for meningeal vessels
3	pituitary fossa
4	sphenoidal sinus
5	frontal sinus
6	orbit
7	nasal bones
8	maxillary sinus
9	anterior nasal spine
10	hard palate
11	maxilla and teeth
12	mandible and teeth
13	mental foramen
14	mandibular canal
15	angle of mandible
16	mastoid process
17	external acoustic meatus
18	petrous ridge
19	groove for sigmoid sinus
20	lambdoid suture

Fig. 11.3 Lateral radiograph of skull. (Courtesy of Dr B. Berkovitz and Dr B. Moxham.)

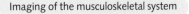

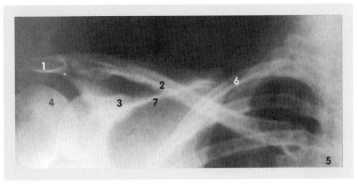

1 Acromion process of scapula
2 Clavicle
3 Coracoid process of scapula
4 Head of humerus
5 Manubrium
6 Ribs
7 Spine of scapula

Fig. 11.4 Radiograph of the right shoulder. (Courtesy of Dr J. Calder and Dr G. Chessell.)

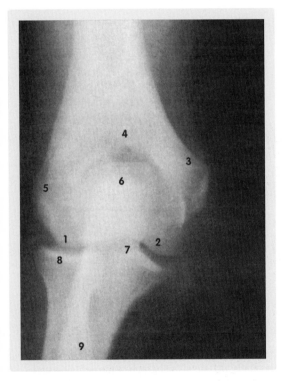

1 Capitulum of humerus
2 Trochlea of humerus
3 Medial epicondyle of humerus
4 Olecranon fossa of humerus
5 Lateral epicondyle of humerus
6 Olecranon process of ulna
7 Coronoid process of ulna
8 Head of radius
9 Radial tuberosity

Fig. 11.5 Anteroposterior radiograph of the right elbow. (Courtesy of Dr J. Calder and Dr G. Chessell.)

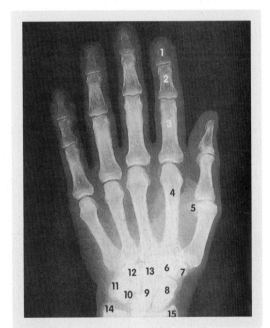

1 Distal phalanx
2 Middle phalanx
3 Proximal phalanx
4 Second metacarpal
5 Sesamoid bone
6 Trapezoid
7 Trapezium
8 Scaphoid
9 Lunate
10 Triquetral
11 Pisiform
12 Hamate
13 Capitate
14 Styloid process of ulna
15 Styloid process of radius

Fig. 11.6 Radiograph of an adult hand. (Courtesy of Drs J. Gosling, P. Harris, J. Humpherson, I. Whitmore and P. Willan.)

217

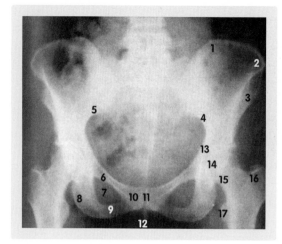

1	Iliac crest
2	Anterior superior iliac spine
3	Anterior inferior iliac spine
4	Pelvic brim
5	Sacroiliac joint
6	Superior pubic ramus
7	Obdurator foramen
8	Inferior ischial ramus
9	Inferior pubic ramus
10	Body of pubis
11	Pubic symphysis
12	Subpubic arch
13	Acetabulum
14	Head of femur
15	Neck of femur
16	Greater trochanter of femur
17	Lesser trochanter of femur

Fig. 11.7 Anteroposterior radiograph of the female pelvis. (Courtesy of Dr J. Calder and Dr G. Chessell.)

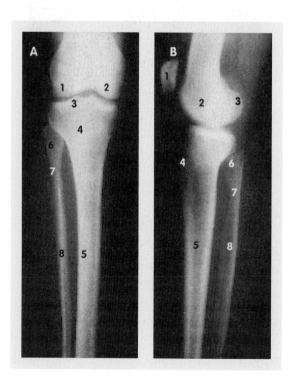

A

1	Lateral femoral condyle
2	Medial femoral condyle
3	Tibial spine
4	Tibial tuberosity
5	Shaft of tibia
6	Head of fibula
7	Neck of fibula
8	Shaft of fibula

B

1	Patella
2	Medial femoral condyle
3	Lateral femoral condyle
4	Tibial tuberosity
5	Shaft of tibia
6	Head of fibula
7	Neck of fibula
8	Shaft of fibula

Fig. 11.8 Anteroposterior radiograph of: (A) the right tibia and fibula; (B) lateral radiograph of the right tibia and fibula. (Courtesy of Dr J. Calder and Dr G. Chessell.)

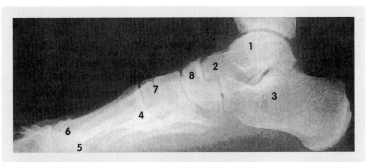

1   Medial malleolus
2   Head of talus
3   Calcaneus
4   Base of first metatarsal
5   Sesamoid bone
6   Head of first metatarsal
7   Cuneiforms
8   Navicular

Fig. 11.9 Radiograph of the right foot and ankle showing longitudinal arches. (Courtesy of Drs J. Gosling, P. Harris, J. Humpherson, I. Whitmore and P. Willan.)

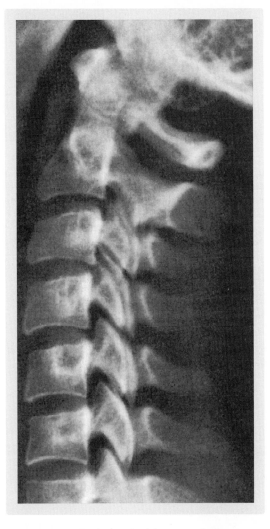

Fig. 11.10 Lateral radiograph of the cervical spine. (Courtesy of Dr A. Greenspan and Dr P. Montesano.)

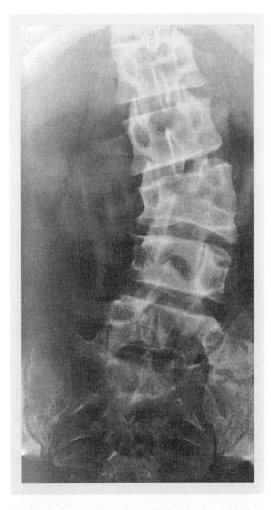

Fig. 11.11 Congenital scoliosis. This case of scoliosis in a 22-year-old man was due to hemivertebrae — a complete unilateral failure of formation. (Courtesy of Dr A. Greenspan.)

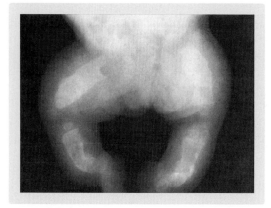

Fig. 11.12 Osteogenesis imperfecta congenita. This infant was born with type II osteogenesis imperfecta, where multiple fractures are present before birth. There is gross deformity of the lower limbs with multiple healing fractures. (Courtesy of Dr T. Lissauer.)

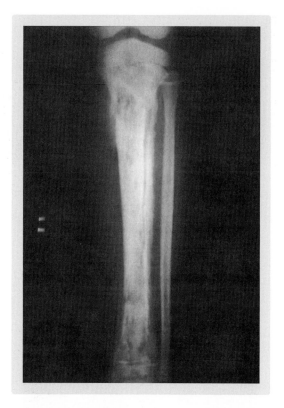

Fig. 11.13 Osteomyelitis. This chronic case shows a periosteal reaction along the lateral shaft of the tibia, and multiple hypodense areas within the metaphyseal region. (Courtesy of Dr T. Lissauer.)

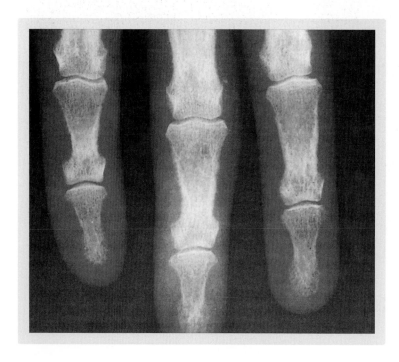

Fig. 11.14 Hyperparathyroidism. The terminal phalanxes show tufting and subperiosteal lesions, characteristic signs of primary hyperparathyroidism. (Courtesy of Dr P. M. Bouloux.)

Fig. 11.15 Radioisotope bone scan showing a generalized increase in technetium uptake with multiple hot spots due to small fractures. The patient had metabolic bone disease caused by vitamin D deficiency. The darker areas indicate increased uptake of technetium, representing altered cell growth. (A) Thoracic spine; (B) pelvis; (C) lumbar spine; and (D) femur and knee joint. (Courtesy of Dr P. M. Bouloux.)

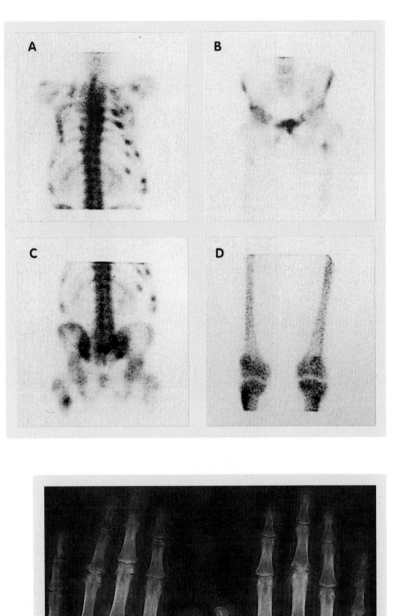

Fig. 11.16 Periarticular osteoporosis with mild ulnar changes in early rheumatoid arthritis. (Courtesy of Dr P. M. Bouloux.)

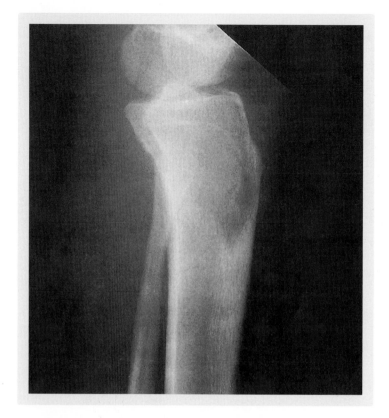

Fig. 11.17 Osteosarcoma in a child. The radiograph shows an infiltrative, poorly demarcated tumour in the metaphyseal region of the tibia. (Courtesy of Dr S. Taylor.)

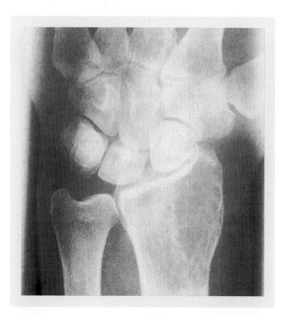

Fig. 11.18 Giant-cell tumour of the radius. Radiograph of the left wrist shows an expanding lytic lesion replacing the distal radius. The lesion is epiphyseal and abuts the adjacent articular surface. There is thinning of the radial cortex but no periosteal reaction and no reactive sclerosis at the proximal extent of the lesion. (Courtesy of Mr W.A. Jones.)

- List the techniques available to determine bone density.
- What are the uses and limitations of the EMG technique?
- Describe the technique of muscle biopsy.
- List the important blood tests in investigating the musculoskeletal system.
- Describe the characteristics of synovial fluid found in osteoarthritis, rheumatoid arthritis and septic arthritis.
- Explain three ways of measuring bone density.
- In which diseases can rheumatoid factor be detected?
- List some methods of assessing muscle function.
- List routine laboratory investigations to assess musculoskeletal function.
- Interpret normal radiographs of the skeleton.
- Spot abnormalities in radiographs of diseased skeletons.
- What skin disorders can be diagnosed by use of a light microscope?
- Differentiate between prick tests and spot tests.
- List the techniques used for biopsy of the skin.
- For what is a Wood's lamp used?

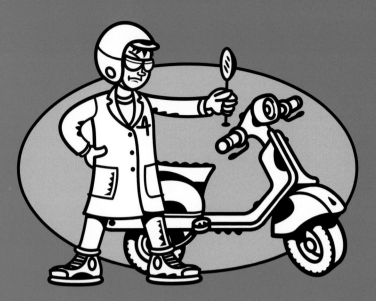

SELF-ASSESSMENT

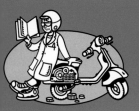

Multiple-choice Questions (MCQs)

Indicate whether each answer is true or false.

Skeletal Muscle

1. In an action potential:

(a) Size is proportional to the stimulus strength.
(b) Initiation occurs when the membrane potential is reduced to a critical value.
(c) Influx of sodium ions is responsible for the rising phase.
(d) There is a transient decrease in membrane permeability of potassium ions.
(e) The duration and size are constant for all cell types.

2. The RMP of a nerve fibre:

(a) Has a higher concentration of potassium ions inside the nerve than on the outside.
(b) When reduced, results in an increase in excitability of the cell.
(c) Has a value of –90 mV in muscle cells.
(d) Is also known as the equilibrium potential.
(e) Is equal to the equilibrium potential of potassium.

3. Neurotransmission at the neuromuscular junction is impaired by:

(a) Hemicholinium.
(b) Suxamethonium.
(c) Adrenaline.
(d) Botulinum toxin.
(e) Edrophonium.

4. Edrophonium:

(a) Is used in the treatment of myasthenia gravis.
(b) May cause constriction of the pupil.
(c) Is an anticholinesterase.
(d) Impairs neuromuscular transmission.
(e) Decreases acetylcholine release at the neuromuscular junction.

5. Chemical synapses differ from electrical in that:

(a) Transmission is more rapid.
(b) Synaptic cleft is larger.
(c) Plasticity may occur.
(d) They are more common in the body.
(e) Amplification of the signal is possible.

6. With regard to saltatory conduction:

(a) It can occur in unmyelinated nerve fibres.
(b) Speed is proportional to the diameter of the nerve fibre.
(c) Speed is proportional to the strength of local circuits.
(d) A large safety factor is demonstrated.
(e) Membrane depolarization does not occur.

7. Conduction velocity:

(a) Increases in the presence of a myelin sheath.
(b) Increases up to a temperature of 60°C.
(c) Decreases with larger fibre diameters.
(d) Is influenced by the strength of local circuits.
(e) May be less than 1 m/s.

8. Striated muscle:

(a) Contains alternating A and Z bands.
(b) Fibres are multinucleate.
(c) Is present in the upper part of the oesophagus.
(d) Fibres are bound together by sarcolemma.
(e) Is the most common type of muscle found in the body.

9. With regard to skeletal muscle:

(a) A smaller stimulus is required to cause local contraction if applied to the Z band.
(b) Distance between the Z bands is constant during contraction.
(c) Each muscle fibre is innervated by only one motor neuron.
(d) APs are propagated in both directions to the ends of the muscle fibre.
(e) The length of the I bands decreases during contraction.

10. With regard to the arrangement of skeletal muscles:

(a) Muscles are arranged in groups.
(b) A muscle may be a member of only one group.
(c) For a given volume of muscle, an oblique arrangement of muscle fibres would result in a greater force of contraction than a parallel arrangement.
(d) Muscle fibres are innervated by muscle spindles.
(e) The origin of a muscle is the attachment site at which there is little movement when the muscle performs its main action.

11. **With regard to the motor unit:**

(a) The muscle fibres innervated by a single motor neuron within a motor unit lie side by side.
(b) The muscle fibres within a motor unit are of the same type.
(c) Muscles involved in fine movement have smaller motor units.
(d) The strength of muscle contraction is increased by recruiting more motor units.
(e) The muscle fibres within a motor unit contract simultaneously.

12. **The following proteins are components of the thin filament:**

(a) Actin.
(b) Desmin.
(c) Calmodulin.
(d) Troponin.
(e) α-Actinin.

13. **With regard to muscle fibre types:**

(a) Speed of contraction is greatest with red fibres.
(b) Red fibres are resistant to fatigue.
(c) Myoglobin is present in red fibres.
(d) White fibres are involved in maintenance of posture.
(e) Glycogen content is high in white fibres.

14. **In skeletal muscle contraction, ATP:**

(a) Is required to cause detachment of myosin heads from the actin filaments.
(b) Is provided by glycolysis.
(c) Is produced by slow synthesis from creatine kinase.
(d) Is necessary for the influx of sodium ions.
(e) Is produced by oxidative phosphorylation.

15. **Upon contraction of skeletal muscle:**

(a) The rise in intracellular calcium ions results from direct entry through the cell membrane.
(b) The calcium ions bind to tropomyosin.
(c) The number of sarcomeres decreases.
(d) The actin and myosin filaments shorten.
(e) The strength of contraction is influenced by initial muscle fibre length.

16. **With regard to muscle function:**

(a) Isometric contraction of skeletal muscle is contraction at a constant tension.
(b) The treppe effect is associated with cardiac contraction.
(c) The force of skeletal muscle contraction increases with frequency of stimulation.
(d) Plasticity may involve altering vascular supply to the muscle.
(e) Most muscles in the body are at optimum length for maximal tension.

17. **Myasthenia gravis:**

(a) May be associated with ptosis.
(b) Occurs most commonly in the fifth decade.
(c) May be managed by thymectomy.
(d) Is inherited in an autosomal recessive manner.
(e) May be transient in newborn babies of female sufferers.

18. **The following statements are correct:**

(a) Gower's sign is a feature of myotonic dystrophy.
(b) Duchenne muscular dystrophy is inherited in an autosomal recessive manner.
(c) Fascioscapulohumeral dystrophy may be associated with winging of the scapulae.
(d) Mitochondrial myopathy may be associated with patients infected with HIV.
(e) Pseudohypertrophy of the calves is a sign of Duchenne muscular dystrophy.

19. **The following statements are correct:**

(a) Idiopathic inflammatory myopathies present in teenagers.
(b) Dermatomyositis is associated with a characteristic purple heliotrope rash.
(c) Viral myositis is strongly associated with herpes simplex.
(d) Duchenne muscular dystrophies usually present in early childhood.
(e) Hypertonia can be caused by lipid disorders.

20. **Recognized side effects of local anaesthetics include:**

(a) Allergic reactions causing sudden collapse.
(b) Stimulation of the central nervous system.
(c) Constriction of blood vessels.
(d) Physical dependency.
(e) Hypertension.

Cardiac and Smooth Muscle

21. **Smooth muscle cells:**

(a) Have a single nucleus located at the widest part of the cell.
(b) Contain myofilaments that can only be seen with an electron microscope.
(c) Cannot be replaced in adult life by the transformation of mesenchymal cells.
(d) Remain a constant size throughout life.
(e) Form tight junctions with each other.

22. **In smooth muscle cells:**

(a) The protein desmin is present.
(b) The protein troponin is present.
(c) Sodium ions are responsible for the AP.
(d) Contraction requires lower ATP contraction.
(e) The protein calmodulin is a component of the thin filament.

23. **The following statements regarding smooth muscle are true:**

(a) The bladder is composed of three circular layers of smooth muscle.
(b) Local tissue factors that affect smooth muscle tone include H^+.
(c) Smooth muscle cells communicate electrically via gap (nexus) junctions.
(d) Organic nitrates increase smooth muscle tone.
(e) Smooth muscle is important in digestion.

24. **In cardiac muscle:**

(a) The AP is initiated in the sinoatrial node.
(b) The AP is shorter than that in skeletal muscle.
(c) The AP demonstrates a plateau phase.
(d) Cells are multinucleated.
(e) Summation of contractions does not occur.

25. **Regarding the AP in ventricular cardiac muscle:**

(a) Calcium ions are responsible for the rising phase of the AP.
(b) The refractory period is longer than that following an AP in skeletal muscle.
(c) The sympathetic nervous system shortens the plateau phase of the AP.
(d) Calcium ions play a part in the AP.
(e) Initiation is neurogenic.

26. **The following statements to do with cardiac muscle are correct:**

(a) Pacemaker tissue is only found in the SA node.
(b) Inotropes increase the force of cardiac contraction.
(c) Starling's law states that the force of contraction is proportional to the initial length of the cardiac muscle fibre.
(d) The RMP of cardiac cells is −90 mV.
(e) The endocardium is thicker than the myocardium.

27. **The following properties hold true for all three types of muscle:**

(a) Rapid stimulation results in summation.
(b) An increase in intracellular calcium concentration is necessary for muscular contraction.
(c) Contraction is controlled by the nervous system.
(d) Membrane depolarization is necessary for APs to occur.
(e) The presence of actin and myosin.

28. **The following statements are correct:**

(a) Intercalated discs are present in skeletal muscle.
(b) Cardiac muscle fibres are cross-striated.
(c) Transverse tubules are found in smooth muscle.
(d) Myofilaments are arranged in an organized way in smooth muscle.
(e) Muscle spindles are present in smooth muscle.

Bone

29. **The skeleton:**

(a) Is derived from the primitive mesenchyme.
(b) Has a solid extracellular matrix.
(c) Consists of bone only.
(d) Is a major storage site for calcium.
(e) Does not contain any red bone marrow in adults.

30. **The human skeleton:**

(a) Is bilaterally symmetrical.
(b) Has an axial part, comprising the bones of the head, neck and trunk.
(c) Has an appendicular part consisting of limb bones only.
(d) Contains active red bone marrow in both children and adults.
(e) Contains bones that all start as a cartilage template.

31. **Cartilage:**

(a) Is an avascular tissue.
(b) Never forms permanent structures.
(c) Can increase in size by appositional and interstitial growth.
(d) Can survive if invaded by ingrowing capillaries.
(e) Of the hyaline type is always covered by perichondrium.

32. **Hyaline cartilage:**

(a) Contains prominent elastic fibres.
(b) Contains a few collagen-like fibres.
(c) Is the precursor of endochondral ossification.
(d) Forms the knee menisci.
(e) Is vascular compared with bone.

33. **Long bones:**

(a) Usually ossify directly from mesenchyme.
(b) Are made wholly of compact bone.
(c) Normally contain yellow marrow in adulthood.
(d) Are organized in Haversian systems.
(e) Are covered with an acellular periosteum.

34. **Endochondral ossification:**

(a) Occurs in all long bones except the clavicle.
(b) Occurs in cartilage that has replaced a membranous model.
(c) Has its primary centres appearing *in utero*.
(d) Is usually complete by the age of 25 years.
(e) Is typical in the bones of the skull.

35. In the development of long bones:

(a) Osteoclasts do not absorb the calcified matrix of the cartilage.
(b) Osteoblasts become osteocytes.
(c) Endochondral ossification extends along the diaphysis.
(d) The epiphyseal plate separates the diaphysis from the metaphysis.
(e) Circumferential growth is by subperiosteal ossification.

36. The epiphyses:

(a) Are all present at birth.
(b) Are formed in hyaline cartilage.
(c) Are not present in all long bones.
(d) Are involved in increasing length and width of long bones.
(e) May occur at sites of muscle attachment.

37. The destruction of bone is associated with the following biochemical changes:

(a) Raised urinary hydroxyproline.
(b) Raised plasma alkaline phosphatase.
(c) Raised plasma acid phosphatase.
(d) Raised plasma calcium.
(e) Lowered plasma phosphate.

38. Osteoporosis differs from osteomalacia in the following ways:

(a) The density of the skeleton is reduced in osteoporosis and not in osteomalacia.
(b) The remaining bone in osteoporosis has a normal histological appearance.
(c) There are gross changes in the epiphyses in osteomalacia.
(d) Pseudofractures are more common in osteoporosis than in osteomalacia.
(e) Excess bone matrix is found in osteomalacia.

39. The following promote fracture healing:

(a) Absence of infection.
(b) Adequate vitamin C.
(c) Good blood supply.
(d) Immediate mobilization.
(e) Treatment with steroids.

40. Metastases in bone show the following characteristic features:

(a) Both bone destruction and new bone formation.
(b) Pathological fractures.
(c) Lowered plasma alkaline phosphatase.
(d) Red marrow affected more than yellow marrow.
(e) Red blood cells in peripheral blood may be of immature forms.

41. Calcium:

(a) Controls neuromuscular excitability.
(b) Acts as an intracellular second messenger.
(c) Is mobilized slowly from cancellous bone to blood.
(d) Absorption in small intestine is enhanced by vitamin D.
(e) Excess in blood is reduced by parathyroid hormone.

42. Cartilage:

(a) Consists of chondroblasts and chondrocytes embedded in a cartilage matrix.
(b) Growth and maturation are mainly towards the periphery of the cartilage mass.
(c) Contains a rich blood supply.
(d) Of the hyaline type is present in the epiphyseal plates.
(e) Of the elastic type is found in the epiglottis.

43. Long bones:

(a) Have a shaft called the diaphysis.
(b) Have two expanded ends called metaphyses.
(c) Contain a central medullary cavity.
(d) Consist of compact bone only.
(e) Are lined by endosteum.

44. Paget's disease of bone:

(a) Is also known as osteitis deformans.
(b) Is a disease of bone resorption.
(c) Commonly presents during the second decade of life.
(d) Affects the small bones of the hand.
(e) Is common in Asian and African populations.

45. Osteomyelitis:

(a) Is inflammation of bone.
(b) Can be pyogenic or tuberculous.
(c) Necrosis of bone leads directly to involucrum.
(d) May lead to the formation of Brodie's abscesses.
(e) Causes acute bone pain and fever.

46. Avascular necrosis:

(a) This is the death of bone following infection.
(b) It is caused by a poor blood supply.
(c) The most common sites are the head of the tibia and the occiput of the skull.
(d) Subchondral infarction may lead to wedge-shaped areas of damage.
(e) Intracapsular fractures predispose to avascular necrosis.

47. Metastatic tumours of the skeleton:

(a) Are more common than primary tumours.
(b) Arising from the breast, kidney, thyroid and lung are lytic.
(c) Arising from the breast are sclerotic.
(d) Can be detected by isotope bone scanning.
(e) If suspected, a full examination should be undertaken.

Joints and Related Structures

48. In synovial joints:

(a) Articular surfaces are always lined by articular cartilage.
(b) Fibrocartilaginous discs usually partially divide the joint cavity.
(c) The hinged type can be exemplified by metacarpophalangeal joints.
(d) The stability of the joint is generally inversely proportional to its mobility.
(e) The hip joint is of the plane type.

49. Carpal tunnel syndrome:

(a) May cause irreversible wasting of the thenar eminence.
(b) Can be detected by Thomas's test.
(c) Causes paraesthesia in the ulnar nerve distribution.
(d) Is caused by compression of the nerve by the extensor retinaculum.
(e) Occurs in pregnant women.

50. Fibrous joints:

(a) Contain fibrous tissue on their articulating surfaces.
(b) Have a joint cavity.
(c) Allow little or no movement.
(d) Of the suture type may become ossified.
(e) Of the syndesmosis type are found in the interosseous membrane of the radioulnar joint.

51. Congenital dislocation of the hip:

(a) Is more common in boys than girls.
(b) Occurs in the left hip more than the right.
(c) Should be corrected in the first week of life.
(d) The acetabulum is abnormally shallow.
(e) May lead to delayed walking and abnormal gait.

52. Cartilaginous joints:

(a) Contain some hyaline cartilage.
(b) Of the primary type are all temporary unions.
(c) Of the secondary type are also united by fibrocartilage.
(d) Are generally very mobile.
(e) Are found in the symphysis pubis, costosternal and manubriosternal joints.

53. Osteoarthritis:

(a) Is commonly due to infection.
(b) Causes Heberden's and Bouchard's nodes.
(c) Features early morning stiffness.
(d) Usually affects joints symmetrically.
(e) Enzymes released from chondrocytes are responsible for cartilage degeneration.

54. A joint:

(a) Allows mobility in direct proportion to its stability.
(b) Has a poor blood supply inside its capsule.
(c) Contains veins and lymphatic vessels in the synovial membrane.
(d) Is supplied by the same nerves as those of the overlying skin and muscles moving the joint.
(e) Does not mediate pain but allows proprioception only.

55. Deformities of the toes:

(a) Hammer toes most commonly develop in the big toes.
(b) Poliomyelitis may cause claw toes.
(c) In a mallet toe, the proximal interphalangeal joint cannot be fully extended.
(d) Bunions may be a consequence of hallux valgus.
(e) Hallux rigidus may cause pain on walking and limited movement.

56. Synovial joints:

(a) Do not always contain a cavity.
(b) Are the most common joint type found in the skeleton.
(c) Of the hinge type allow biaxial movement.
(d) Of the condyloid type are found at the base of the fingers and toes.
(e) Of the ball and socket type allow the greatest range of movement.

57. HLA B27 may be associated with the following:

(a) Rheumatoid arthritis.
(b) Osteoarthritis.
(c) Reiter's syndrome.
(d) Behçet's syndrome.
(e) Ankylosing spondylitis.

58. Rheumatoid arthritis:

(a) Is more common in males.
(b) May be complicated by septic arthritis.
(c) Most commonly affects the distal interphalangeal joints.
(d) Is associated with destruction of cartilage.
(e) Patients may demonstrate the presence of ANAs.

59. Gait:

(a) Osteoarthritis of the hip causes limping.
(b) Myogenic gait is caused by weak gluteal muscles.
(c) Leg circumduction may be caused by abduction deformity.
(d) Ankylosis may cause an arthrogenic gait.
(e) A neurogenic gait may be caused by cerebellar ataxis.

60. Regarding the painful arc syndrome

(a) Shoulder adduction causes pain in the midrange, but not at extremes of movement.
(b) The syndrome can be caused by tearing of the supraspinatus tendon.
(c) The syndrome can be caused by infraspinatus tendonitis.
(d) The clinical symptoms may be confused with those of subacromial bursitis.
(e) The disorder should be treated by surgery.

61. Adhesive capsulitis:

(a) This disorder is also known as 'frozen shoulder'.
(b) It affects the acromioclavicular joint.
(c) Gross changes are seen on X-ray.
(d) It may be preceded by minor trauma.
(e) If rested, recovery will occur within a few hours.

62. Epicondylitis:

(a) Affecting the lateral epicondyle is known as tennis elbow.
(b) Lateral epicondylitis affects the common flexor tendon.
(c) The pain of medial epicondylitis may be exacerbated by resisted active flexion of the wrist.
(d) Tennis elbow causes pain that radiates down the extensor aspect of the forearm.
(e) Golfer's elbow may be treated by steroid injections.

63. Regarding the differences between gout and pseudogout:

(a) Gout is caused by calcium pyrophosphate crystals.
(b) The presence of pseudogout is demonstrated by brick-shaped crystals.
(c) Gout is caused by hyperuricaemia.
(d) Pseudogout commonly presents in those over 60 years.
(e) Renal disease is a complication of gout.

64. Reactive arthritis:

(a) Occurs after genital infection with *Candida*.
(b) Occurs after gastrointestinal infection with *Escherichia coli*.
(c) Has an association with HLA B27.
(d) Reiter's syndrome is an example of reactive arthritis.
(e) May lead to severe spondylitis.

The Functioning Musculoskeletal System

65. In motor control:

(a) The three main central controls are the cerebral cortex, brainstem and spinal cord.
(b) The cerebellum and basal ganglia are independent of the cerebral cortex in coordinating movement.
(c) The pyramidal tracts mostly stay on the same side from the motor cortex down the spinal cord.
(d) Muscle spindles are modified muscle fibres called extrafusal fibres.
(e) Golgi tendon organs lie in series with extrafusal muscle fibres.

The Skin

66. Collagen:

(a) Is formed by undifferentiated mesenchymal cells.
(b) Is normally embedded in ground substance.
(c) Has a breakdown product called hydroxyproline, excreted in the urine.
(d) Type III is found in the basement membrane of most cells.
(e) Fibres are mostly located intracellularly.

67. In connective tissue:

(a) Ground substance is not part of the extracellular matrix.
(b) There is a low matrix:cell ratio.
(c) There may be undifferentiated mesenchymal cells present.
(d) Elastic fibres are arranged in random sheets.
(e) Proteoglycans are protein chains bound to branched polysaccharides.

68. Skin:

(a) Makes up 16% of the total body area.
(b) Has a surface area of 25 m².
(c) Is composed of three layers.
(d) Hair is a derivative structure of skin.
(e) Is derived from ectoderm and mesoderm.

69. The dermis:

(a) Is composed of four layers.
(b) The skin is composed of keratin in varying stages.
(c) Keratin is produced by melanocytes.
(d) Keratinocytes absorb the energy of ultraviolet radiation.
(e) The outermost layer of the skin is the stratum spinosum.

70. Regarding the layers of the skin:

(a) The stratum basale is composed of 90% keratinocytes.
(b) Merkel cells aid the diffusion of nutrients.
(c) The keratinocytes in the stratum spinosum are columnar.
(d) Keratinocytes lose their nuclei in the stratum granulosum.
(e) Keratinocytes become cornified at the stratum corneum.

71. Regarding the physiology of the skin:

(a) Cell turnover takes around 21 days.
(b) The keratinocytes take 14 days to mature fully.
(c) The dermis is situated directly below the epidermis.
(d) Dead corneocytes are reabsorbed by the skin.
(e) The subcutaneous level is made up of loose connective tissue and fat.

72. Regarding hair:

(a) The main function of hair is to conserve warmth.
(b) Follicles are most dense on the face and the scalp.
(c) Follicles are derived from the dermis and the epidermis.
(d) The three types of hair are terminal, vellus and telogen.
(e) There are four different stages of hair growth.

73. Regarding the nails:

(a) The nail is composed of a nail bed, nail matrix and a nail plate.
(b) The nail bed is composed of dividing keratinocytes.
(c) The fingernails grow at 0.1 mm/24 h.
(d) Beau's lines are horizontal lines in the nail caused by systemic illness.
(e) Clubbing of the nails is a common indicator of systemic illness.

74. Regarding the glands:

(a) Sebaceous glands produce saliva.
(b) The sebaceous glands are sensitive to androgens.
(c) There are around 2.5 million sweat glands in the skin.
(d) Eccrine glands are found in mucous membranes.
(e) The ducts of apocrine glands empty out into the hair follicles.

75. Regarding nerves in the skin:

(a) The densest concentration of nerve endings is found in the hands, face and genitalia.
(b) Free sensory nerve endings detect pressure.
(c) Free sensory nerve endings contain neurotransmitters such as substance P.
(d) Meissner's corpuscles are sensitive to touch.
(e) Merkel cells are derived embryologically from the neural crest.

76. Regarding melanocyte function:

(a) Melanocytes are found within the stratum corneum of the epidermis.
(b) They produce melanin, a brown pigment.
(c) Melanin helps to protect the skin against ultraviolet light.
(d) Melanocytes are stimulated by photo-oxidation.
(e) Melanocytes act as free radical scavengers.

77. Regarding fibroblast function:

(a) Fibroblasts produce and secrete the components of the extracellular matrix.
(b) Collagen has a brick-like structure.
(c) Collagen makes up 80% of the dry weight of the dermis.
(d) There are 15 different types of collagen present in the skin.
(e) Elastin is produced by fibroblasts.

78. Regarding hypersensitivity reactions of the skin:

(a) The skin can exhibit two out of the four main types of hypersensitivity response.
(b) Type I hypersensitivity is an immediate response.
(c) Type II hypersensitivity is a reaction to immune complex disease.
(d) Immune complexes are formed by the combination of antigen and antibodies in the blood.
(e) Tissue damage caused by type IV hypersensitivity reactions is maximal at 48–72 h.

79. Regarding terminology of skin disorders:

(a) A macule is a raised area of colour change.
(b) A nodule is an elevation less than 5 mm in diameter.
(c) A plaque is an elevation greater than 5 mm in height.
(d) An excoriation is a superficial linear abrasion caused by scratching.
(e) Dyskeratosis is a process in which keratinocytes mature late.

80. Psoriasis:

(a) Is an inflammatory dermatosis with a chronic course.
(b) Palmoplantar pustulosis is the most common form.
(c) Flexural psoriasis is not characterized by scales.
(d) Psoriasis affects 1 in 50 people in the western world.
(e) Active, psoriatic skin has a cell turnover rate that is twice as slow as that of normal skin.

81. Psoriasis may be treated with:

(a) Lassar's paste.
(b) Acetretin.
(c) Calcipotriol.
(d) The Ingram regimen.
(e) Dithranol.

233

82. Contact eczema:

(a) Contact dermatitis is a more severe condition than eczema.
(b) Atopic eczema affects 10–15% of European children.
(c) Family history is positive in 35% of patients with atopic eczema.
(d) Eczema may induce hyperactivity in children.
(e) Medicated bandages are impregnated with ichthammol paste.

83. Dermatitis:

(a) *Pityrosporum ovale* is associated with seborrhoeic dermatitis.
(b) Pompholyx is associated with hand dermatitis.
(c) Asteatotic dermatitis develops in childhood.
(d) Discoid dermatitis may be precipitated by emotional distress.
(e) Generalized exfoliative dermatitis is also known as erythroderma.

84. Urticaria:

(a) Presents insidiously.
(b) Is characterized by oedema.
(c) Can be chronic or acute.
(d) Wheals leave scars upon healing.
(e) Dermographism may be present.

85. Skin eruptions:

(a) Wickham's striae are associated with lichen sclerosus.
(b) Lichen sclerosus has a male: female ratio of 10:1.
(c) Lichen nitidus is a common lichenoid eruption that features tiny monomorphic papules.
(d) A pityriasis rosea eruption is usually preceded by a 'herald patch'.
(e) Parapsoriasis lesions may be pre-malignant.

86. Photodermatoses:

(a) Polymorphic light eruption is the most common photodermatosis.
(b) Chronic actinic dermatitis is a rare condition affecting elderly women.
(c) The wheals of solar urticaria appear within minutes of sun-exposure.
(d) Patients with xeroderma pigmentosum may exhibit photosensitivity.
(e) Sunlight benefits rosacea.

87. The normal skin flora includes:

(a) Staphylococci.
(b) Streptococci.
(c) Escherichia.
(d) Corynebacteria.
(e) Propionibacteria.

88. Bacterial infections:

(a) Erythrasma eruptions will not fluoresce under Wood's light.
(b) Trichomycosis axillaris affects hair.
(c) Impetigo is highly contagious.
(d) Ecthyma leads to ulcer development.
(e) Scalded skin syndrome is caused by a phage 32 staphylococcal infection.

89. Viral infections:

(a) Viral warts are caused by infection with human papilloma virus.
(b) Molluscum contagiosum mainly affects children and teenagers.
(c) Herpes simplex type 1 primary infection is genital.
(d) Herpes zoster occurs in a dermatomal distribution.
(e) Neonatal infection with herpes simplex is commonly fatal.

90. Fungal infections:

(a) Tinea cruris affects the foot.
(b) Dermatophyte fungi reproduce by producing spores.
(c) *M. canis* is passed on from family pets.
(d) *T. mentagrophytes* causes tinea barbae.
(e) Hypothyroidism may predispose to *Candida albicans*.

91. Scabies:

(a) Is caused by *Sarcoptes scabiei hominis*.
(b) The skin takes 4–6 weeks to react to the infestation.
(c) 'Norwegian scabies' is a common infestation in institutions.
(d) The male mite burrows down into the skin at a rate of 2 mm a day.
(e) Burrows are usually found on the wrists, ankles, nipples and genitalia.

92. Acne vulgaris:

(a) Results from chronic inflammation of the stratum corneum.
(b) It affects males more than females.
(c) Primary infection of the pilosebaceous duct by staphylococci may occur.
(d) Acne may lead to severe psychological sequelae.
(e) Comedomes may leave 'ice-pick' scars.

93. Alopecia:

(a) Affects 80% of men by age 70 years.
(b) Can be caused by warfarin.
(c) Pathognomonic 'exclamation mark' hairs occur in tinea capitis.
(d) May be caused by syphilis.
(e) Can be caused by diet deficiencies.

94. Nail disorders:

(a) Paronychia congenita causes nail thinning and discoloration.
(b) Nail–patella syndrome is inherited in a Mendelian dominant fashion.
(c) Malignancy may cause subungual haematoma.
(d) Splinter haemorrhages may be indicative of infective endocarditis.
(e) Infection may predispose to ingrowing toenails.

95. Leg ulcers:

(a) Affect 1 in 1000 people.
(b) Venous ulcers are caused by valve incompetence.
(c) Arterial ulcers may be accompanied by eczema.
(d) Vasculitis ulcers are 'punched-out' lesions.
(e) Neuropathic ulcers commonly occur in diabetics.

96. Disorders of pigmentation:

(a) Vitiligo is associated with pernicious anaemia, thyroid disease and Addison's disease.
(b) Albinism has a prevalence of 1 in 5000.
(c) Phenylketonuria leads to increased melanin synthesis.
(d) Chloasma may be induced by puberty.
(e) Amiodarone may cause pigmentation.

97. Pemphigus:

(a) May prove fatal.
(b) Ninety per cent of patients have circulating IgE autoantibodies.
(c) Affects both sexes equally.
(d) In one-half of patients presents as an eruption of shallow blisters around the mouth.
(e) Steroid treatment must be continued for several years.

98. Seborrhoeic warts:

(a) Are malignant.
(b) Are also known as a basal cell papilloma.
(c) Are composed of basal keratinocytes.
(d) Can grow up to 6 cm in diameter.
(e) Must be treated.

99. Malignant melanoma:

(a) This is the most lethal of skin tumours.
(b) The incidence of malignant melanoma is increasing.
(c) Individuals with multiple melanocytic naevi are at increased risk.
(d) The most common site in the female is the back.
(e) The male: female ratio is 1:5.

100. Cutaneous signs of diabetes mellitus include:

(a) Rosacea.
(b) Necrobiosis lipoidica.
(c) Eruptive xanthomas.
(d) Ulcers.
(e) Kaposi's sarcoma.

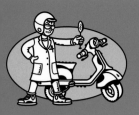

Short-answer Questions (SAQs)

1. List the location and the function of the five main types of collagen.

2. Draw the AP produced in nerve fibres. Explain the ions involved at each stage.

3. Write brief notes on fracture healing and how it may be delayed.

4. Draw a sarcomere: (a) in relaxed muscle; (b) during contraction.

5. Draw a normal synovial joint.

6. List the extra-articular features of rheumatoid arthritis.

7. What are the five changes that may occur in bone secondary to osteoarthritis?

8. List the components of the stratum basale.

9. What are the common skin changes in pregnancy?

10. Which conditions does sunlight benefit?

11. A 35-year-old man presents with a polyarthritis of the terminal interphalangeal joints and dactylitis of the second toe. Upon examination, the patient is found to have a rash on the scalp. Describe the epidemiology of the underlying disorder.

12. A 40-year-old publican presents with a recent history of hot, red and painful knee. There is no previous history of joint disease or trauma; there were no other systemic complaints. What are the two main differential diagnoses and how would you distinguish between them?

13. A 50-year-old woman presents with a 2-month history of progressive, unrelenting night pain of the back associated with cachexia. What systems should be examined?

14. A 24-year-old man presents with a 5-month history of lower back pain. The pain is worse upon rest, and his back is particularly stiff in the morning. His lumbar spine movement is reduced in all planes. What is the likely diagnosis, what blood tests should be taken and what changes may be apparent on X-ray?

15. An 18-year-old woman developed a red, pruritic eruption on her forehead. Her chemist advised the use of a topical anti-histamine. 24 h after applying the cream her face became severely swollen. What is the diagnosis and how can it be confirmed?

16. A 72-year-old woman with rheumatoid arthritis presents with tingling over the fingers of her left hand. The thumb, index and middle fingers were most severely affected, and sometimes the symptoms woke her during the night. What is the most likely diagnosis, what are the structures affected and which tests should be performed?

17. A 78-year-old woman fell onto the side of her hip and presented with severe pain in her left lower limb. The leg was externally rotated and shortened. What is the diagnosis and treatment for this lady, and what is the most severe complication?

18. A 68-year-old man presented with a history of aching legs, with a worsening of pain at the end of the day. Recently, he had also noticed pain and stiffness in his neck. He noticed that his legs were initially stiff in the morning, but this wore off after about 15 min. What is his diagnosis, prognosis and what may his X-rays show?

19. A 14-year-old boy presented with a generalized eruption of scaly, oval, mildy pruritic papules and plaques on his trunk. The pattern of the eruption was parallel to the lines of the ribs, radiating away from the spine. What is the diagnosis, how long will the eruption persist, and what may the patient have noticed a few days before the eruption began?

20. A 27-year-old man presents with a knee that recurrently 'gives way'. He first noticed the problem after twisting his knee whilst playing football; he recalls hearing a popping sound at the time. What is the diagnosis, and what test should be performed to confirm it? What may this injury cause in the future?

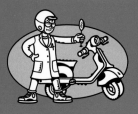

Essay Questions

1. List the events occurring at the NMJ on arrival of an AP at the nerve terminal, and discuss the drugs that may influence this process.

_____

2. Describe the ionic basis of the RMP and how this is maintained.

_____

3. Compare the cardiac AP with that seen in skeletal muscle and explain how any differences may be related to function.

_____

4. Discuss the role of vitamin D, PTH and calcitonin in calcium metabolism.

_____

5. Compare and contrast intramembranous ossification with endochondral ossification.

_____

6. Describe the microstructure of skeletal muscle.

_____

7. Describe the epidemiology, pathology and clinical features of osteoporosis.

_____

8. What are the clinical manifestations of osteoarthritis in the wrist and hand? Compare these with the 'rheumatoid hand'.

_____

9. Write an essay on the microscopic arrangement of bone.

_____

10. Describe the epidemiology, pathology and clinical features of Duchenne muscular dystrophy.

11. Classify the different types of bone tumour.

_____

12. Compare the blood supply, lymphatic drainage and nerve supply of bone with that of cartilage.

_____

13. Describe the major differences between cardiac, skeletal and smooth muscle.

_____

14. What are the stages of keratinocyte maturation? Describe the cell changes in each stage.

_____

15. Compare the different treatments for psoriasis.

_____

16. Differentiate between basal cell carcinoma and squamous cell carcinoma.

_____

17. What are the differences between common, plantar and genital warts?

_____

18. Describe the different clinical presentations of _Trichophyton_ infection.

_____

19. What are the clinical manifestations of _Sarcoptes scabiei hominis_ infestation.

_____

20. Describe the differing stages of hair development.

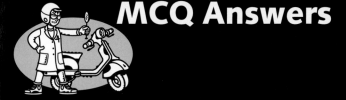

1. (a) F—The all-or-none law states that once an AP has been initiated the size is constant for a given type of cell and that altering the stimulus strength does not affect this.
    (b) T—Initiation does occur when the membrane potential is reduced to a critical value.
    (c) T—Influx of sodium ions is responsible for the rising phase.
    (d) T—There is a transient decrease in membrane permeability of potassium ions.
    (e) F—The size and duration of the AP within different cells is variable.

2. (a) T—The concentration of potassium ions is higher inside the nerve than on the outside.
    (b) T—The RMP does result in an increase in excitability of the cell when reduced.
    (c) T—The RMP does have a value of –90 mV in muscle cells.
    (d) T—The RMP is also known as the equilibrium potential.
    (e) T—The RMP is equal to the equilibrium potential of potassium.

3. (a) T—Neurotransmission at the NMJ is impaired by hemicholinium.
    (b) T—Neurotransmission at the NMJ is impaired by suxamethonium.
    (c) F—Adrenaline is a stimulant.
    (d) T—Neurotransmission at the NMJ is impaired by botulinum toxin.
    (e) F—Edrophonium is a short-acting anticholinesterase which enhances transmission.

4. (a) T—Edrophonium is used in the treatment of myasthenia gravis
    (b) T—Edrophonium may cause constriction of the pupil
    (c) T—Edrophonium enhances transmission at the NMJ
    (d) F—Edrophonium enhances transmission at the NMJ.
    (e) F—Edrophonium decreases reuptake of neurotransmitter at the NMJ.

5. (a) F—There is a synaptic delay of 1–5 ms in chemical transmission, which does not occur with electrical transmission.
    (b) T—The synaptic cleft is larger in chemical synapses.
    (c) T—Plasticity may occur in chemical synapses.
    (d) T—Chemical synapses are more common.
    (e) T—Amplification of the signal is possible at chemical synapses.

6. (a) F—Saltatory conduction only occurs in myelinated nerve fibres.
    (b) T—Speed is proportional to the diameter of the nerve fibre in saltatory conduction.
    (c) T—In saltatory conduction, speed is proportional to the strength of local circuits.
    (d) T—A large safety factor is demonstrated in saltatory conduction.
    (e) F—Membrane depolarization is more rapid as saltatory conduction occurs at a greater velocity in saltatory conduction.

7. (a) T—Conduction velocity does increase in the presence of a myelin sheath.
    (b) F—Above 40°, conduction velocity decreases until there is heat block.
    (c) F—Large fibres increase the conduction velocity.
    (d) T—Conduction velocity is influenced by the strength of local circuits.
    (e) T—Conduction velocity may be less than 1 m/s.

8. (a) F—It contains alternating A and I bands.
    (b) T—Striated muscle fibres are multinucleate.
    (c) T—Striated muscle is present in the upper part of the oesophagus.
    (d) F—Sarcolemma is another term for the cell membrane of a muscle cell.
    (e) T—Striated muscle is the most common type of muscle found in the body.

9. (a) T—In skeletal muscle, a smaller stimulus is required to cause local contraction if applied to the Z band.
    (b) T—In skeletal muscle, the distance bewteen the Z bands is constant during contraction.
    (c) T—In skeletal muscle, each muscle fibre is innervated by only one motor neuron.
    (d) T—In skeletal muscle, APs are propagated in both directions to the ends of the muscle fibre.
    (e) T—In skeletal muscle, the length of the I bands decreases during contraction.

10. (a) T—In skeletal muscle, muscles are arranged in groups.
    (b) F—A muscle may be a member of more than one group.
    (c) T—For a given volume of muscle, an oblique arrangement of muscle fibres would result in a greater force of contraction than a parallel arrangement.
    (d) F—Muscle fibres are innervated by muscle spindles.
    (e) T—The origin of a muscle is the attachment site at which there is little movement when the muscle performs its main action.

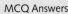

11. (a) F—The muscle fibres innervated by a single motor neuron are spread out within the motor unit.
    (b) T—In the muscle unit, the muscle fibres within a motor unit are of the same type.
    (c) T—Muscles involved in fine movement have smaller motor units.
    (d) T—The strength of muscle contraction is increased by recruiting more motor units.
    (e) T—The muscle fibres within a motor unit contract simultaneously.

12. (a) T—Actin is a component of the thin filament.
    (b) F—Desmin is a contractile filament with smooth muscle.
    (c) F—Calmodulin is an intracellular protein found in the cytoplasm of smooth muscle cells.
    (d) T—Troponin is a component of the thin filament.
    (e) T—α-Actinin is a component of the thin filament.

13. (a) F—Conduction speed is greatest in white fibres.
    (b) T—Red fibres are resistant to fatigue.
    (c) T—Myoglobin is present in red fibres.
    (d) F—White fibres are involved in the performance of brief, strong muscle contractions, e.g. jumping.
    (e) T—Glycogen content is high in white fibres.

14. (a) T—ATP is required to cause detachment of myosin heads from the actin filaments.
    (b) T—ATP is provided by glycolysis.
    (c) F—ATP is produced by rapid synthesis from creatine kinase.
    (d) T—ATP is necessary for the influx of sodium ions.
    (e) T—ATP is produced by oxidative phosphorylation.

15. (a) F—The rise in intracellular calcium ions results from entry through Ca^{2+} channels in the sarcoplasmic reticulum, along a concentration gradient.
    (b) F—The calcium ions bind to troponin C.
    (c) F—The length of the sarcomeres decrease because of the sliding of actin filaments. The number of sarcomeres stays the same.
    (d) F—The actin and myosin filaments slide along each other during muscle contraction; they do not shorten.
    (e) T—In skeletal muscle, the strength of contraction is influenced by initial muscle fibre length.

16. (a) F—Isometric contraction of skeletal muscle is contraction in muscle with a constant length.
    (b) T—The treppe effect is associated with cardiac contraction.
    (c) T—The force of skeletal muscle contraction increases with frequency of stimulation.
    (d) T—Plasticity may involve altering vascular supply to the muscle.
    (e) T—Most muscles in the body are at optimum length for maximal tension.

17. (a) T—Myasthenia gravis may be associated with ptosis.
    (b) F—Occurs most commonly in the third decade.
    (c) F—Is associated with antibodies to the ACh receptor.
    (d) T—When associated with a thymoma.
    (e) T—Myasthenia gravis may be transient in newborn babies of female sufferers.

18. (a) F—Gower's sign is a feature of Duchenne muscular dystrophy.
    (b) F—Duchenne muscular dystrophy is inherited in an X-linked recessive manner.
    (c) T—Fascioscapulohumeral dystrophy may be associated with winging of the scapulae.
    (d) T—Mitochondrial myopathy may be associated with patients infected with HIV.
    (e) T—Pseudohypertrophy of the calves is a sign of Duchenne muscular dystrophy.

19. (a) F—Most patients with idiopathic inflammatory myopathies usually present in middle age.
    (b) T—The rash is usually found on the eyelids.
    (c) F—Viral myalgia most commonly follows a respiratory infection.
    (d) T—The average age of presentation is 2 years old.
    (e) F—Lipid disorders usually cause hypotonia.

20. (a) T—Side effects of local anaesthetics include allergic reactions causing sudden collapse.
    (b) T—Side effects of local anaesthetics include stimulation of the central nervous system.
    (c) F—Local anaesthetics are administered with vasoconstrictors to prevent the drug diffusing away from the required site too quickly. Local anaesthetics do not act as vasoconstrictors themselves.
    (d) F—Local anaesthetics do not cause physical dependency.
    (e) F—Local anaesthetics cause hypotension.

21. (a) T—Smooth muscle cells have a single nucleus located at the widest part of the cell.
    (b) T—Smooth muscle cells contain myofilaments that can only be seen with an electron microscope.
    (c) F—Mesenchymal cells can be adapted in adult life to replace smooth muscle cells.
    (d) F—Change size when they contract.
    (e) T—Smooth muscle cells form tight junctions with each other.

22. (a) T—In smooth muscle cells, the protein desmin is present.
    (b) F—Actin, myosin and desmin are the only contractile proteins present in smooth muscle.
    (c) F— Calcium ions are responsible for the AP.
    (d) T—In smooth muscle cells, contraction requires lower ATP contraction.
    (e) F—Calmodulin is an intracellular protein found in the cytoplasm of smooth muscle cells.

23. (a) F—The three layers: inner longitudinal layer, middle circular layer and outer longitudinal layer.
    (b) T—Carbon dioxide and Ca^{2+} are also local tissue factors that produce smooth muscle contractions.
    (c) T—Smooth muscle cells communicate electrically via gap (nexus) junctions.
    (d) F—Organic nitrates decrease smooth muscle tone.
    (e) T—Smooth muscle facilitates peristalsis.

24. (a) T—In cardiac muscle, the AP is initiated in the sinoatrial node.
    (b) F—The AP is 100 times longer than that in skeletal muscle.
    (c) T—The AP demonstrates a plateau phase.
    (d) F—Cells have a large, central nucleus.
    (e) T—Summation of contractions does not occur.

25. (a) T—Calcium ions are responsible for the rising phase of the AP.
    (b) T—The refractory period is longer than that following an AP in skeletal muscle.
    (c) T—The sympathetic nervous system shortens the plateau phase of the AP.
    (d) T—Calcium ions play a part in the AP.
    (e) F—Self-initiation occurs via pacemaker cells.

26. (a) F—Pacemaker tissue is also found in the AV node, bundle of His and Purkinje fibres.
    (b) T—Inotropes increase the force of cardiac contraction.
    (c) T—Starling's law states that the force of contraction is proportional to the initial length of the cardiac muscle fibres.
    (d) F—The RMP of cardiac cells is –55 mV.
    (e) F—Myocardium composes the bulk of the heart: it is thickest in the ventricles.

27. (a) F—Rapid stimulation results in summation only in skeletal muscle.
    (b) T—An increase in intracellular calcium concentration is necessary for muscular contraction.
    (c) F—Control of contraction varies between muscle types.
    (d) T—Membrane depolarization is necessary for APs to occur.
    (e) T—The presence of actin and myosin.

28. (a) F—Intercalated discs are present in cardiac muscle.
    (b) T—Cardiac muscle fibres are cross-striated.
    (c) F—Transverse tubules are found in skeletal muscle.
    (d) F—Myofilaments are disorganized in smooth muscle.
    (e) F—Muscle spindles are not present in smooth muscle.

29. (a) T—The skeleton is derived from the primitive mesenchyme.
    (b) T—The skeleton has a solid extracellular matrix.
    (c) F—Consists of bone and cartilage.
    (d) T—The skeleton is a major storage site for calcium.
    (e) F—Yellow bone marrow can revert to red under stress.

30. (a) T—The human skeleton is bilaterally symmetrical.
    (b) T—The human skeleton has an axial part, comprising the bones of the head, neck, and trunk.
    (c) F—The appendicular part consists of limb bones and those forming the pectoral and pelvic girdles.
    (d) T—The human skeleton contains active red bone marrow in both children and adults.
    (e) F—Contains bones that all develop from the same embryonic cellular connective tissue, the mesenchyme.

31. (a) T—Cartilage is an avascular tissue.
    (b) F—Hyaline cartilage is immensely strong and forms permanent structures.
    (c) T—Blood is carried into the centre of tissue by cartilage canals: mature cartilage is an avascular tissue.
    (d) F—Blood is carried into the centre of tissue by cartilage canals: mature cartilage is an avascular tissue.
    (e) F—Articular hyaline cartilage.

32. (a) F—Elastic cartilage has prominent elastic fibres.
    (b) T—Hyaline cartilage contains a few collagen-like fibres.
    (c) T—Hyaline cartilage is the precursor of endochondral ossification.
    (d) F—The knee menisci are formed from fibrocartilage.
    (e) F—Is avascular compared with bone.

33. (a) F—No bone ossifies directly from mesenchyme; the cells must differentiate, chondroblasts, etc. first.
    (b) F—Long bones have a thin outer layer of compact bone.
    (c) T—Long bones normally contain yellow marrow in adulthood.
    (d) T—Long bones are organized in Haversian systems.
    (e) F—Periosteum is not acellular.

34. (a) T—Endochondral ossification occurs in all long bones except the clavicle.
    (b) T—Endochondral ossification occurs in cartilage that has replaced a membranous model.
    (c) T—Endochondral ossification has its primary centres appearing *in utero*.
    (d) T—Endochondral ossification is usually complete by the age of 25 years.
    (e) F—The bones of the skull undergo intramembranous ossification.

35. (a) F—Osteoclasts absorb the calcified matrix of the cartilage.
    (b) T—Osteoblasts become osteocytes.
    (c) T—Endochondral ossification extends along the diaphysis.
    (d) F—The epiphyseal plate separates the epiphysis from the metaphysis.
    (e) T—Circumferential growth is by subperiosteal ossification.

36. (a) F—Are not all present at birth.
    (b) T—The epiphyses are formed in hyaline cartilage.
    (c) F—Are present in all long bones.
    (d) F—Are involved in increasing only the length of long bones.
    (e) T—The epiphyses may occur at sites of muscle attachment.

37. (a) T—The destruction of bone is associated with raised urinary hydroxyproline.
    (b) T—The destruction of bone is associated with raised plasma alkaline phosphatase.
    (c) F—Associated with decreased plasma acid phosphatase.
    (d) T—The destruction of bone is associated with raised plasma calcium.
    (e) T—The destruction of bone is associated with lowered plasma phosphate.

38. (a) F—The density of the skeleton is reduced in both osteoporosis and osteomalacia.
    (b) T—The remaining bone in osteoporosis has a normal histological appearance.
    (c) T—There are gross changes in the epiphyses in osteomalacia.
    (d) F—Pseudofractures are more common in osteomalacia than in osteoporosis.
    (e) T—Excess bone matrix is found in osteomalacia.

39. (a) T—Absence of infection promotes fracture healing.
    (b) T—Adequate vitamin C promotes fracture healing.
    (c) T—Good blood supply promotes fracture healing.
    (d) F—Immediate immobilization.
    (e) F—Use of steroids is not necessary in fracture management.

40. (a) T—Metastases in bone show both bone destruction and new bone formation.
    (b) T—Metastases in bone cause pathological fractures.
    (c) F—Increased plasma alkaline phosphatase.
    (d) T—Metastases in bone affect red marrow more than yellow marrow.
    (e) T—Metastases in bone may cause immature red blood cells in peripheral blood.

41. (a) T—Calcium controls neuromuscular excitability.
    (b) T—Calcium acts as an intracellular second messenger.
    (c) F—Calcium is mobilized quickly from cancellous bone to blood.
    (d) T—Calcium absorption in small intestine is enhanced by vitamin D.
    (e) F—Parathyroid hormone is responsible for raising low blood calcium levels to normal.

42. (a) T—Cartilage consists of chondroblasts and chondrocytes embedded in a cartilage matrix.
    (b) F—Growth and maturation take place either at the centre (interstitial growth) or at the periphery (appositional growth).
    (c) F—Mature cartilage is an avascular tissue.
    (d) T—Hyaline cartilage is present in the epiphyseal plates.
    (e) T—Elastic cartilage is found in the epiglottis.

43. (a) T—Long bones have a shaft called the diaphysis.
    (b) F—The expanded ends are called epiphyses.
    (c) T—Long bones contain a central medullary cavity.
    (d) F—Long bones consist of cancellous and compact bone.
    (e) T—Long bones are lined by endosteum.

44. (a) T—Paget's disease of bone is also known as osteitis deformans.
    (b) F—It is a disease of bone formation and resorption.
    (c) F—Commonly presents in patients aged over 40 years.
    (d) F—Affects the tibia, femur, vertebrae, humerus and skull.
    (e) F—Is rare in the Asian and African populations.

45. (a) F—It is infection of bone.
    (b) T—Osteomyelitis can be pyogenic or tuberculous.
    (c) F—Necrosis of bone leads directly to sequestrum. Involucrum is the formation of new bone.
    (d) T—Osteomyelitis may lead to the formation of Brodie's abscesses.
    (e) T—Osteomyelitis causes acute bone pain and fever.

46. (a) F—This is the death of bone without infection.
    (b) T—Avascular necrosis is due to a poor blood supply.
    (c) F—The most common sites are the head of the femur and scaphoid.
    (d) T—Subchondral infarction may lead to wedge-shaped areas of damage.
    (e) T—Intracapsular fractures predispose to avascular necrosis.

47. (a) T—Metastatic tumours of the skeleton are more common than primary tumours.
    (b) T—Metastatic tumours that arise from the breast, kidney, thyroid and lung are lytic.
    (c) T—Metastatic tumours that arise from the breast are sclerotic.
    (d) T—Detects areas of increased bone turnover.
    (e) T—To detect primary tumour.

48. (a) F—Articular surfaces are always lined by hyaline cartilage.
    (b) F—Fibrocartilaginous discs usually partially divide the joint cavity in fibrous joints.
    (c) F—Metacarpophalangeal joints are condyloid joints.
    (d) T—The stability of the joint is generally inversely proportional to its mobility.
    (e) F—The hip joint is a ball and socket joint.

49. (a) T—Carpal tunnel syndrome may cause irreversible wasting of the thenar eminence.
    (b) F—Tineal's or Phalen's test is used to detect carpal tunnel syndrome.
    (c) F—Causes paraesthesia in the median nerve distribution.
    (d) F—Is caused by compression of the nerve by the flexor retinaculum.
    (e) T—Also in cases of myxoedema and rheumatoid arthritis.

50. (a) T—Fibrous joints contain fibrous tissue on their articulating surfaces.
    (b) T—Fibrous joints do not have a joint cavity.
    (c) T—Fibrous joints allow little or no movement.
    (d) T—Fibrous joints of the suture type may become ossified.
    (e) T—Fibrous joints of the syndesmosis type are found in the interosseous membrane of the radioulnar joint.

51. (a) F—The female: male ratio is 8:1.
    (b) T—Congenital dislocation of the hip occurs in the left hip more than the right.
    (c) T—Congenital dislocation of the hip should be corrected in the first week of life.
    (d) T—In congenital dislocation of the hip, the acetabulum is abnormally shallow.
    (e) T—Congenital dislocation of the hip may lead to delayed walking and abnormal gait.

52. (a) T—Cartilaginous joints contain some hyaline cartilage.
    (b) F—Primary cartilaginous joints are usually permanent.
    (c) T—Cartilaginous joints of the secondary type are also united by fibrocartilage.
    (d) F—Cartilaginous joints usually permit very little movement.
    (e) T—Cartilaginous joints are found in the symphysis pubis, costosternal, and manubriosternal joints.

53. (a) F—It is due to degeneration of cartilage.
    (b) T—Osteoarthritis causes Heberden's and Bouchard's nodes.
    (c) T—This resolves after a short period, unlike the early morning stiffness of rheumatoid arthritis.
    (d) T—A unilateral pattern may also be seen.
    (e) T—Enzymes released from chondrocytes are responsible for cartilage degeneration.

54. (a) F—The more unstable a joint becomes, the more mobile it is.
    (b) F—Joint capsules have a good blood supply.
    (c) T—A joint contains veins and lymphatic vessels in the synovial membrane.
    (d) T—A joint is supplied by the same nerves as those of the overlying skin and muscles moving the joint.
    (e) F—Joints mediate both pain and proprioception.

55. (a) F—Hammer toes most commonly develop in the second toes.
    (b) T—Poliomyelitis and rheumatoid arthritis may cause claw toes.
    (c) F—In a mallet toe, the distal interphalangeal joint cannot be fully extended.
    (d) T—Protective bunions develop where shoes rub.
    (e) T—Hallux rigidus may cause pain on walking and limited movement.

56. (a) F—Synovial joints always contain a cavity.
    (b) T—Synovial joints are the most common joint type found in the skeleton.
    (c) F—Hinge-type joints allow monoaxial movement.
    (d) T—Synovial joints of the condyloid type are found at the base of the fingers and toes.
    (e) T—Synovial joints of the ball and socket type allow the greatest range of movement.

57. (a) F—HLA B27 is not associated with rheumatoid arthritis.
    (b) F—HLA B27 is not associated with osteoarthritis.
    (c) T—HLA B27 may be associated with Reiter's syndrome.
    (d) F—HLA B27 is not associated with Behçet's syndrome.
    (e) T—HLA B27 may be associated with ankylosing spondylitis.

58. (a) F—Male: female ratio is 1:3.
(b) T—Rheumatoid arthritis may be complicated by septic arthritis.
(c) F—Commonly affects the proximal interphalangeal joints.
(d) T—Rheumatoid arthritis is associated with destruction of cartilage.
(e) T—Patients with rheumatoid arthritis may demonstrate the presence of ANAs.

59. (a) T—Caused by shortening of bone.
(b) T—Myogenic gait is caused by weak gluteal muscle.
(c) T—Leg circumduction may be caused by abduction deformity.
(d) T—Fixed flexion deformity may also result in this gait.
(e) T— As may hemiparesis, parkinsonism, cerebal palsy, footdrop and bilateral leg spasticity.

60. (a) F—Shoulder abduction causes pain in the midrange: between 45 and 150°.
(b) T—The syndrome can be caused by tearing of the supraspinatus tendon.
(c) F—The syndrome can be caused by supraspinatus tendonitis.
(d) T—The clinical symptoms may be confused with those of subacromial bursitis.
(e) F—The first line of treatment should be hydrocortisone injection and then surgery.

61. (a) T—Adhesive capsulitis is also known as 'frozen shoulder'.
(b) F—It affects the glenohumeral joint.
(c) F—No changes are seen on X-ray.
(d) T—It may be preceded by minor trauma.
(e) F—Recovery includes the stages of pain, stiffness and then recuperation. The lesion may take months to heal.

62. (a) T—Epicondylitis affecting the lateral epicondyle is known as tennis elbow.
(b) F—It affects the common extensor tendon.
(c) T—The pain of medial epicondylitis may be exacerbated by resisted active flexion of the wrist.
(d) T—Tennis elbow causes pain that radiates down the extensor aspect of the forearm.
(e) T—As may tennis elbow.

63. (a) F—Pseudogout is caused by calcium pyrophosphate crystals; gout is caused by monosodium urate crystals.
(b) T—Gout crystals are needle-shaped.
(c) T—Gout is caused by hyperuricaemia.
(d) T—Gout presents in those aged 20–60 years.
(e) T—Renal disease is a complication of gout.

64. (a) F—Occurs after genital infection with *Chlamydia*.
(b) F—Occurs after gastrointestinal infection with *Salmonella*, *Campylobacter* or *Shigella*.
(c) T—Reactive arthritis has an association with HLA-B27.
(d) T—It is characterized by a triad of arthritis, urethritis/cervicitis and conjunctivitis.
(e) T—Reactive arthritis may lead to severe spondylitis.

65. (a) T—In motor control, the three main central controls are the cerebral cortex, brainstem and spinal cord.
(b) F—The cerebral cortex ultimately coordinates movement.
(c) F—80% of fibres decussate as they descend.
(d) F—Muscle spindles are modified muscle fibres called intrafusal fibres.
(e) T—Golgi tendon organs lie in series with extrafusal muscle fibres.

66. (a) F—Is produced from topocollagen, a substance synthesized by the endoplasmic reticulum of matrix-secreting cells.
(b) T—Collagen is normally embedded in ground substance.
(c) T—Collagen has a breakdown product called hydroxyproline, excreted in the urine.
(d) F—Type III is found in the connective tissues of organs.
(e) F—Collagen is the main fibre found of the extracellular matrix of connective tissue.

67. (a) F—The three main components of connective tissue are cells, fibres and ground substance.
(b) F—There is a high matrix:cell ratio.
(c) T—There may be undifferentiated mesenchymal cells present.
(d) T—Elastic fibres are arranged in random sheets.
(e) T—Proteoglycans are protein chains bound to branched polysaccharides.

68. (a) T—Skin makes up 16% of the total body area.
(b) F—Has a surface area of 1.8 m².
(c) T—Skin is composed of three layers.
(d) T—Hair is a derivative structure of skin.
(e) T—Skin is derived from ectoderm and mesoderm.

69. (a) T—The dermis is composed of four layers.
(b) T—The skin is composed of keratin in varying stages of maturation.
(c) F—Keratin is produced by keratinocytes.
(d) F—Melanocytes absorb the energy of ultraviolet radiation.
(e) F—The outermost layer of the skin is the stratum corneum.

70. (a) T—The stratum basale is composed of 90% keratinocytes.
    (b) F—Merkel cells appear to have a role in sensation.
    (c) F—The keratinocytes in the stratum spinosum transform from columnar to polyhedral.
    (d) T—Keratinocytes lose their nuclei in the stratum granulosum.
    (e) T—Keratinocytes become cornified at the stratum corneum.

71. (a) F—Cell turnover takes around 28 days.
    (b) T—The keratinocytes take 14 days to fully mature.
    (c) T—The dermis is situated directly below the epidermis.
    (d) F—Dead corneocytes are shed from the surface of the skin.
    (e) T—The subcutaneous level is made up of loose connective tissue and fat.

72. (a) F—The main function of hair today is sexual attraction.
    (b) T—Follicles are most dense on the face and the scalp.
    (c) T—Follicles are derived from the dermis and the epidermis.
    (d) F—The three types of hair are terminal, vellus and lanugo.
    (e) F—There are three different stages: anagen, catagen and telogen.

73. (a) T—The nail is composed of a nail bed, nail matrix and a nail plate.
    (b) F—The nail matrix is composed of dividing keratinocytes.
    (c) T—The fingernails grow at 0.1 mm/24 h.
    (d) F—Beau's lines are transverse lines in the nail caused by systemic illness.
    (e) T—Clubbing of the nails is a common indicator of systemic illness.

74. (a) F—Sebaceous glands produce sebum.
    (b) T—The sebaceous glands are sensitive to androgens.
    (c) T—There are around 2.5 million sweat glands in the skin.
    (d) F—Eccrine glands are found all over the skin, especially in the palms, soles, axillae and forehead, but are not present in mucous membranes.
    (e) T—The ducts of apocrine glands empty out into the hair follicles.

75. (a) T—The densest concentration of nerve endings is found in the hands, face and genitalia.
    (b) F—Free sensory nerve endings: pain, itch and temperature.
    (c) T—Free sensory nerve endings contain neurotransmitters such as substance P.
    (d) T—Meissner's corpuscles are sensitive to touch.
    (e) T—Merkel cells are derived from the neural crest.

76. (a) F—Melanocytes are found within the stratum basale of the epidermis.
    (b) T—They produce melanin, a brown pigment.
    (c) T—Melanin helps to protect the skin against UV.
    (d) T—Melanocytes are stimulated by photo-oxidation.
    (e) F—Melanins act as free radical scavengers.

77. (a) T—Fibroblasts produce and secrete the components of the extracellular matrix.
    (b) F—Collagen has a cable-like structure that provides tensile strength.
    (c) T—Collagen makes up 80% of the dry weight of the dermis.
    (d) F—Out of the 15 different types of collagen, five are present in the skin.
    (e) T—Elastin is produced by fibroblasts.

78. (a) F—The skin can exhibit all four main types of hypersensitivity response.
    (b) T—Type I hypersensitivity is an immediate response.
    (c) F—Type III hypersensitivity is a reaction to immune complex disease.
    (d) T—Immune complexes are formed by the combination of antigen and antibodies in the blood.
    (e) T—Tissue damage due to Type IV hypersensitivity reaction is maximal at 48–72 hours.

79. (a) F—A macule is a flat area of colour change.
    (b) F—A nodule is an elevation more than 5 mm in diameter.
    (c) F—A plaque is an elevation less than 5 mm in height.
    (d) T—An excoriation is a superficial linear abrasion due to scratching.
    (e) F—Dyskeratosis is a process in which keratinocytes mature early.

80. (a) T—Is an inflammatory dermatosis with a chronic course.
    (b) F—Plaque is the most common form.
    (c) T—Flexural psoriasis is not characterized by scales.
    (d) T—Psoriasis affects 1 in 50 people in the western world.
    (e) F—Active, psoriatic skin has a cell turnover rate that is 20–30 times faster than that of normal skin.

81. (a) T—Coal tar preparation.
    (b) T—Retinoid.
    (c) T—Vitamin D analogue
    (d) T—Psoriasis may be treated by the Ingram regimen.
    (e) T—Dithranol is an effective treatment.

82. (a) F—Contact dermatitis and eczema are names for the same condition.
    (b) T—Atopic eczema affects 10–15% of European children.
    (c) F—Family history is positive in 65% of patients with atopic eczema.
    (d) T—Eczema may induce hyperactivity in children.
    (e) T – Also with coal tar.

83. (a) T—*Pityrosporum ovale* is associated with seborrhoeic dermatitis.
    (b) T—Pompholyx is associated with hand dermatitis.
    (c) F—Asteatotic dermatitis develops in old age.
    (d) T—Discoid dermatitis may be precipitated by emotional distress.
    (e) T—Generalized exfoliative dermatitis is also known as erythroderma.

84. (a) F—Lesions present acutely, appearing and disappearing within 24 h.
    (b) T—Urticaria is characterized by oedema.
    (c) T—Urticaria can be chronic or acute.
    (d) F—Wheals leave no residual scar.
    (e) T—Demographism may be present in urticaria

85. (a) F—Wickham's striae are associated with lichen planus.
    (b) F—Lichen sclerosus has a male: female ratio of 1:10.
    (c) F—Lichen nitidus is a rare condition.
    (d) T—A pityriasis rosea eruption is usually preceded by a 'herald patch'.
    (e) T—Parapsoriasis lesions may be pre-malignant.

86. (a) T—Polymorphic light eruption is the most common photodermatosis.
    (b) F—Chronic actinic dermatitis affects elderly men.
    (c) T—It only takes a few minutes for the effects of sunlight to appear on the skin on patients with solar urticaria.
    (d) T—Photosensitivity is a symptom of xeroderma pigmentosum.
    (e) F—Sunlight aggravates rosacea.

87. (a) T—The presence of Staphylocci is a normal finding.
    (b) F—The presence of Streptococci indicates pathology.
    (c) F—The presence of Escherichia indicates pathology.
    (d) T—The presence of Corynebacteria is a normal finding.
    (e) T—The presence of Propionibacteria is a normal finding.

88. (a) F—Erythrasma eruptions will fluoresce under Wood's light.
    (b) T—Trichomycosis axillaris affects hair.
    (c) T—Impetigo is highly contagious.
    (d) T—Ecthyma leads to ulcer development.
    (e) F—Scalded skin syndrome is caused by a phage 71 staphylococcal infection.

89. (a) T—Viral warts are due to infection with human papilloma virus.
    (b) T—Molluscum contagiosum mainly affects children and teenagers.
    (c) F—Herpes simplex type 2 primary infection is genital.
    (d) T—Herpes zoster occurs in a dermatomal distribution.
    (e) T—Neonatal infection with herpes simplex is commonly fatal.

90. (a) F—Tinea cruris affects the groin.
    (b) T—Dermatophyte fungi reproduce by producing spores.
    (c) T—Mainly kittens and puppies.
    (d) T—*T. mentagrophytes* causes tinea barbae.
    (e) T—Hypothyroidism may predispose to *Candida albicans*.

91. (a) T—Scabies is caused by *Sarcoptes scarbiei hominis*.
    (b) T—The skin takes 4–6 weeks to react to the infestation.
    (c) T—'Norwegian scabies' is a common infestation in institutions.
    (d) F—It is the female mite that burrows down into the skin, not the male.
    (e) T—Burrows are usually found on the wrists, ankles, nipples and genitalia.

92. (a) F—Results from chronic inflammation of the pilosebaceous duct apparatus.
    (b) F—It affects both sexes equally.
    (c) F—Primary infection of the pilosebaceous duct is by *Propionibacterium acnes*.
    (d) T—Acne may lead to severe psychological sequelae.
    (e) F—'Ice-pick' scars are left by cysts.

93. (a) T—Alopecia affects 80% of men by age 70.
    (b) T—Alopecia can be caused by warfarin.
    (c) F—Pathognomonic 'exclamation mark' hairs occur in alopecia areata.
    (d) T—Alopecia may be caused by syphilis.
    (e) T—Including protein, iron and zinc deficiency

94. (a) F—Paronychia congenita causes nail thickening and discoloration.
    (b) T—Nail–patella syndrome is inherited in a Mendelian dominant fashion.
    (c) T—Malignancy may cause subungual haematoma.
    (d) T—Splinter haemorrhages may be indicative of infective endocarditis.
    (e) F—Ingrowing toenails are usually caused by ill-fitting shoes and incorrect cutting of the nail.

95. (a) F—Leg ulcers affect 1% of the population.
    (b) T—Venous ulcers are caused by valve incompetence.
    (c) F—Eczema occurs alongside venous ulcers.
    (d) T—Vasculitis ulcers are 'punched-out' lesions.
    (e) T—Due to diabetic neuropathy.

96. (a) T—Vitiligo is associated with pernicious anaemia, thyroid disease and Addison's disease.
    (b) F—Albinism has a prevalence of 1 in 20 000.
    (c) F—Phenylketonuria leads to decreased melanin synthesis.
    (d) F—Chloasma may be induced by pregnancy or the oral contraceptive pill.
    (e) T—As may phenothiazines, minocycline, clofazimine, chlorpromazine and antimalarials.

97. (a) T—Pemphigus may prove fatal.
    (b) F—90% of patients have circulating IgG autoantibodies.
    (c) T—Pemphigus affects both sexes equally.
    (d) T—In one-half of patients pemphigus presents as an eruption of shallow blisters around the mouth.
    (e) T—Steroid treatment must be continued for several years.

98. (a) F—They are benign.
    (b) T—Seborrhoeic warts are also known as a basal cell papilloma.
    (c) T—Seborrhoeic warts are composed of basal keratinocytes.
    (d) T—Seborrhoeic warts can grow up to 6 cm in diameter.
    (e) F—Seborrhoeic warts may resolve without treatment.

99. (a) T—Malignant melanoma is the most lethal of skin tumours.
    (b) T—The incidence of malignant melanoma is increasing.
    (c) T—Individuals with multiple melanocytic naevi are at increased risk.
    (d) F—This is the most common site in the male; in the female it is the leg.
    (e) F—The male: female ratio is 1 : 2.

100. (a) F—Rosacea is not a sign of diabetes mellitus.
     (b) T—Necrobiosis lipoidica may occur in diabetes mellitus.
     (c) T—Eruptive xanathomas may occur in diabetes mellitus.
     (d) T—Neuropathic ulcers are a common feature of diabetes mellitus.
     (e) F—This is a common lesion in AIDS.

1. Refer to Fig. 1.7.

2. Refer to Fig. 2.13.

3. Fracture healing involves several stages. These include:
   - A haematoma forming at the fracture site, which then forms into a procallus; this procallus is converted into a fibrocartilaginous callus.
   - The fibrocartilaginous callus forming an osseous callus (trabecular lamellar bone); remodelling takes place by osteoclasts.
   - Delay; this can be caused by several factors, including malalignment, movement during healing, poor blood supply, and soft tissue interposition in the fracture gap.

4. Refer to Fig. 2.8.

5. Refer to Fig. 5.2.

6. Refer to Fig. 5.8.

7. The five changes that may occur in bone secondary to osteoarthritis include:
   - Eburnation, i.e. thickening and polishing of subarticular bone owing to bone–bone articulation.
   - Disuse muscle atrophy caused by immobility of a joint.
   - Synovial hyperplasia resulting from inflammation.
   - Subchondral cyst formation.
   - Formation of osteophytes.

8. The stratum basale is composed of the following:
   - Keratinocytes (90%), which are either dividing or non-dividing.
   - Melanocytes (5–10%).
   - Infrequent Merkel cells.

9. The common skin changes in pregnancy include:
   - Increased pigmentation (especially in the nipples).
   - Proliferation of melanocytic naevi.
   - Development of spider-naevi and abdominal striae (stretchmarks).
   - Pruritus.
   - Telogen effluvium may also occur in the postpartum period.

10. Sunlight benefits the following conditions:
    - Acne.
    - Psoriasis.
    - Parapsoriasis.
    - Pityriasis rosea.
    - Atopic eczema.

11. The clinical features are consistent with psoriatic arthropathy presenting in a pattern of distal arthritis. Psoriatic arthritis affects 5% of all patients with psoriasis; psoriasis affects 2% of the western world. It is less common in Africa and Japan. The sex incidence is equal, and the disease may start at any age, although the peak onset is between 20 and 30 years.

12. The history points towards either septic arthritis or gout, though there are no risk factors to favour septic arthritis, and a suggested risk of excessive alcohol consumption that is one of the risk factors for gout. Joint aspiration with culture and microscopy of the synovial fluid, and a full blood culture, will aid in diagnosis.

13. The history is suggestive of secondary bone metastases. A search for the primary tumour must be undertaken, including examination of the lungs, thyroid, kidney, breast and large bowel. The prostate must also be examined in men.

14. The most likely diagnosis is ankylosing spondylitis. You should test for the presence of HLA B27. An X-ray may show:
    - Squaring of the vertebral bodies.
    - Syndesmophyte formation.
    - Anterior longitudinal and interspinous ligaments may become ossified, resulting in a 'bamboo spine' appearance.
    - Calcification of the intervertebral discs.

15. The history is indicative of an acute allergic reaction to the anti-histamine cream (medicament dermatitis). This can be confirmed by performing a patch test with the cream.

16. The most likely diagnosis is carpal tunnel syndrome, which affects the median nerve. The nerve becomes compressed with the carpal tunnel, which leads to wasting of the thenar eminence and loss of power in the hand. The symptoms of the syndrome may become aggravated when Tinel's test or Phalen's test is performed. The treatment is by surgical decompression.

17. The diagnosis is almost certainly a complete fracture of the neck of the femur, which, in a lady of this age, is treated by complete hip replacement. The most severe complication in this age group is death, with a 50% mortality rate within 12 months. A close second is avascular necrosis, which only occurs with an intracapsular fracture.

18. The history is indicative of osteoarthritis, the structural failure of a joint. It is a progressive, degenerative disease, and this man's symptoms are likely to become worse over time. His X-ray findings may show loss of joint space, sclerosis, osteophyte formation and subchondral cysts, or they may show nothing: disease severity does not correlate well with X-ray signs.

19. This eruption is caused by pityriasis rosea and will usually clear spontaneously within 1–2 months. It is usually preceded by a 'herald patch', a single lesion which erupts a few days before the main rash appears.

20. The history points towards a diagnosis of anterior cruciate ligament injury. A positive anterior drawer sign or Lachmann's sign will confirm the diagnosis. The patient should be warned that this injury presents a long-term risk of osteoarthritis development.

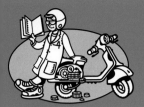

Index

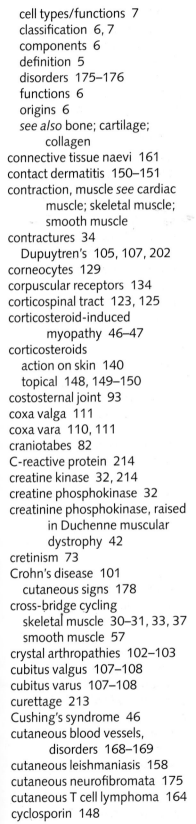

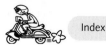

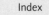

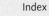

osteoporosis 67, 73, 81–82
  management 82
  periarticular 221
osteoprogenitor cells 67, 68
osteosarcoma 86–87, 198, 222
osteosclerosis 83, 88
oxidative phosphorylation
  cardiac muscle 50
  skeletal muscle 32

P
'pacemaker potential' 52
pacemaker tissue 49, 50
Pacinian corpuscles 134
Paget's disease of bone (osteitis
    deformans) 87, 88–89
Paget's disease of the nipple,
    cutaneous signs 177
Paget's sarcoma 88
pain
  back 100, 183, 185, 187
  bone 77, 84, 87, 194
  forefoot 116
  knee 113–114
  muscle 194
  referred see referred pain
painful arc syndrome 109
palmoplantar pustulosis 145,
    146
palpation
  abdomen 206–207
  cervical spine 199
  elbow 201
  feet 205
  hands 202
  hip 203
  joints 198
  knee and ankle 204
  lumbosacral spine 200
  lymph nodes 208
  shoulder 201
  skin 208
  thoracic spine 199
  thorax 206
  wrist 201
pannus 98–99
papillomatosis 145
papule 143–144
papulosquamous eruptions
    152–153

parakeratosis 145, 146
paralysis, botulism 40
paramyotonia congenita 45,
    194
paraplegia, Pott's 120
parapsoriasis 153
parasympathetic nerves,
    activation, heart rate
    51–52
parathyroidectomy 83
parathyroid hormone (PTH)
  calcium level regulation 69,
    71, 72
  increased see
    hyperparathyroidism
paronychia
  acute bacterial 168
  chronic 168
paronychia congenita 167
patch tests 214
patella, recurrent dislocation
    113–114
pathology/disorders
  bone 74–76
  skeletal muscle 40–47
pectus carinatum (pigeon chest)
    205
pectus excavatum (funnel chest)
    205
pediculosis (lice) 157–158
pellagra 153
  cutaneous signs 177
pelvic tilt 119
pelvis, radiograph 218
pemphigoid 173
pemphigus 172–173
penis, balanitis 153
pericardium 49–50
perichondrium 61, 68
perimysium 16
periodic paralyses 45–46
perioral dermatitis 165
periosteal arteries 64–65
periosteal nerves 66
periosteum 63, 64
peristalsis 54, 55, 57
periungual fibromas 168, 175
Perthe's disease 80, 111
pes cavus (hollow foot) 114,
    115

pes planus (flat foot) 114, 115
Peutz–Jager syndrome 172
Peyronie's disease 105
phaeomelanin 136
phenylketonuria 172
phosphate, depletion 82
phosphodiesterase inhibitors 51
phosphorylation 23
  smooth muscle myosin 57
  see also oxidative
    phosphorylation
photodermatoses 153–154
pigmentation, drug-induced
    172
pigmentation disorders 172
pilocarpine hydrochloride
    99–100
pinta 155
pitted keratolysis 154
pitted nails 169
pituitary dwarfism 73
pityriasis rosea 152–153
pityriasis versicolor 153
pivot joints 94, 95
plane (gliding) joints 94, 95
plantar digital neuritis (Morton's
    metatarsalgia) 116–117
plaque 143–144
plaque psoriasis 145, 146
polyarteritis nodosa 171
polyarticular arthritis 183
  causes 183
  diagnosis 183, 185
polymorphic light eruption 153
polymyositis 46, 99
popliteal cyst 114
porphyria 153
port-wine stain 161
postsynaptic disorders,
    neuromuscular junction
    40–42
postsynaptic membrane 27–
    28
  disorders 40–42
  drugs acting at 29
postural reflexes 124
posture 124, 126
  control 124, 126
  normal 119
postviral fatigue syndrome 47

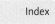

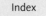